HOW GOOD IS THAT?

The Story of a Reluctant Heroine

Jane & Mike Tomlinson

POCKET BOOKS

LONDON • SYDNEY • NEW YORK • TORONTO

To Suzanne, Rebecca and Steven

First published in Great Britain by Simon & Schuster UK Ltd, 2008
This edition published by Pocket Books, 2009
An imprint of Simon & Schuster UK Ltd
A CBS COMPANY

1 3 5 7 9 10 8 6 4 2

Simon & Schuster UK Ltd
1st Floor
222 Gray's Inn Road
London
WC1X 8HB

www.simonandschuster.co.uk

Simon & Schuster Australia
Sydney

Pictures 1–11 © Ryan Bowd

A CIP catalogue for this book is available
from the British Library.

ISBN: 978-1-84739-072-1

Typeset in Sabon by M Rules
Printed by CPI Cox & Wyman, Reading, Berkshire RG1 8EX

Also by Jane & Mike Tomlinson

The Luxury of Time
You Can't Take It With You

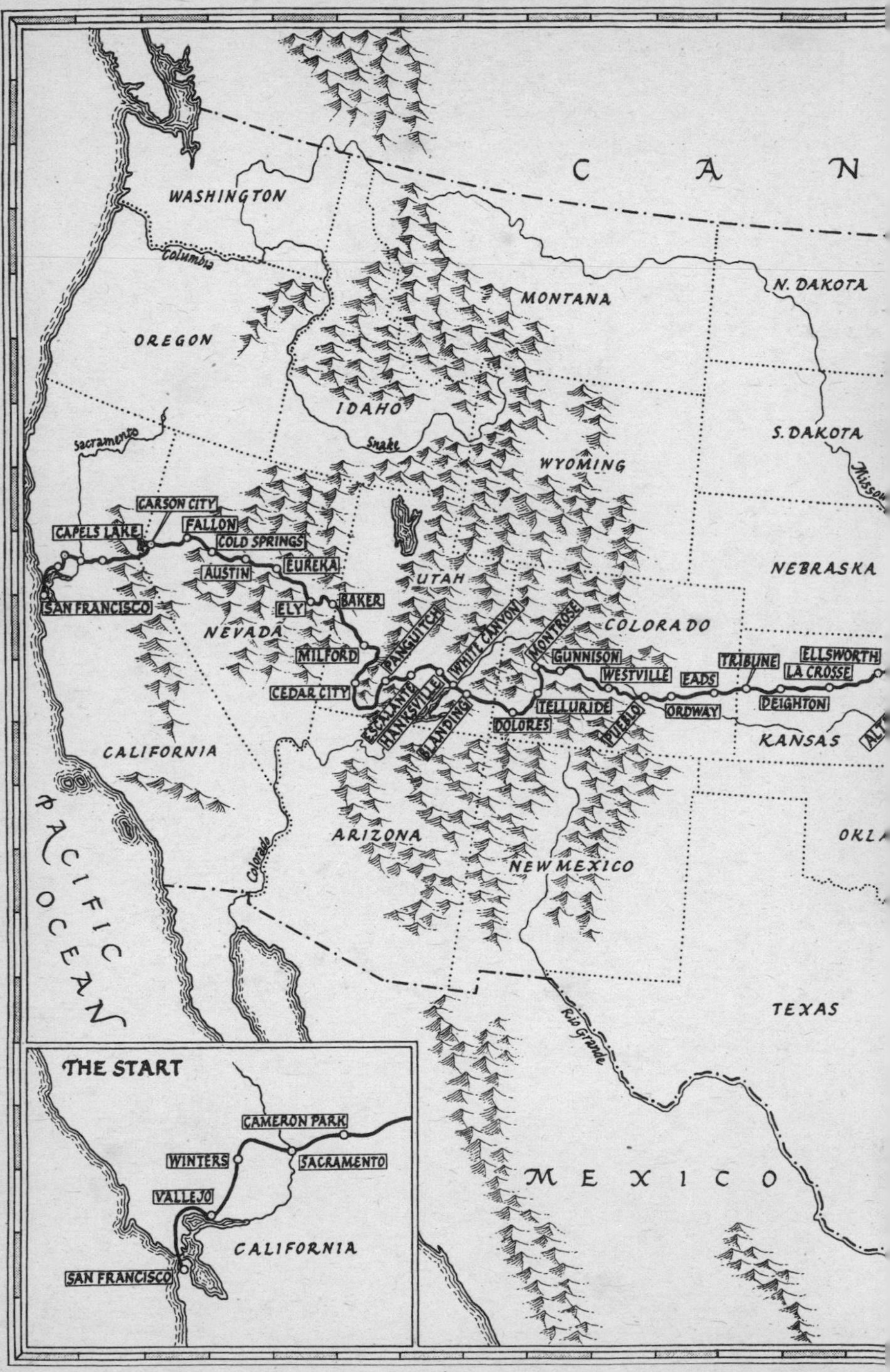

C A N
WASHINGTON
Columbia
MONTANA
N. DAKOTA
OREGON
IDAHO
Sacramento
Snake
S. DAKOTA
WYOMING
Missouri
CARSON CITY
FALLON
CAPELS LAKE
COLD SPRINGS
AUSTIN
EUREKA
NEBRASKA
UTAH
SAN FRANCISCO
ELY
BAKER
NEVADA
COLORADO
PANGUITCH
WHITE CANYON
MONTROSE
GUNNISON
TRIBUNE
ELLSWORTH
MILFORD
WESTVILLE
EADS
LA CROSSE
CEDAR CITY
ESCALANTE
HANKSVILLE
BLANDING
TELLURIDE
DOLORES
PUEBLO
ORDWAY
DEIGHTON
KANSAS
CALIFORNIA
PACIFIC OCEAN
ARIZONA
Colorado
NEW MEXICO
OKLA
TEXAS
Rio Grande
MEXICO
THE START
CAMERON PARK
WINTERS
SACRAMENTO
VALLEJO
CALIFORNIA
SAN FRANCISCO

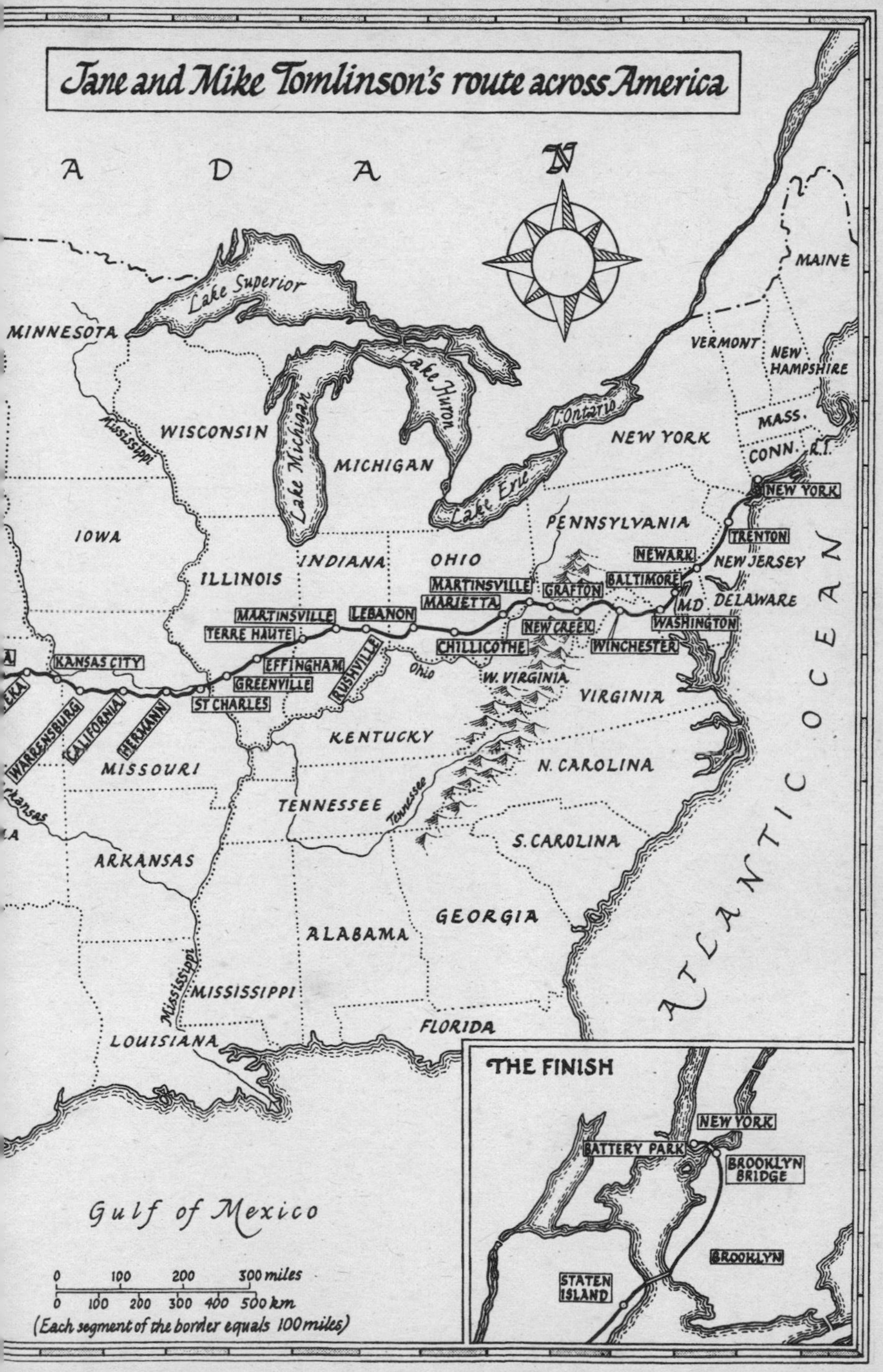

Jane and Mike Tomlinson's route across America
A D A
N
Lake Superior
Lake Michigan
Lake Huron
L. Ontario
Lake Erie
MINNESOTA
WISCONSIN
MICHIGAN
NEW YORK
MAINE
VERMONT
NEW HAMPSHIRE
MASS.
CONN.
R.I.
NEW YORK
PENNSYLVANIA
TRENTON
NEWARK
NEW JERSEY
BALTIMORE
MD
DELAWARE
WASHINGTON
IOWA
ILLINOIS
INDIANA
OHIO
MARTINSVILLE
GRAFTON
MARIETTA
MARTINSVILLE
LEBANON
TERRE HAUTE
NEW CREEK
CHILLICOTHE
WINCHESTER
KANSAS CITY
EFFINGHAM
GREENVILLE
RUSHVILLE
Ohio
W. VIRGINIA
VIRGINIA
ST CHARLES
WARRENSBURG
CALIFORNIA
HERMANN
KENTUCKY
MISSOURI
N. CAROLINA
TENNESSEE
Tennessee
S. CAROLINA
ARKANSAS
GEORGIA
ALABAMA
MISSISSIPPI
Mississippi
LOUISIANA
FLORIDA
ATLANTIC OCEAN
Gulf of Mexico
0 100 200 300 miles
0 100 200 300 400 500 km
(Each segment of the border equals 100 miles)
THE FINISH
NEW YORK
BATTERY PARK
BROOKLYN BRIDGE
BROOKLYN
STATEN ISLAND

CHAPTER 1

Sunday, 25 June
Rothwell, Leeds

JANE

Lying in bed waiting for the alarm to sound I tried to find a position that stopped the pulling sensation down my left thigh. At least the pain in my hip had calmed over the last couple of days. I just hoped that the long flight ahead wouldn't make me too stiff.

I knew I shouldn't be setting off, but the tickets and our accommodation were paid for. How could I not try? I laid back, my head sinking into the soft feather pillows, the covers warm around my body. My eyes closed and opened as the alarm clock beeped. I pushed myself upright and turned it off, snapping it shut in its case. Swinging myself from my bed, I walked to my suitcases and slid the small black clock into the top of one of them.

I'd split my cycling gear and my off-the-bike clothes between the two cases – just in case baggage handlers at the airport mislaid one of them. My bike was packed in its long cardboard box and was downstairs in the middle of our living room floor.

'Do you want a cup of tea, Mike?' I asked the humped figure lying motionless at the other side of the bed.

'That would be lovely, thanks.' He lifted himself slightly, turning his head to the window before resting back into the comfort of the bed.

Turning the light on and waiting for the kettle to boil I looked around the kitchen. It would be many weeks before I saw my home again. The room I was standing in would be half the size of our living accommodation for the next nine weeks on our long trip across America. I wondered how we would all manage in such a tight space.

I carried the hot tea upstairs, turning more lights on as I moved back through the house. I placed Mike's cup beside him and went through to Steven's room.

'It's time to get up, Steven. We're going on a plane this morning.' Steven sat bolt upright. He yawned, his mouth opening widely. I moved towards him and placed my little finger on his bottom lip. His mouth snapped shut.

'Oh Mum, you spoilt my yawn.' I laughed at his scrunched up face, indignant with shock. Then his lips spread and he laughed with me.

'We're off to America,' I said. 'Come on, get dressed and don't forget to brush your teeth.' He nodded and crept down the small ladder from his bed before sitting in the corner to put on his clothes.

I walked through to Suzanne's room. 'Suzanne,' I whispered. 'We're just getting dressed. You asked me to call you.' She opened one eye and squinted at me as I stood in the doorway with the landing light behind. My shape threw a long shadow across her room.

'Thank you. I'll get up in a minute.' Her hands reached up and tousled her hair, tangled with sleep. 'Leave the door open,' she called as I moved to close it behind me.

I pulled on the clothes I'd laid out the night before and in the bathroom washed my face and brushed my teeth. I could hear Mike moving clumsily around the bedroom.

I knocked on Rebecca's door. 'We're going in half an hour, Becks,' I called. I could see her still figure covered by her quilt.

'Yeah, thanks,' she grunted at me and turned her head towards the wall.

Downstairs, my coffee had gone cold. Taking out a travel bag, I checked my medication: bottles of oral morphine, painkillers, warfarin, iron tablets, hand cream, mouthwash and numerous smaller prescribed drugs all designed to control pain or the side effects of disease or treatment. There was three months' supply and even I was surprised by the amount – there was enough to fill a family picnic bag. I checked the letters from the doctors which gave permission for me to travel with so many controlled drugs then heard movement on the stairs. Steven appeared at the kitchen door.

'Do you want a drink of milk?' I asked. He nodded, his eyes still half closed with sleep, and I gave him a glass.

'Are you excited?' I asked. His eyes widened and his cheeks rounded out as he smiled, his face becoming animated with the thought of the adventures ahead.

I climbed the stairs and lifted the heavy rucksack from my bedroom and took it back to the kitchen. Unzipping it and zipping it again, I did one last check of my reading books, our passports and travel information and insurance documents.

Mike clumped down the stairs with a suitcase.

'Will you bring them all down so I can make sure we don't miss any?' I called.

'That's what I was doing,' he snapped.

'Thank you.' I returned to the living room redundant, my back and hip pain preventing me from helping.

'Right, that's everything,' he said, dumping the last bag in the hall.

I mentally ticked off the cases. Packing for a ten-week trip with all the cycling kit, phones, satellite units, GSP, laptops and maps without exceeding the baggage quota had been a challenge.

'Where's Steven's bag?' I asked.

'It should be there. I've brought down everything from our room.'

'Steven's bag's in his room,' I said and Mike stomped upstairs.

Suzanne pulled her dressing gown around her. Her face was full and her arms encircled her expectant abdomen. It protruded under her white towelling dressing gown. Her face was pale without make-up, the tiredness showing after long days travelling to and from work. She put her arm round me and I hugged her back, reaching past the bulge of six months' pregnancy.

'You look after yourself,' I said.

'You too,' she said, laughing at me. 'You don't have to make yourself ill doing this. No one will mind if you don't finish.'

'I might,' I said. 'Let us know if you get the lease on the house, won't you?'

Tom, her partner, and Suzanne had been looking for a house to settle into once we were back from America. They were excited about the last one they had seen. I hoped there would be no problems for them.

A rumble along the road outside announced the arrival of our taxi. I unlocked the door and watched as the driver opened his.

'Right, how we gonna manage this? You've got a bike in a box?' he asked.

Mike stepped forward. 'Yeah, mate. I'll bring that out first, and then there are four suitcases and two bags.'

The driver's eyes closed briefly. 'Right, let's see if the bike will fit back here first.'

Mike slid the bike box out of the house, and the two men handled it into the back of the people carrier where it fitted snugly. The suitcases jigsawed together and the two large bags full of T-shirts for the ride sat on the back seat.

'Plenty of room,' the driver said. 'Anything else?'

'No.' I shook my head. I counted the six bags. Mike, Steven and I had our rucksacks and our coats.

The porch light of our next-door neighbours glowed yellow and there was a rattle of the keys in the lock. Cynthia and Terry stood in their nightclothes, dressing gowns firmly closed against the chill of the early morning.

Cynthia stepped forward, looking her usual regal self despite her attire, her hair still shaped carefully round her head.

'We just wanted to say goodbye,' she said, as her arms enveloped me into the warmth of her body. 'Good luck. Look after yourself.'

I stepped back a little and saw her eyes fill with tears ready to fall down her cheeks.

'Don't you go crying, you'll set me off,' I said in as stern a voice as I could manage, but my voice cracked with fear and I could feel the heat of tears in my eyes. Suzanne was crying now and I felt so close to joining them but dare not let myself. I was too frightened of what might be ahead to allow myself the luxury of tears. I might not get into the taxi to start the journey.

Suzanne held me tight. 'You don't have to do this you know,' she said again, as the tears slid down her face. I lifted my finger and caught a tear before it ran to her lips.

'I know,' I whispered. 'Look after yourself, won't you?' I raised my voice, 'And no falling out you two.' I turned to Rebecca. 'I'll see you soon, just make sure you get to that exam and don't pack too much stuff.'

'Yes, Mum,' she said and hugged me tightly. 'Good luck.'

'Come on, Jane,' Mike called as he stepped away from Suzanne and Rebecca. Steven gave them a final hug and we climbed into the taxi ready for our journey to Manchester airport. I waved at the foursome standing outside our house, turning my head and raising my hand as we neared the end of the road. I scrunched the tissue in my hand and then wiped the tears that were falling freely from my eyes.

'What am I letting myself in for? Why am I doing this?' I thought. 'Ten weeks of hardship – why did I agree to this? How on earth is this going to happen?'

Mike turned and looked at me. 'What are you crying for?' he asked. 'It's going to be a huge adventure, isn't it, Steven?'

Steven nodded his head eagerly, his whole body moving. 'Yes, Dad.'

Sunday, 25 June
New York

MIKE

'You'd better have this,' Jane said. 'It's Steven's passport – put it with the travel documents.'

'Yes, dear, I think I can manage,' I said. The queue through

US immigration at JFK snaked round the hall and inevitably we were at the end of it. In the frantic, elbowing, jostling and pushing of passengers exiting the aircraft, we'd held back knowing that with Steven and my mum in tow it would be easier. There were only four immigration booths manned. I reached inside my pocket and flicked open my mobile – 7.15 p.m. I mentally deducted five hours.

'Ten hours in and already you're stressed. I knew despite the promises, you'd be frantic,' Jane said.

'What promises?' I said.

'When we had that discussion with Ryan.'

My mind switched back to a year earlier and a scene in our kitchen where Ryan, Jane and I sat round the table late one Sunday night. We'd known Ryan since 2003 when Jane had competed in the Half Ironman in Somerset. He'd been the PR for the event and had gone on to compete with Jane in the Florida Ironman a year later. He lived and worked in Leeds so we'd kept in touch throughout and he was helping us to put together the ten kilometre race we were planning for the city.

'So what do you reckon, Ryan? Are you up for cycling across America with Jane next summer?' I asked. Jane was looking at Ryan, shaking her head as if a secret signal had been arranged.

Oblivious, Ryan beamed. 'Awesome, absolutely awesome, we could get sponsors. Gatorade would definitely help.' Ryan's voice didn't hide his enthusiasm. 'It's one of those things that I've always fancied doing. Awesome.'

'I'll take that as a yes then,' I said. Jane put her head in her hands.

'Well, you still need Martyn,' said Jane. 'I'm not going without there being at least three riders.'

'Already sorted,' I smirked.

'Bastard.' But Jane couldn't hide the sparkle in her eyes. I had no doubt that she had no desire to ride across America or even visit it, but it was the challenge that was the attraction. 'I'm not going without you and Steven, and the girls if they want to come,' she said. I nodded. 'What about support?'

'I was going to ask Sparks if they'd free Cassie and Michael to help.'

'But I don't think they'd want to do that,' she said. 'It's a shit job.'

'Cassie's already said she'd be up for it in principle.'

'Is there anyone you haven't discussed this ride with, Mike?' Jane said. 'Family? Friends? Media? Casual acquaintances?' She looked at me, her eyes widening.

'Cassie and Michael would be ideal, organised and thorough.'

She drew a deep breath. 'What about work, yours and mine?'

'Not a problem.' Ryan smiled.

There was a look of resignation on Jane's face as logistical questions were raised and answered. I'd meticulously looked into every aspect of Jane's anticipated worries.

'I think I can get a main sponsor,' Ryan said.

'I really think we could raise a million in total from both sides of the Atlantic, but most importantly it would allow us to set up the Leeds 10k,' I said.

'So where are we going from and to?' Jane asked. I glanced at Ryan. It was the first indication that Jane might have accepted that she'd be doing the ride after all. I smiled.

'New York to San Francisco, Brooklyn to the Golden Gate,' I said.

'Awesome,' said Ryan. It was hard not to be bowled along with his youthful exuberance.

'It's bloody miles, bloody miles,' Jane laughed. But I could see we were on our way.

Over the months that passed, Jane busied herself with planning the route, ordering map after map from the American Adventure Cycling Association. Ryan worked on sponsorship and I worked on the logistics. Very few things changed from that original conversation in the kitchen except – after a meeting with a documentary film maker – it was decided to go from west to east as we'd receive better media coverage if we finished the ride in New York.

Ryan and Jane were confirmed as two of the riders. They

would be joined by Martyn Hollingsworth, a Sky cameraman who had been with Jane on her very first John o'Groats to Land's End bike ride and then had filmed her again on the 'Rome to Home' one she'd done with her brother, Luke. Martyn was a down-to-earth Yorkshireman and he and Jane had hit it off from the start. He was a welcome addition to the team.

Unfortunately, Cassie resigned from Sparks in the spring. Michael Creighton, one of the charity's events managers, would join us for three weeks at the start of the trip and two weeks at the end. But the main support would be Cindy, an American lady who'd been recommended to us by one of the charities. She had no previous experience of this kind of event but she would join us for the duration, providing drinks, food and general support throughout the trip.

This was far from ideal. Having done two previous long-distance endurance events, we knew that tensions would continually reach breaking point on the journey, even among people who were well used to each other. Having a stranger in the mix could be a recipe for disaster.

One thing Jane insisted upon was that Steven and I would accompany her throughout. And after discussing it with Rebecca, she decided she would join us for a month after her A levels, departing early to be in Leeds for her results in case she needed to go through the clearing process for university. Jodie, her friend from school, would come with her. Meanwhile, my mother Alice would travel with us to San Francisco to see Jane start the trip as well as visit family friends. The final member was Rob Davidovitz, a Sky News producer who would assist Martyn.

'What time does the flight to San Francisco go, Michael?' I said.

'Three forty, New York time,' he said calmly. Michael would be twenty-four in two days. He was fresh-faced and had a pleasant manner that I felt would be reassuring during the first three weeks of the adventure.

'At this pace we're going to struggle to meet the connection,' I said.

'Chill out, Mike,' said Jane, as she juggled the rucksack on her shoulders.

I reached over to her. 'I'll take that for a while,' I said.

Jane smiled. 'Just concentrate on looking after Steven, and put his passport in with the travel documents not just your fleece pocket, otherwise we'll have you screaming "I've lost his passport" in a minute.'

As we inched forward, I put my laptop bag down and tugged the blue travel wallet out from the bottom of it. I kept my passport out and flicked through the thirty-two watermarked pages, looking at the immigration stamps. Singapore and Adelaide from April 2001; the holiday we'd always promised ourselves if Jane's cancer became incurable. By then she'd already outlived the initial prognosis in September 2000 by two months. New York, September 2003: a treat from GMTV to Jane as recognition of her charity work. November 2004: the Florida Ironman and exactly a year later the New York marathon. Memories flooded back – snorkelling on the Barrier Reef; a wetsuit-clad Jane wading out from the sea during the Ironman and the meal at Mr Kay's Chinese restaurant in New York after the marathon.

'Mike, honestly, put your passport away properly,' said Jane, clearly agitated. I slipped it back in the inside pocket of my fleece.

'You've created a lot of memories in the last six years,' I said.

'Yes, but we don't need you getting stranded at JFK as one of them,' she replied. The queue moved slowly. Bored children began to play up, testing their parents' patience. Upon reaching the front, Steven, Jane and I stood behind the yellow line awaiting the economical nod that would be our signal to move through. Two minutes later, without a word spoken, fingerprints and photos were taken and we were behind another yellow line five yards further on. I looked behind me. Mum was being sent back to the queue.

'What's wrong?' I asked.

'I've not filled the bottom section in,' she said, clearly flustered. She scrambled through her handbag looking for a pen.

Precious minutes slipped away as for a second and third time she was admonished for the gaps in information on the form.

'Welcome to America. Have a nice day,' I whispered to Jane. I moved to retrace my steps through immigration but the officer pointed a finger at me to get back in the line.

'I don't know what's wrong, Michael,' Mum said. I could see fellow passengers watching her, hoping that their own progress through immigration would not be slowed by what was happening to Mum.

I tutted as I watched her fumbling with the forms.

'At what point are *we* going to need our kids to look after us?' I said. Jane looked at me and I immediately realised my faux pas.

Thirty minutes later, we were saying goodbye to Jane and Ryan who were staying in New York so Jane could appear on the NBC breakfast show *Today*.

It is one of the most popular shows in America and we hoped it would kick-start the American fundraising. Martyn and Rob had travelled independently to New York. Michael, Steven, Mum and I were running/walking to the connecting flight to San Francisco. Mum, already into her eighth decade with shoes that Nike wouldn't recommend, moved remarkably quickly alongside Michael.

However, there was no need to rush. To compound the miserable day the flight was delayed by two hours. My only consolation was that England had progressed in the World Cup by beating Ecuador and on the early part of the flight we'd sat enthralled as Holland and Portugal, our next opponent, seemingly self-destructed under an avalanche of red and yellow cards.

After the seven-hour flight, we landed in San Francisco at 7 p.m. local time, a good twenty hours after leaving Leeds. Rather than stand there trying to identify the generic standard-sized Samsung black cases from the two hundred others on the carousel, I decided to collect the bike from the oversized luggage area. The top of the brown cardboard bike box had been severed, which made the message the box bore, 'This Package is Recyclable', seem inappropriate somehow. Ryan and Jane had protected the bike frame by wrapping an old duvet around it, and so the faded patterns of our old bedding were now on display to everyone in the arrivals lounge. A squashed Continental bike spares box littered the area, sharing space with spare tyres. An airport worker passed by, kicking an inner tube box back towards the bike. 'Oi, careful with that, arsehole,' I yelled, unable to control my annoyance. My stomach churned as it dawned on me the bike could be damaged.

The specialised Roubaix bikes, which we'd bought for the 'Ride Across America', were road bikes designed specifically for the most gruelling of professional races in northern France – the Paris–Roubaix. After the First World War the annual race was given the nickname L'Enfer du Nord or Hell of the North, because the route closely follows the trench lines. I'd seen many images of the cyclists caked in spring mud, riding for many miles over rough terrain, cobblestones and older roads. The route is changed yearly to avoid newly surfaced roads.

It seemed an ideal bike to choose for Jane because it would provide suspension to her fragile spine while allowing her to reach road bike speeds. And while they cost hundreds of pounds each, there was no question that we needed to spend that kind of money to ensure Jane was as comfortable as she could be.

Like a child fishing around in a bran tub my hand groped inside the bike box, pulling away at the duvet. As the bike appeared I could see the buckled front wheel and felt sick.

'Fuck,' I said through clenched teeth, quickly deciding I didn't want to see any more, and began packaging the bike back up. Nothing could be done until the cyclists arrived from New York anyway but without the financial support of a bike manufacturer, spares could be difficult to obtain and expensive.

Michael appeared at my left shoulder.

'Shit,' he said when he saw the bike. I rubbed my forehead, my fingers loosening the taut skin.

'What a fucking disgrace. Baggage handlers, eh?' I forced a smile. 'I'm going to have a word.'

But as I could have predicted, that word was futile, and I

was dismissed with a shrug and 'tough shit' attitude. So much for have a nice day.

As I returned to the carousel, our bags were circling in solitude. Suzy, our American friend, had appeared and was embracing my mum. Suzy and her dad Jim were both residents of San Francisco and had insisted on collecting us and taking us to our rented house. My mum would stay with her while in the USA.

Within minutes we'd been steered outside and were sharing the airport concourse with returning fishermen from Alaska and students coming home. With a flurry of lights from huge four-by-fours, open-top pickups and RVs there was no disguising, this was California.

We ushered Steven into Jim's car while Michael and I loaded the boot. In no time we were travelling on a road where you needed binoculars to see all the lanes and with no clue as to our destination or navigation, we settled into a conversation recapping the past three decades since I'd last seen Jim.

Until the Ironman competition, the Murphy family had been my only meaningful experience of Americans. We'd been introduced in a somewhat fateful way thirty-five years ago when one of Suzy's letters to her grandma became trapped inadvertently in a letter to my mum from America. My ten-year-old sister Janet had started writing to Suzy, who was eleven at the time, and we'd been in touch ever since.

'Have you booked a campground for Independence Day weekend?' asked Jim.

'Should we?' I said.

'Hell yes, all the RVs will be out. Everyone celebrates kicking the British asses out of the country.'

'I'd never quite thought of it like that,' I said.

'You should get spots booked all weekend, especially if you're in National Parks. Boy, does it get busy.'

Michael and I looked at each other. In the weeks leading up to departure I'd been feeling overwhelmed. Despite our arrival here, I knew we'd left many loose ends untied. My stomach rumbled from lack of food and nerves. I could have sat and wept. For eight months prior to leaving the UK, Jane and I had felt increasingly under pressure as our plans systematically fell apart. Jane's health was deteriorating daily, we'd had untold difficulties obtaining health insurance, there were no confirmed media outlets . . . the list went on. The stress had continued to mount and our arrival in the USA had only confirmed how inadequately prepared we were.

Jim gave us a monologue of his RV experiences and by the time we arrived at the rented house, my spirits had never been lower; the brooding darkness only adding to the melancholy atmosphere. Russ, the house caretaker, had left some provisions on the kitchen table – which were quickly consumed – and some maps, instructions and contact numbers.

Steven was quickly settled down and I looked at my watch. It was 10 p.m. and I wanted to speak to Jane. But it was 1 a.m. in New York.

Monday, 26 June
New York

JANE

The sound of a car engine gently ticking over woke me. My head felt heavy, my mouth dry, my eyes stung with tiredness as I forced them partially open. I could see an orange glow creeping across the floor. The window was in the wrong place, the curtains weren't pulled across fully and were letting in an acid yellow light which made a sharp triangle across the black shadow.

My head felt full and fluffy, a cotton wool stuffiness pushing my reason away, and I lay back more awake, still unable to figure the noise. My eyes opened again on the red dot glowing above me. The noise suddenly quietened and there was a sound in the room like several doors closing at once onto their latches.

I pushed myself up the bed and felt to the side of me. There was no familiar companion there, only empty coldness. I fumbled in the strangeness of the darkened hotel room trying to find a light switch. I forced myself upright but still couldn't find any way to light the room. I pulled back the covers and stood by the bed. My left thigh pulled tight and my heel arched from the floor. A cord of coolness ran down my left leg through the muscles, knotting my calf.

Limping towards the glow of the hallway lighting, which crept dimly under the room door and showed me where the bathroom was, I could make out the bank of switches by it.

I clicked one and pushed the bathroom door open, my eyes blinking back the brightness. I stepped forward, feeling the coldness of the floor tiles on my feet. The muscles from my painful left side clenched even tighter. There was the plastic click of many shutters and the noise in the room of an engine started again as the air conditioning clicked on.

The sweat on my body, cool now, made my pyjama top cling to my skin. I pulled it off and stood half-naked, shaking from the cool air in the room.

I grabbed one of the thick hotel gowns down from behind the bathroom door and wrapped myself in the fluffy towelling. My hair clung in wet tendrils to my head, creeping damply across my face. I reached for a hand towel and tried to dry it, rubbing roughly at my head.

My mouth was so dry. I wiped my hand across my lips and stepped back into the bedroom. Beside my now lit bedside lamp was a small bottle of water. It tasted stale, warmed from my clenched fist the day before. I glugged the contents down, trying to slake my thirst. I looked at the bed, the sheets crumpled from my unsettled sleep.

The journey from Manchester to New York had meant long hours of confusion at the airports and interminable queues through passport control. Finally, a car had deposited us outside a hotel overlooking Central Park. After the constant noise of the airport lounges and the thrum of the aircraft carrying us across the Atlantic, it felt wonderful to be in the peace of the gilded lobby.

I sat on the bed. The pain had been decreasing over the last couple of weeks but the flight and the cramped seating had negated all the exercise and all the physio I'd done with my therapist Alison, even though I had walked and stretched for the duration of the journey.

I lay my head on the pillow but sat upright immediately, my face scrunching with disgust. The pillow was soaked with the sweat of the night's pains. The bed sheets were similarly damp where my body had lain.

I couldn't find any comfort. I sat in the chair rocking myself gently to ease the pain in my back and legs. The clock below the large screen television showed 3.30 a.m. and I sat in my private discomfort, rocking and rocking, still hoping the pain would ease. My shoulder tightened in small despair as I thought about what lay ahead of me. Maybe the pain would subside when I'd had a few days' rest in San Francisco. Maybe it would be all right. There was no way I could face nine weeks of this if I was cycling every day.

How was I going to do it? Everybody showed such faith in me. I couldn't even voice the small fear I had of failure. No, we would be setting off from San Francisco on Friday and nine weeks and 4000 miles later we'd be arriving back here in New York. Say it quickly and it doesn't sound too far – or too mad.

I pulled the pages of physiotherapy diagrams and instructions from my rucksack. Stick men with feet up and feet down. I followed the routine, stretching my back, my neck, my legs, forcing some of the tightness from the long flight from my body. My muscles reacted but the pain remained. I glanced at my watch, still on UK time, and worked out that I still had one dose of Coproximol left that I could take. I swallowed the pills quickly before they could leave the bitterness in my mouth. I stood and tugged the heavy curtains back from the window. Outside, I could see a blank grey roof beneath me and air-conditioning units jutting from the wall. One was dripping and I watched the false rain, following it down to the flat roof below where it made a dark puddle, just a black smudge visible against the otherwise dusty grey.

Perhaps a hot-water bottle would help. The ache was growing duller in my lower thigh. In my suitcase I found the cream hot-water bottle and undid the stopper. It smelt of old rubber. With no kettle to boil I returned to the bathroom and ran the hot water into the basin until I could no longer bear to hold my hand under it. I filled the bottle, holding it against my side. I squeezed the air from it till the water showed and then screwed the black stopper firmly in place.

The advantage of being alone meant I could sleep on the cool dryness of the other side of the bed. I threw the damp pillow to the floor and arranged the remaining pillows, two for beneath my head and one to support the warm bottle beneath my leg. Before I climbed into the bed I made my way back to the bathroom and pulled a hand towel from the rack to wipe the sweat from my face and neck. The bed was too high to climb into and I crawled forward and eased myself between the covers. The heavy gown still enveloped my body and I enjoyed the comfort it brought. I clicked off the light and could see the clock showing 4.00 a.m. Closing my eyes I hoped sleep would return, if not it would soon be a respectable enough time to knock on Ryan's door. Company and talk can take pain away or keep it at bay whereas hours alone allow it to grow enormously, taking over everything else.

I awoke to light shining through the opened curtains, which threw the far side of the room into an alien relief.

I pushed myself from the bed. There was a piece of paper on the floor by the door and I grunted with discomfort as I bent to retrieve it. 'Gone for a run, meet you at 9.00 a.m. in the lobby, Ryan.'

The clock below the television said 7.30 a.m. At least I'd rested well. I yawned, stretched my neck and shoulders trying to release the tightness and glanced around the room at the littered nightclothes. Opening the wardrobe, I manoeuvred the hangers from the metal loops and threaded my tops on to them, hoping that they might dry out a little in the course of the day.

After a hot bath, I opened my suitcase and found some muscle rub. I sat on the floor massaging it into the muscles in the backs of my calves and my thighs. Loosing the gown, which fell to the floor, I rubbed some of the warming cream into the rear of my pelvis at the top and at the base of my back, still trying to ease the tightness.

That done I went through the stretching routine again. It was difficult to get my stiff unwieldy body to obey so I managed as best I could, finishing sitting upright in the chair turning my head first one way, then the other, going through the sequence shown me by Alison.

My body felt less tight as I struggled to my feet. Looking through my meagre clothes choice I pulled out a skirt and vest top. Dressed, I felt more normal, less at odds with where I was, what I was here to undertake.

I pulled the rucksack open and looked through the details for the next day. I was just thinking about leaving the hotel to look for breakfast when the phone rang and made me start.

'Hi, Jane. I thought you'd be up by now,' Ryan's voice echoed in my ear.

'Yeah. What are you up to?' I asked.

'That's why I was phoning. I'm going to get on with some work this a.m. if that's okay.'

I nodded to myself. 'That's fine. Do you want to meet up for lunch?'

'Yeah. Is twelve thirty all right with you?'

'Fine by me. If I go past a Starbucks this morning, do you want me to fetch you back a latte?'

'That would be fantastic, thanks.'

I replaced the receiver and pushed my feet into soft pumps and headed off to find some breakfast.

Martyn guffawed loudly, his laugh echoing along the corridors of the NBC studios early the following morning.

'What have they done to you? You don't even look like Jane.'

'What?' I said, startled by his wide gesturing as he pointed to my face. 'They've made your face a different shape, and done something American to your hair.'

I laughed. The women in make-up had been very pleasant and had not been over generous with the cosmetics.

'This is quite natural, actually,' I said to Martyn. 'They didn't want to plaster me with make-up.'

'That's not natural,' Martyn replied, 'you look like every other American woman off the television. I can't believe what they can do with make-up. Doesn't it bother you when they make you up to look like someone else?'

I shrugged my shoulders. 'It used to. But not any more. It's not really me out there on the television. At least it doesn't feel like me, it's just somebody's idea of what you should be like. This is me here. I don't like being on the television but the charity wouldn't make any money if I didn't make the effort, so I kind of just pretend it's not happening.'

'Does it make you nervous?' Ryan asked.

'Not as much as it did,' I said. 'I hate the thought of it, the intrusion, but it's not so bad now I'm here and it will be over soon and we can get on with the ride proper.'

'Jane.' The producer called me. 'Can we take you downstairs now?'

I followed him down and we made our way through the building. Ryan walked with me and Martyn followed with his camera, filming the NBC *Today* experience for his documentary. We crossed the road, heading for the stage which was surrounded by a live audience. One man was very vocal and kept calling out comments to gain attention. Once the cameras had left him, he was moved on by some black-suited men, only to turn round and head back towards the stage when they had left his side.

We waited at the side of the stage. A technician came and helped me attach a microphone to my top. Ryan's bike was wheeled to the area in front of the stage and a man stood holding it as I was called there. The black bike was emblazoned with our website www.janesappeal.com in white. It was very striking, a good crisp image. 'Ryan, you need to come and hold the bike,' I called as a man fidgeted behind me. Ryan bounded forward and stood behind me holding his bike, his lean frame covered with his cycling top bearing the logo with our appeal and our main supporters Leeds Metropolitan University and Yorkshire Bank.

'So what does this ride involve?' the presenter Campbell Brown asked. She was much taller than me and power-dressed in tight white trousers and jacket. Her confident poise and questioning already had me slightly on the back foot. The interview was outside in the open air at the Rockefeller Center and a stiff breeze was causing my hair to ruffle. Ryan stood motionless behind us as if employed only to be a human bike stand.

'Ryan, Martyn and I are setting off from San Francisco on Friday and hopefully in nine weeks' time, on 1 September, we'll cycle across Brooklyn Bridge into New York City,' I said.

'How far is that?'

'About four thousand miles. We'll be averaging about seventy miles a day.'

'Well, good luck with that and we hope to follow you.'

'Thank you,' I nodded.

A woman at the back called out, 'Awesome, man. Go Jane go.'

I smiled and then we were being shown off stage. I breathed deeply and dropped my hands to my sides, feeling my shoulders droop lower as I relaxed.

'Well done,' Ryan said.

I shook my head a little. 'Thank you. I'm glad that's over with. We'd better get back to the hotel so we can pack up your bike.'

Monday, 26 June
Oakland, California

MIKE

The guidebooks had promised that the Sutro Tower, a distinctive three-pronged orange and white antenna tower on Mount Sutro in San Francisco, would be visible throughout the city, but today all we could see were misty clouds hanging low in the air. Suzy had told us that the climate was usually very mild throughout the year but the cold currents of the Pacific Ocean would conflict with the Californian mainland summer heat to create a fog which blanketed the city. Even though we'd been warned, the temperature took us by surprise – it was cooler than we were used to, even at home.

'Which direction do we need to head?' asked Michael, his T-shirt and shorts a sign of his optimism that things would brighten up.

'Well, if this map is to be trusted,' I said, looking at the San Francisco City Series map that the caretaker had left us, 'this must be Geary, so we go right.' We were standing there for a second, studying the map, when a middle-aged man in baggy overalls who looked like he'd just finished a night shift loped towards us.

'Yo man, you lost?' he smiled.

'Just wondering which bus to get to the centre of town,' I said.

'That's your bus,' he said, pointing to a single-decker bus 200 yards away.

'Thanks.'

'You Australian?' he asked.

'British.'

'Enjoy San Francisco!' he said with just a tinge of disappointment in his voice.

'Australian?' Michael said. 'It must be the hat,' referring to the Tilley I was wearing.

The bus pulled up on the opposite side of the road.

'It's here, Dad!' shouted Steven and we walked up to it and climbed on board.

'Are you all right, Mike? You seem distracted,' Michael said.

'I'm fine,' I said, nudging Steven further down the bus. 'Sit there, Steven,' I said and pointed to a vacant seat by the pushchair area, next to an elderly gentleman.

As I reached for my wallet, the driver waved his hand.

'It's free, sir,' he said.

'Free, perfect. Why?'

'Clean Air Day, the city's big on promoting it; so all the transport's free today.'

With its propensity for thick fog, I could understand why air quality could be a big issue in the city. The bus seemed enormous, twice the length of a British bus. Looking at the man next to Steven, I said, 'I'm terribly sorry to bother you, which stop would be the most convenient to catch the BART?'

'Is that an Australian accent?' he asked, holding out his hand. 'I'm Doug.'

'British, Mike,' I said, shaking his hand. Doug was a good sixty-five, wiry, tidily dressed, with a vice-like grip.

'Are you on holiday in San Francisco?' he asked.

'Not exactly. We're supporting a team of cyclists who are cycling across America, one of whom is my wife; Steven's mum.'

'D'yall hear that?' he exclaimed in a booming voice to his fellow passengers. 'This boy's mum is cycling across the country.'

'Where you heading, boy?' an elderly lady said, her bony frame perched uncomfortably on the edge of her seat.

Steven looked up at me for confirmation that it was okay to talk. 'New York,' he said.

'Wow,' Doug said. 'That's incredible. You British are mad. That must be four thousand miles. In this heat? Which way are you going?'

'Nevada, Utah,' I said.

'Woah,' he exclaimed, giving out a huge laugh. 'No way, man, not in this heat, it's gotta be one ten in the desert. You hearing this?' he said, scanning the bus.

'Colorado, Kansas and Missouri, then across to New York,' Michael said.

'Your wife's doing this?' he said, looking up at me. 'Why not you? What are you going to be doing?'

'We're the support team in an RV, aren't we, Steven?'

'You're not going to Chicago, are you?' a female voice shouted from behind.

'No.'

'Good, don't go to Chicago, it's dangerous, you'll get killed, you listen here, don't go there, it's a bad place. A very bad place.'

Various mutterings from throughout the bus seemed to echo the sentiment. Michael and I exchanged a quizzical look.

'We'll tell you where to get off,' Doug said, as we rolled through the suburbs. By the time we alighted on Powell Street it was to a crescendo of good luck and best wishes from the other passengers.

Powell Street was a hub of tourist activity: a cable car was climbing the hill with passengers standing on footplates adding an extra yard to the width; a Japanese man was leaning wide with one hand grasping the pole, the other a digital camera.

In contrast, the Bay Area Rapid Transport (BART) rail service was intimidating by its quietness, the ticket barriers were open and unattended. By the time we alighted at the Coliseum/Oakland Airport station the sun was out and the temperature was threatening three Fahrenheit digits. Oakland is the eighth largest city in California, standing across the bay from San Francisco and is the more famous city's poor relation. In 2006 it was ranked eighth most dangerous city in the USA and it was easy to see why. Groups of steroid-enhanced youths in baseball shirts loitered on corners, watching us curiously.

'Let's get out of here,' I said to Michael, as we studied the street map. I clutched Steven's hand.

'Probably best not to hang around,' Michael nodded and, studiously avoiding eye contact, we strode purposefully in the direction of the main road.

'Yo, have you any change?' asked a six-foot wide youth. I shrugged and quickly stuffed the map in my pocket. My heart was pounding and it was a relief to be on a main road with vehicles.

In the absence of a pavement, we walked underneath the BART line on a dusty gravel road. It was lonely, but I was glad to settle for that. A goods train rumbled in the background, its horn punctuating the silence. Fortunately, within minutes we were in sight of the RV rental company. I made a mental note to catch a taxi here the following week.

All summer, the thought of having to drive a thirty-foot RV across the USA had turned my blood cold. We'd been offered a free upgrade to a thirty-five-foot rig which luckily I'd refused, and my palms were sweating as we wandered past the enormous parked vehicles.

'Shit, Michael, don't we need an HGV licence for these?' I said.

'You'd think so. It's all right though, John says they'll be straightforward to drive.'

A family of unfeasibly hairy, toned and tanned Swedish tourists was unpacking an RV. Several suitcases, a box of food and cleaning equipment littered the car park and the father, sweeping brush in hand, was encouraging the sporty looking children to help.

'I reckon these are ours,' said Michael, pointing over to two pristine RVs parked next to each other.

We went through to reception where, after signing the necessary paperwork, I had the payment blocked on both my Visa and MasterCard credit cards. At least it proved that my fraud protection tools were working, although it was frustrating as I'd advised my credit card companies that we'd be in the United States for ten weeks. Eventually we managed to find someone in the UK with sufficient credit to complete the transaction.

We were shown the art of 'dumping' – emptying out the RV sewers – and 'hooking up', which meant connecting water and electricity to the RV. Then, bemused, we were escorted to the RVs we'd spotted earlier.

'You're not driving this are you, Dad?' Even Steven sounded nervous. 'Please tell me you're not, Dad.'

The young, bored, female Hispanic assistant spoke at speed and in an accent which was impossible to follow as she explained how to use the various gauges, caps, sockets, pipes and compartments.

'Okay, y'all have a good day, questions?' she said, but never waited for an answer. Could I detect a glint of mischievousness as she left the three of us bemused and befuddled?

Thankfully, we didn't need to drive the RVs straight away and had a few days to stock them up. We took a taxi to the airport where we hired an enormous black people mover with blacked-out windows and headed to a Wal-Mart. We piled up three trolleys until our heads were hidden behind piles of bedding, water purifiers, cans of food, every conceivable item a household would need. We paid up and went out to the car park.

'Dad!' said Steven, as we started loading up.

'What's up?'

'Dad, it won't all fit in,' he said.

Michael smiled. 'We'll see, Steven, we'll see.'

'It won't, I can just tell.'

We weren't about to be beaten. As we crammed tins of vegetables, cartons of juice and boxes of cereals into every conceivable corner of the car, it looked like Steven might have a point. But as we placed him in his booster seat, holding on to cans and boxes, we finally filled the car. We'd only been in San Francisco for sixteen hours. I silently hoped that things would improve once we were on the move.

Tuesday, 27 June
New York to San Francisco, California

JANE

I pushed my forehead against the small oval window and stared down at the landscape below. We moved through pithy clouds that wisped away from us, the long wing of the plane slicing through the nothingness of white as it swirled around and disappeared.

We passed over road grids cutting up and dividing the masses of habitation. There was an occasional azure glint – small jewels of pools in the gardens far beneath us.

I moved slightly, so that the side of my head rested against the clear plastic and moved my feet trying to find a comfortable place in the tiny area I was to exist in for the next five hours. I shut my eyes and tried to rest. I was exhausted with travel, my body not accustomed to the change in time zones and weary from too little sleep and the nervous tension that kept overtaking me.

Ryan typed busily away on his laptop, glancing over at me as I shuffled once again.

'Are you okay?' he asked.

'Yes,' I replied. 'I just wish we were there then maybe I could get rid of this tightness.'

'I know what you mean. I'll be relieved to be in San Francisco,' he said. I nodded and leant back in my seat, closing my eyes once more and trying to will the time to pass.

We were passing over ridges that dipped into valleys and rose to high crests, dipping and rising again; high green masses that resembled from this height the 3D maps that are on display on school open days. Judging by how long we'd been in the air, I assumed they must be the Appalachians; the height unnerved me and a shudder passed through my body as I thought of cycling over them in several weeks' time.

I sat back in my seat. I couldn't really believe I was here. A thought passed through my mind back to when we were planning the ride just days before Christmas. It seemed so remote now.

Mike and I were leaving my oncologist Dr Perrin's office. It was only four thirty in the afternoon but it was already cold and dark, the street lamps lit and penetrating the darkness.

'I think we should carry on trying to sort out the American ride,' Mike said, his words steaming from his mouth in the crisp air. He turned to look at me. 'What do you think?'

'I don't think I'll be going,' I said and continued to walk.

'I think we should carry on planning and see how you are. It will give you something to aim for,' Mike said.

'I don't need a ridiculous bike trip to aim for,' I replied.

There was a pause. 'Even so, it's something positive to work towards,' he said. I bit back an acidic comment and walked on in silence. It was typical of Mike to still want to go ahead even though Dr Perrin had told me that the cancer was in my liver and I might just have twelve months of life left.

Through the winter I had struggled to try to stay fit, running several times a week, but the chemotherapy left me tired and the pain in my left buttock just wouldn't go away. It got so severe that I could hardly walk, but with the help of a good physiotherapist I was gradually able to mobilise myself and by the end of February had started venturing out on the bike for small distances.

I kept waiting for Mike to see how ridiculous the nine-week American venture was, but still the planning continued. Ryan had agreed to cycle with Martyn and me. Martyn would film the whole trip and there would be just three of us on bicycles. Ryan's enthusiasm was catching and I would alternate between excitement and despair at the prospect of the summer in America. Ryan procured funding for the trip from Leeds Metropolitan University and Yorkshire Bank and started researching suitable bikes.

Spring became warmer and my training rides became longer and longer. My confidence grew as my legs became stronger and the bike moved quickly under their power. Still, I wasn't sure that ten weeks away from home was something I would relish. As we moved towards early summer the American trip started to become true. I hadn't spoken of my doubts and I couldn't now extricate myself from the complex plans that had been put in place.

So now here I was in the plane. The mountains beneath us had become rolling flat plains; long stretches of green broken up by a uniform grid of roads.

'Why don't they stick a road from corner to corner,' I thought as I followed the route of one long right angle. I shuffled once more on my seat and placed a tiny pillow beneath my left thigh. Still the pain ran down my leg, cramping my calf. I was filled with a sudden overwhelming urge to get out of the plane. If I could just press a button, hear the ping as if on a bus and get off and go home.

The desire to get out of the plane grew and grew. I looked around, agitated, my eyes following the service crew as they moved slowly through the body of the plane. My stomach bubbled through nerves and hunger. I picked up the in-flight magazine and flicked through it till I came to the route.

I traced our route and figured we were halfway now. My

back teeth met as I ground them together in my anxiety and I glanced once more out of the window. The plains were becoming corrugated, land bunching together in small undulating hills. As we continued the undulations grew and the height of the hills became higher and higher, until they were small mountains covered in green. Trees soared above them, obscuring any roads. The mountains grew higher still until you could see where the tree line ended, the height too great for the majestic vegetation.

The bubbling in my stomach grew. I ground my teeth and my breath came and went raggedly from my body. I could feel heat rising up my neck through my face, prickling into my hair as the panic I was trying to keep at bay gradually overtook the whole of my body.

I turned my head from Ryan and pushed my forehead hard against the window, clenching my teeth to try to regain control. My shoulders shook with the effort and tears escaped from beneath my closed lids and rolled slowly down my cheeks.

I pulled the small blanket up higher towards my ears in my effort to disguise my emotions. I tried to still the flow of tears. I heard movement a couple of rows back and could hear Martyn's voice.

'Oh, no. He's going to come and film me now,' I thought. 'He can't film me now.' I held my breath, puffing out my cheeks, and scrubbed at my eyes to brush the tears away. In my edgy state I tugged at my ear lobes, rubbing the flesh between finger and thumb, and pulled at my fringe.

'Jane, have you seen out of the window?' Martyn asked, his small camera trained on my face.

'Yes,' I said, nodding fiercely at the same time, trying to sound positive. 'Those hills sure are big.'

'Big? They're enormous,' Martyn said and barked a nervous laugh. 'How the bloody hell are we going to cycle over those?'

'I don't know,' I said. I could hear my voice tremble and the tears returned, finding their own path down my face and dripping off my chin.

'Are you all right?' Martyn asked.

'Oh yea, fine,' I replied. 'I've been looking at the in-flight catalogue. Have you seen what you can buy? I particularly like the solar-powered air-cooling hat.'

'What?' Martyn replied. I flicked through the magazine, shaking my head and laughing at Martyn and his expression.

'Here, here it is.' I pushed the magazine towards him which showed a picture of a small hat with a solar panel and a fan attached to it.

'That,' Martyn said, 'that just looks absolutely fantastic.' He laughed. 'I'll definitely have to get one of those.'

I bent forward now, laughing at the ridiculous notion. Ryan removed his earphones. 'What?' he bawled.

'I want one of those hats,' I said, 'if you want me to cycle over those mountains. I deserve one when we get to the other side.'

Ryan looked and a smile split his face. 'I think if we get to the other side, you should definitely have one of those.'

Wednesday, 28 June
San Francisco, California

MIKE

Steven, with his newly acquired Canadian baseball hat donated by Ryan's parents, drew some funny looks from the locals in San Francisco, but at least no one mistook us for Australians.

Jane's thighs were prominent in her fawn combats and she was carrying a little more weight, which was good, as she'd be burning up calories at a rate of knots. She'd arrived the night before and it had been impossible for me to mask my shock when I saw her. Her cheeks were swollen – a result of the chemo's steroids – but they gave a mistaken picture of good health.

There was a sadness in her demeanour, an air of resignation that the cancer had won a premature victory. Although its steady march to triumph was so graphically displayed every three months on her scans, its steady trot had turned into a gallop and there was a sense that the final rout had started.

'Can we walk back through the Golden Gate Park?' asked Jane. We were walking through the city's Haight-Ashbury area, a rather bohemian part of town filled with street cafés and second-hand shops.

'Why?' I asked.

'Do you need to ask?' she said, wishing to delay the 'start' of the trip.

I walked along beside her. 'I think we should tell everybody that the ride may not start,' I offered.

'Who is everybody?' asked Jane.

'Support team, riders, media, the kids.'

'Whatever you think is best. You deal with it, Mike.'

'Are we going home?' Steven asked.

'I dunno,' I said.

'What about Becca?' he asked.

'Mum's going to try riding her bike this afternoon. If she can't, we might ring Becca tonight and say for her and Jodie not to travel.'

'Oh.'

'What do you think we should do?' I asked.

'Whatever's best for Mum.'

'At least someone cares,' Jane said.

I felt a stab of guilt watching Jane as she hobbled across Stanyon Street to the park entrance. My heart sank, a feeling of self-loathing came across me. Was this my fault? We cut across an overgrown area, just away from the normal paths, but soon turned back when we came across discarded syringes. Because of its temperate climate, San Francisco attracts a disproportionate number of homeless people and it looked like many of them had chosen the park for the night's stay. A scruffy African American who was as wide as he was tall began hollering, 'I'm gonna fucking kill y'all, you're fucking dead, motherfuckers,' and Steven gripped my hand tighter.

'What a shit hole,' I said to Jane, steering Steven away. We walked around the edge of the park, the disgruntled grunt from our obese colleague fading away. Within minutes we were walking down Kennedy Drive surrounded by tourists, rollerbladers and cyclists. We ambled through the incredible floral displays and stunning greenery, saying little.

Ryan and Michael were in the ground-floor garage assembling the bikes when we got back to the house. All the tools, spares and components were laid out with precision on the floor.

'Good day, sir,' Ryan said as I descended the steep concrete stairs with caution. 'Hiya little man,' he said – to Steven thankfully. 'I've got something for your scrapbook upstairs.'

Steven beamed. The house had the feel of a transit camp, boxes of energy bars were stacked in the hall, laptops covered the kitchen work surfaces, cases filled the living room. Meanwhile, Jane looked increasingly agitated, quite unsure of what to do with herself.

I followed her to the calm of our bedroom.

'Ryan's nearly finished your bike. When are you going out on it?'

'I don't know.'

'How's your back and pelvis?' I asked.

Six years ago, when the doctors had delivered their first prognosis, they'd told us that if Jane managed to live any length of time, her bones would become more fragile. She'd be liable to fractures in the longer bones and her spine could also be a major issue.

But, of course, at the time, and given only six months to live, we were only concerned about the tumour in her lung. We never ever thought the bone cancer would have a chance to come into play.

Ironically, however, as the disease in her visceral organs was kept at bay, the bone disease continued to advance. And because the scans were showing more areas of cancer, other small fractures were increasingly hard to detect.

I couldn't help but think I was to blame for some of her current problems. Back in January I'd mixed up the dates for the Brass Monkey Half Marathon in York and Jane had taken part in it at very short notice.

She returned home afterwards struggling to move her leg.

'I've done something to my pelvis,' she said. 'It happened early in the run, I got to six miles and then had to give up.'

There was a hint of tears bubbling under the surface, it was most unlike her.

However bad things had been previously, Jane had never pulled out of any event so I was all too aware that this was serious. Over the following four months, Jane's training had suffered and if it hadn't been for the work of Alison Rose, her physiotherapist, there's no doubt that she would have abandoned the American ride. Even now, there was still a hint of a limp as Jane walked, but the real problems came when she needed to sit down on the bike.

Back in the basement, Ryan and Michael were finishing assembling the bikes so I took the opportunity to cajole Jane into recording her first weekly piece into camera. Steven set up the tripod and positioned the camcorder.

'Can I do the interview, Mum, Dad?'

'It's for TV so we need to get it right,' I said.

'I would!' he said, his cow eyes pleading to be given a chance. It had been a boring day for a nine-year-old so Jane and I exchanged glances.

'Go on then,' Jane said. 'You need to write yourself some questions and a script.' Steven enthusiastically grabbed a pen and notebook and bustled off into the dining room. Minutes later he was back.

As he wound up the interview and started to disassemble the equipment he asked: 'Can I do them every week?'

'We'll see,' Jane said, 'but if you do, it's just for us.'

'I understand,' Steven said, his face beaming as if waking up on Christmas morning.

Wednesday, 28 June
San Francisco, California

JANE

'Will you put my bike together first?' I asked Ryan.

He nodded. 'I'm changing the wheel that's bent with the one from Martyn's bike. He'll never notice.'

He opened the nearest large box and started pulling out bike parts, placing spares to one side of the basement garage. The floor was starting to fill with mechanical parts, saddles, pedals, pumps, tyres. The doorbell sounded and I started cautiously up the stairs.

'I hope that's my mum and dad,' said Ryan. 'Dad said he'd give me a hand today.' We looked at the three bikes and enough spare stuff for 4000 miles, which was starting to take over the small space.

'I think you'll need it,' I said and carried on upwards.

It was indeed Ryan's parents.

'It's so good to finally meet you,' his mother said.

'And you,' I said. 'Your son's a real credit to you.'

We negotiated the space left in the hall, picking our way past boxes of Gatorade, and moved towards the kitchen. I made them a drink then Ryan and his dad headed for the garage stairs, leaving his mum and me in the kitchen area.

'Is there any way I can help?' she asked.

'No, I think we're good.'

We moved into the front part of the house and I retrieved glasses and cups and opened the dishwasher and started stacking the dirty crockery away into it.

'Actually, there is something you can help me with,' I said and she turned and smiled at me, her head held to one side. 'I'm not sure how to work the washing machine.'

Her smile turned into an open-mouthed chuckle.

'Yeah, sure. Where's the machine?'

'Downstairs,' I said, and headed for the steps.

Ryan's mum followed me. She gave me an idiot's guide to the washer and dryer and before long I had the tumble dryer working and Ryan's clothes in the washing machine.

'Jane, Jane!' I could hear Mike calling as footsteps thundered overhead. I could also hear Steven's voice but not what he was saying. I called back and the door opened above. 'Are you down there?'

'Yes,' I called back, 'I'm just going out to try the bike.' Ryan had rebuilt my bike and made some adjustments to the saddle.

I was just about to go out and see if I could bear to sit on it and indeed if I could turn the pedals without too much pain. Mike started to make his way down the steps.

'I'll come outside and make sure you're okay,' he said.

'No,' I said hastily, 'I'd rather you didn't watch.'

'Oh.' His eyes closed briefly while he composed his face and a small droop of his features and shoulders passed by. 'Don't feel you have to set off tomorrow if you're in too much pain or too ill,' he said. 'Nobody expects you to set off. I can ring Rebecca and tell her not to come.'

'No. Don't do that,' I said. 'It's too early to stop them coming and it'll be fine.'

'Jane, you can barely walk.'

'I know that, but I'm sure I'll start to feel better soon. If I can get on the bike it will help I'm sure. I just feel all curled up and my muscles feel tight, the cycling will stretch them.'

'I know that whatever I say won't make any difference but it's complete madness to be thinking of setting off,' Mike said.

I raised my shoulders and then dropped them, turning away from Mike as I punched the button that started the shuttered door rolling upwards. Ryan had been present throughout our exchange but had kept silent. He stood and wheeled my bike out as the shutter rose and pushed the bike to the side of the road. I stepped forward and took the bike from him.

The rental house was on a road that ran down to one of the major highways into town, so I headed uphill. Try as I may, I couldn't get my foot into the strapping of the pedal. I was too stiff and each time I tried, I veered madly across the road. Eventually, I gave it up as a bad job and sat my feet on the straps instead.

In a low gear, I pushed the pedals and made it to the next junction, signalling to turn left.

I was relieved to find I could sit in the saddle. It was uncomfortable but the position of my posterior meant that the sorest parts of my pelvis had little or no direct pressure through them. My groin area was stiff and pedalling was difficult but not impossible. My foot slipped forward and the pain shot through my leg and up my back, forcing hot tears to rise in my eyes. I raised my hand and smeared them away. This wasn't going to work. I brought the bike to a halt and realised how frail my body felt. Setting off slowly again, I very shortly stopped. I had come to another junction. Each time I stopped, putting my foot down became more and more problematic, pushing off jerked my back and pelvis.

'Shit, shit, shit,' I muttered, as I cycled in a loop heading back to the house. Gliding down the hill I saw Mike standing next to Ryan by the garage door. Mike's face was creased with concern, his eyes narrow, his lips small, his mouth scrunched as he watched me climbing off the bike clumsily and forcing my leg over the crossbar.

'This is ridiculous,' Mike said. 'You can't even get on and off the bike. How are you going to cycle four thousand miles?'

I shook my head at him. 'Don't, Mike.'

I wheeled the bike towards the garage and Ryan stepped up to take it from me.

'How was it?' he asked quietly.

'Bloody awful,' I replied but added, 'I could sit on the saddle at least. It's my muscles in my leg that are really tight so I can't put much force through the left side; my right leg's fine though.'

I hobbled slowly up the stairs and lowered myself on to a chair. I was sitting there slumped with my head in my hands, trying to slow the hot tears that surged from my eyes and down my face, when Mike appeared.

'You can't set off like this,' Mike said. I took a deep breath, my chest expanding, my shoulders rising, and sat and looked at Mike, waiting for him to speak again. 'What are you going to do?' he asked.

'I don't know,' I replied. 'There are so many people here, they have gone to so much trouble to cover the start that I think I have to set off tomorrow.'

'You don't have to, we could just go home now.'

'No. We came to cycle across America and I'm not going home without even trying.' I leant over and pulled a map towards me. 'I won't make it up the route we planned across town. So we could cycle round the coastline instead. It's only ten miles or so. I think I can cope with that and then if I have to delay the first proper stage, we can set off a couple of days late. But we should set off from Golden Gate Bridge tomorrow as planned.'

'I don't agree with you. But you're right to not be going up those hills. They're bloody awful to walk up.'

'I could do with a little encouragement,' I said. 'It wouldn't be so bad if I could go for a proper cycle ride, but that's impossible here. There are junctions every couple of hundred feet so it's impossible to get up any momentum. What time is it anyway?'

Mike glanced at his phone. 'Three o'clock.'

'Oh bugger, I need to get changed for this Consulate thing. Will you sort Steven out if I get a quick bath?'

'Yeah, of course.' He stood and went through to the dining area. 'Stevie!' he called, 'you need to get changed, mate.' I could hear a chair being scraped back as Steven stood up.

'What for, Dad?' he asked.

'We're going out to a party to meet some people.'

'Do I have to?' Steven asked.

'Dave and Phil will be there,' Mike said, referring to Dave Harrison and Phil Iveson from Yorkshire Television, who were here to report on the ride's first week. Both had been covering us for over five years so were friends first and media people second.

'Yeaaah,' shouted Steven.

An hour later, we drove to a plush residential area near the city centre, where we came to a large house with brightly lit windows shining out on the dull afternoon. The Consul had invited us but as we entered the building, a man came over to Mike.

'I'm so sorry but the Consul can't be here, his mother's ill,' he said apologetically.

'Oh, I'm so sorry to hear that,' I said. 'It's been so kind of you to look after us.'

A tall man appeared with a tray and offered me a drink. I took a glass and looked at him.

'That's Pimms,' he said. 'I hope you enjoy it.'

He walked towards Ryan, Phil and Dave, and offered them drinks. I took a sip, the refreshing crystal ting hitting my tongue.

I looked around and recognised Anna from the Consulate staff, who'd shown us around the small park area that was overlooked by the Golden Gate Bridge. She'd checked out the best route from there to the ferry terminal. She came over. 'I'm so glad you could come, there are some journalists who would like to talk to you. I think they want to film something in the garden, would you do it?'

I nodded and looked around for Mike.

Stepping outside, I shivered, my back tightening with the chill in the air. Phil was setting the camera up, turning a bright light towards Dave, and I closed my eyes against it. The wind caught leaves on the path and they swirled upwards and then rattled in a corner.

'How's it going?' Dave asked. I drew a short breath and clenched my jaw. I shook my head slowly.

'I'm really sore and so tired,' I said.

'We won't take too long,' he said. 'Just a few words about tomorrow.'

Dave looked towards Phil, who nodded, and Dave crouched down, bending his leg to lessen the height difference between us.

'So, Jane, after months of preparation the big day is looming. How are you feeling?' He turned the microphone towards me.

'I'm very nervous. The travelling has been really hard and has made me very achy but tomorrow morning we're going to cycle just a few miles around the Bay in San Francisco and I'm looking forward to it. It's a long way to New York – four thousand miles.'

'Do you think you can do it?'

I smiled. 'We just have to take it a day at a time but yes, I'm hopeful that in nine weeks' time we'll be cycling across Brooklyn Bridge into New York.'

Dave turned and talked into the camera. 'Rockies', 'desert' and other words stuck in my mind but I didn't follow all he said.

Then the lighting from the camera was extinguished.

'We'd better get you back inside,' Dave said.

'Is there anything you need?' Phil asked.

'No, thanks.' I shook my head and we made our way towards the small gathering inside the house.

'We wish Jane well and hope she'll come back to visit us and spend a little time in San Francisco,' Anna said. They handed a T-shirt to Steven and a box of candies to me.

'I'll make sure these get the attention they deserve,' I smiled. 'Thank you for all your help and support and I can only wish for a safe and successful journey,' I said.

As we said our goodbyes, Mike noticed his mother Alice with a tray of finished glasses.

'Mum, what are you doing now?' he asked.

'I'm just taking these glasses to the kitchen.'

'You can't do that,' I said.

'I've already taken one lot in and said hello to the people in there, they're all very nice and the kitchen's huge.'

I shook my head at her, laughing. 'What are you like?'

Alice smiled at me and I followed her into the hall shaking hands with people as we went.

Day 1 – Thursday, 29 June
Golden Gate Bridge to Fisherman's Wharf
11.2 miles – 2 hrs 19 mins

MIKE

It was a dank start to the day but by the time we arrived at Lincoln Field, most people were there – staff and their relatives from the Consulate, a splattering of British and American media, Ryan's mum and dad, my mum and Suzy's mum. The three new bikes, resplendent with their black finish, looked wonderful with the appeal web address clearly visible.

Like most media events, the start would be something of a visual trick; Jane, Martyn and Ryan were to be filmed starting from the city side of the Golden Gate Bridge as expensive filming permits were required if we were to set off from the very western point in the National Recreation Area on the opposite side.

So, there would be a formal TV start, then after a mile, all three cyclists would double back over the bridge and begin the ride properly – and for free.

I was very apprehensive. Yesterday's trial ride by Jane had proved nothing. There was still every chance that the first day would also be the last even though, in comparison to what lay ahead, it was simply a leisurely joy ride to enable the media to get some terrific shots of San Francisco. Already, our original plans had been thwarted. Jane had hoped to ride up Lombard Street, the self-appointed most crooked street in the world, but it would have been too much strain on her back. All did not bode well for the Rockies.

Martyn approached me, his white cycling top the perfect advertisement for a whiter-than-white washing powder.

'Good morning, Mike.' He looked studious with his camera positioned loosely over his shoulder. 'How are you?'

'Okay and you?'

'Excited. I can't believe we're here. I can't believe that we're gonna get the chance to set off.' He hunched his shoulder, repositioning the camera slightly before looking back. 'There's a glint in Jane's eye this morning,' he said.

'I know.' I had seen the same sparkle that only came out when Jane was about to compete. Like a mischievous child's slight grin, it was a characteristic that had been missing from her for months. It was the first suggestion of hope that Jane might be able to give this ride a decent stab.

I watched Jane as I had for the last few years with a mixture of pride and concern. From the moment the extraordinary adventure started in May 2001 with a 5km race right through to the Ironman competition in Florida, her fragile grip on life had become ever more perilous.

Her characteristics were never defined by the disease; they simply provided a stage for them to be displayed. Her strength, her courage – from the moment she left her hospital bed in her dressing gown a few days after the mastectomy in 1990 for an interview to study radiography, she had not been defined by a few rogue cells.

I watched her as she strutted around the quayside making

final preparations to her bike – adjusting panniers, the saddle position – and flitting between media interviews. It was the same guts that had seen her shovelling down food and vitamin supplements when going through bouts of extreme nausea while on chemotherapy. She knew that if she didn't, she would become even more ill.

The endurance events had not extended her life, she'd merely channelled her energies into them and not allowed herself feelings of melancholy. The weight of her illness could challenge the most positive thinker, and it occurred to me how ironic it was that we were starting this incredible ride on a bridge where, at the last count, at least 1200 people had jumped to their death since it opened in 1937.

As she removed a yellow waterproof cycling jacket and wheeled the bike slowly between the cameramen and reporters to reach the designated starting point, the muscles in her neck tightened and a wave of apprehension flickered across her face. It was a relief to see her finally mount the bike and slowly increase her cadence as she made her way to San Francisco.

It was two hours before we met up again at Fisherman's Wharf, a busy tourist attraction halfway between the Golden Gate and Bay bridges. The idea had been for Jane to stop at the Vallejo ferry terminal and to reconvene the next morning in Vallejo at the San Francisco ferry terminal, thereby avoiding the need to travel by boat which could affect her balance.

But as we arrived at the Wharf, crammed with tourist attractions, restaurants and shops, there were no less than forty-seven named piers over the period of a mile. And we'd left all the phones back at the house.

The sun was beating down hard and the temperature was a good twenty degrees higher than it had been at Golden Gate Bridge.

As I came across Jane she had a tuna salad baguette wrapped in paper in one hand, a bottle of orange juice in the other. She looked fresh and relaxed – a striking contrast to us, the support crew who had been running up and down the Wharf trying to find her.

'How are you?' I asked, as she sat on a bench with Alcatraz behind her, the Bay basking in sunshine.

She didn't need to answer, she looked better than she had in months. 'Good,' she said between chomps. 'There wasn't too much pain, I should be okay to set off properly tomorrow.'

CHAPTER 2

Day 2 – Friday, 30 June
Vallejo, California (Calif.) to Winters, Calif.
59.5 miles – 5 hrs 41 mins
Total covered – 70.7 miles

JANE

For the first part of our journey, we decided to follow the Adventure Cycling Association's Western Express route. We figured it would take us along the more quiet roads away from the main interstate highways with their fast moving traffic. But as we headed towards the outskirts of Benicia, the so-called quiet roads seemed to be filled with tall trucks passing dizzyingly close by. Their large wheels were as high as I was on the bike and as they sped past, they would pull the bikes towards them with a rush of wind. It was terrifying.

Ahead of me, Martyn looked back from his bike and I could see him wobble slightly, his mouth wide open in horror as another truck sped by. I concentrated on the road ahead, stiffening my body each time I heard a truck approach behind me so I could brace the bike ahead of the pull.

In convoy, we cycled on for five miles until, thankfully, we passed the point where the heavy vehicles left the highway. Their destination was a large quarry, Syar, set back from the road. The noise of their chugging engines faded into the background as they descended into the deep cuts in the hillside, their glaring yellow white contrasted against the grey green scrub of the surrounding landscape.

Martyn slowed down as Ryan and I caught him up on the small incline.

'That was not good,' he said, shaking his head. 'I couldn't believe how close that last bloke came to you. He was inches from your bike.'

'Hopefully it will be quieter now,' I said.

I pulled my green Gatorade water bottle from its cradle and sucked at the white lip. Martyn did the same and showered himself with water. I laughed.

'How do you use these things?' he asked, brushing splashes from his shirt. 'I keep doing that and getting water all over me.'

Ryan had been observing us and checked his watch.

'Come on troops, we've got to keep going.'

We followed the road and caught a glimpse of blue to our right. Lake Herman. The climb from Vallejo had been gradual, the small hills taking us gently upwards with the small downwards slopes taking the sting from the slight ascents.

I looked at the road behind and caught a glimpse of two other cyclists. Both had black bikes and black panniers at the front and rear wheels. They cycled side by side and I could see by the sway of the bike, a foot side to side with each cadence, the effort they were putting in.

'Look!' I shouted to Martyn and Ryan. 'We've got company.'

'That looks like hard work,' said Ryan. 'I'm glad we aren't having to carry our own equipment.'

He reached forward, standing up from his saddle, and lightly eased up the next small hill. I leant back, switched to a lower gear and circled my legs faster, trying not to lose the momentum from the last dip.

My left hip was still sore, my right leg stronger than the left and I found myself putting more effort through that right side in order to stop the pain becoming unbearable. My mouth was open, my breathing harsh.

We had only been going for thirty minutes and already the tightness in the long muscles in my back, stomach and thighs was easing, making the eternal turning movement more relaxed and natural.

I neared the crest and the two cyclists on the black bikes passed wide on my left. 'Hi there!' I called.

One of the men, bareheaded and with a V of sweat forming down his T-shirt, turned his head to me but turned away again without returning the greeting. Steadily, they forced their heavy bikes onwards, pulled away from me and disappeared round the corner ahead.

I reached the blind spot minutes later and was pleased to see the sweet downhill. I crouched as low on my bike as my stiffness allowed and felt the air rush past me, catching in the bright yellow fabric of my coat and tugging it from my body, blowing it out wide.

The rush of speed allowed me to crest the next hill with ease and I sat on the tail of the two strangers who still hadn't spoken a word. At the next hill I stopped for a moment at the top alongside Ryan and Martyn and we looked out over the dark blue water that lay ahead of us – Suisun Bay, which lies at the entrance of the Sacramento–San Joaquin river delta. Out before us was the mothball fleet, a collection of US navy and merchant ships dating back to the Second World War.

The excitement of starting had numbed some of my pain, but as we neared Rockville after twenty-five miles cycling the base of my back was aching and my left side tightened, twisting my knee if I put too much strain on it.

After passing through Rockville, the three of us stopped to shelter under a tree by the roadside. The sun was high in the sky, we were all hot and hungry and in desperate need of a break. I pulled a banana from my rear pocket and unpeeled it as Martyn set up his camera to take some shots of the route.

'It's greener than I thought it would be today,' I said, looking out at the fruit trees that studded the grass.

'I thought we'd be cycling through industrial estates today. This is much better,' Martyn said. 'What I'd do for a Starbucks though,' he smiled and Ryan's head rose.

'I think we may have had our last Starbucks for a while,' he said.

We stood looking over the fruit orchard in front of us.

'Should we ring Michael and Cindy to see if they've found anywhere for tonight,' said Ryan, pulling his phone out of his bag. Michael and Cindy were providing support for the first few days. There was only one RV on the road which four of us would sleep in. (Martyn would be staying in hotels.) With four adults sharing such a confined space I suspected our patience might be tested. Mike had stayed in San Francisco with Steven, waiting for Rebecca and Jodie to arrive a few days later and they would then set off to join us at Carson City on Monday. I would then move into Mike's RV.

Dialling, he held the phone to his ear. It wasn't long before I could hear the murmuring of Cindy's voice on the other end of the phone.

'Yes,' said Ryan. 'How far? Is that definite?' I couldn't make out what she was saying on the other end of the line. 'We'll ring you when we're nearer and get directions then,' said Ryan and finished the call.

'Have they found somewhere?' I asked.

'Yeah, they're sitting outside an In-N-Out Burger Bar. Cindy says there's a place not far from Winters, but that they'll have to stay in the spot once they have found somewhere or they'll lose the site.'

'That's not a problem,' I said. 'At least we'll have somewhere to sleep.'

'She says it's a couple of miles off route.'

I shrugged my shoulders. 'It doesn't matter. That's why today wasn't too long.' I looked at the mileage on the bikes and saw that it was just over forty miles.

'How far have we got to go now?' he asked.

I unfolded my map and studied the route for a few seconds. 'I reckon about fifteen miles.'

'About an hour and we'll be done,' said Ryan. He stretched his legs while standing astride his bike. 'If you don't mind, I'm going to put my foot down and stretch out a bit – I feel tight after last night.'

Ryan had slept on a pull-out bed, thanks to the amount of people who had ended up sleeping at the house.

'Go ahead, I'm fine back here,' I said and he set off, slipping into a higher gear and pulling away from Martyn and me. We climbed back on to our bikes but Martyn quickened his pace too and soon it felt like I was cycling alone across America, just catching glimpses of my companions in the distance.

'This isn't so bad,' I thought, taking another slug of my energy drink, the sweetness warming my mouth, making me grimace.

The road meandered through a green valley. Orchards full of trees, their boughs heavy with fruit, coloured into dusky reds with plums and crisp greens and reds with apples. Long lush grass grew below. The staccato hiss of the sprinkler systems as they threw their rainbow arcs across the road gave us welcome relief from the heat, which was becoming more fierce as we passed midday.

I met Martyn and Ryan at a crossroads about five miles from Winters. We were heading along Putah Creek Road.

'Another twenty minutes and we'll be finished for the day,' Ryan said.

Martyn looked at me and a grin cracked his face.

'Twenty minutes for you maybe, but it's gonna take me thirty,' I said.

Martyn nodded, his bike was heavy with camera gear and mine was just heavy beneath my tired legs and aching back.

Ryan's face dropped a little. 'Come on, guys, we can do it in twenty.'

I shook my head. 'I probably could, but I'll pay the price tomorrow. This isn't just about today you know.'

We set our eyes forward and pushed the bikes onwards. In less than half an hour we stopped, nearly missing a small road across a wooden bridge spanning the Putah Creek which led into Winters.

The whole town looked like a set from an old Western film. At the first main street was a low wooden building with a veranda all the way around it. I could see a colourful board hanging from the metal railings.

'That looks like somewhere we might get a coffee,' I said and we parked up and wandered over.

The cool of air conditioning made us all stop in our tracks. 'Shall we sit inside?' Ryan asked and we turned to retrieve our cycling gear from outside.

There was a dresser to the side filled with local jams, bottles of cider and traditional root beer. On a leather sofa two people lounged, leaning forward to their companions at the other side of a wooden table. I shivered a little as my body cooled, goose pimples rising on my bare arms.

As Martyn ordered the drinks, I decided to phone our backup team.

'Hi Jane!' Cindy's American twang reverberated in my ear from the phone. 'Wow, you've made some good time there. Was it good cycling? How you feeling?'

'We're fine,' I said. 'Have we got somewhere to park tonight?'

'Yeah, we sure have,' she said. 'We can't move else we'll lose our spot. But it's not far from where you are.'

'That's okay, don't worry about it. We'll have some lunch here then we'll come and find you guys. Can you give us some directions?'

I scrambled in my black bag for a pen and wrote the directions on a serviette.

'We'll be about an hour or so,' I said.

Martyn looked at his phone as a text message came in. 'Rob's on his way here to meet us,' he said. 'He's booked into a small bed and breakfast.' Rob, who worked for Sky News, first joined us for part of the John o'Groats to Land's End ride, then had been the producer for the whole of the 'Rome to Home' journey. He always seemed to be in good humour, providing practical help, and because he'd been on two of these journeys had an insight into predicting what as cyclists we might need. Minutes later Rob walked through the door.

'What a lovely town,' he smiled, joining us at our table. 'I'll be all right if they're all like this. Have you seen the saloon across the road? It's just like the Wild West.'

'Where've you been?' asked Martyn.

'I've just left Cindy and Michael. They're about five miles down the road,' Rob said. 'It's a lovely spot.'

I raised my eyebrows. 'Cindy said it was about two miles away.'

'Well,' Rob hesitated, looking at Martyn. 'I've just clocked it in the car and it's just over five.'

'No chance of a lift?' Ryan joked.

The thought of another five miles didn't upset any of us particularly. We'd only covered just over fifty miles and our legs still felt relatively fresh.

Rob gave us accurate directions to the campsite and we headed out of town, stopping at a small parade of shops which to our amazement had a well-stocked bike shop with some good-looking road bikes hanging in racks.

Velo City Bikes had its own branded cycle shirts and I was tempted to buy one but while the boys went shopping, I had the unenviable job of bike sitting.

Sitting on a bench, I glanced at Ryan and Martyn in the shop chatting with a bearded man behind the counter. I turned away and allowed my mind to wander, closing my eyes to keep the glare of the sun from them.

My face was starting to feel more than a little warm when Ryan and Martyn reappeared. 'It should be a good start tomorrow,' Martyn said. 'Apparently Winters is a "platinum rated" bike city.'

'What does that mean?'

'It's got cycle paths and it's *real bike friendly*.' Martyn drawled the last words in a bad imitation of an American accent.

'I've never cycled in a *platinum rated bike city*,' I said. 'Did they have any of the white leg warmers, Ryan?'

'No,' he said. He had been cursing himself for turning some down earlier in the year. White leg warmers would have been useful in Utah and Nevada as they would reflect the sun's rays to prevent us from overheating. We had dark ones already, but the heat in the desert would make them impractical.

'Come on, we need to get out of this sun,' I said, as Ryan passed me a tube of sun cream and I rubbed some into my arms and face and the back of my neck. 'I think I might use my buff tomorrow,' I said, referring to the multifunctional headwear that can be worn in a number of different styles to protect the cyclist against the sun, cold, wind or dust. 'It'll hopefully keep the sun off my neck. I can feel it's really warm there. You should get yourself one.'

Ryan frowned and shook his head forcefully. 'I don't care how useful they are. I'm not wearing one of those.'

It doesn't matter how many miles you have cycled – it could be eight or eighty, but the last few always get your legs. The last five miles hadn't seemed like much but as I watched Ryan and Martyn ease along, side by side, chatting, I envied their fitness. The two weeks enforced rest before we came out to the USA had made my leg muscles slacken and it was with great effort that I forced myself along the last stretch towards our stop for the night.

Turning right, we entered the Shingle Springs Camping Site.

'That's got to be ours,' Ryan called back to me. Ahead was parked a large white RV with scenes of fields and lakes painted across it. It would become a familiar logo on our trip.

'Hiya, you guys.' Cindy stretched and stood up from her camping armchair. 'What was that like?'

I stepped from my bike. 'Not bad. A good day's cycling,' I said.

'Is this a great spot or what?' she asked.

'It's really pretty,' I agreed.

'There's peacocks and all sorts down there and some critters in cages back down that hill. Isn't it just great?' she said.

I nodded and smiled and wheeled my bike to the back of the van and rested it against the image of a family on horseback.

Cindy gave me a quick tour, showing me the toilet block and some possums in cages which we assumed belonged to the campsite owners.

I gathered up my clothes and a couple of towels and headed

off to shower and change. When I came back Ryan was still clad in his cycling gear. He and Michael were putting together the cycle rack.

'It must just go here,' Michael said, pushing a black metal bar against the back of the van. 'That'll do anyway.' He pulled against the rack. 'It's not going to move from there.' He started putting the tools back into the boxes and turned to me.

'The bed's made up in the back if you need to rest,' he said.

'Ryan, where do you want to sleep?' I asked.

Ryan stepped into the van and we both looked around the small space that would be home for all five of us over the next few days. Ryan chose the bed over the cab so there wasn't very much headroom for him.

'I'd like that one there, if that's okay,' I said, looking at the double bed in the separate room at the back of the RV. 'I can rest if I need to up there when we're done for the day.'

Just looking at the bed made me realise how tired I was. 'I could do with a lie down,' I said.

'Yeah, get some rest, Jane,' Ryan said and I needed no further prompting.

I have no idea how long I was out for but I woke with a start. Sitting upright, I looked around. There were windows to three sides, a small closed curtain and a narrow space either side of the bed about a foot wide which was crammed with bags and suitcases.

I pulled the covers back and eased my legs up. My back had stiffened while I'd slept, and I moved slowly and carefully. I couldn't swing my legs out of the bed, there was no room, so I slid my whole body down the length of the bed towards the curtained entrance leading to the rest of the RV.

'Hiya,' Cindy said, as I appeared in the doorway. 'How yer doing there, girl?'

I opened my eyes wide and stared at her, not fully awake yet. 'Okay, I think,' I replied. 'What time is it?'

She glanced at her watch. 'Ten of six.'

'What?' I scrunched my face trying to understand what that meant.

'Oh, you . . .' she said and held her hands palm up. 'Ten to six. Is that how you say it in England?'

'Oh, right. Yes,' I said. 'What are we doing about food tonight?'

'Rob said he'd fetch us about now,' she said.

I stepped out of the RV and slumped into one of the folding chairs we had brought with us.

'How's the legs?' Ryan asked.

'Not too bad,' I replied. 'I'm hungry though, is there anything to eat?'

I turned to Michael, who thought for a moment. 'Not much. How about a banana or better yet an energy bar? We've got loads of those.'

'No, a banana would be good.'

Michael moved. 'No, don't get up just tell me where they are,' I said.

'No, believe me, it'll be easier to find them myself.'

He tossed me a banana.

'Ryan?' he said, holding one up. Ryan nodded and caught it. We sat munching on them.

'I've given the bikes a once over and they seem okay. I've lubricated the chains so we're ready for the off first thing,' Ryan said.

'Tomorrow doesn't look too bad,' I said, 'but it's the climb the next day I'm worried about.'

Ryan nodded slowly. 'Oh, yeah, it's the biggie up to Carson's Pass. That'll be tough. We'll just have to see how far we can get. There's no point killing ourselves over it. If we can't get all the way up we'll just have to stop.'

'At least it'll put some hills in our legs for later,' I said.

There was still no sign of Rob and I was starting to feel shaky and in need of proper food.

'Are you sure he's coming?' I asked Cindy.

'I'll give him a call,' she said, and wandered away in search of reception for her phone. I could hear her voice but couldn't make out the words. After a few seconds, she walked back towards us.

'Rob's on his way back to San Francisco,' she said. 'He left his wallet at the hotel.'

'Oh no, poor Rob,' I said. 'Never mind, we'll just have to cook something here.'

Michael scratched his head. 'We've not got a lot of food in,' he said.

'I thought you'd loaded the van,' Ryan said. 'There must be something.'

Mike shrugged. 'Sorry, folks.'

I shook my head. 'We'll just have some soup or something or a sandwich will do.'

'Sorry,' Michael said softly, 'there's no bread.'

A stiff silence hung in the air. I sat looking at Cindy and Mike, unable to think of anything much to say. I'd cycled just short of sixty miles and they hadn't even thought to buy bread.

'It's a good job we had lunch,' I said, trying to paste a smile on my face and not lose my temper. Ryan looked at me and shook his head. I took a deep breath and exhaled slowly. 'I think I might take a short walk,' I said and got up and walked away, down the dirt road that led to the entrance to the campsite. 'Better to get away from everyone before I lost my temper,' I thought. Tiredness and hunger never made my words well thought out. Better to say nothing.

MIKE

The rap on the front door of our rented house broke the steady rhythm pounding in my skull. It was Wesley, a reporter from Leeds who worked for the Press Association and was here to cover the ride's start. However, this morning our attention would be focused on watching England's World Cup quarter final against Portugal.

'Come in, Wes,' I called, dragging myself off the settee and towards the door. 'Do you want a tea or coffee?' It was seven thirty in the morning in San Francisco so it seemed strange to be getting up to watch England play.

'Tea would be good, thanks,' said a smiling Wesley, following me into the kitchen area. Despite having arrived from the UK a few days later than the rest of us, he looked remarkably fresh and relaxed, casually dressed in a black T-shirt and blue jeans. His short cropped hair and stocky build were set off nicely against a pleasant, easy going manner.

'I gather Jane did well yesterday,' he said. 'You must be relieved.' I nodded. I'd missed her this morning and was already looking forward to meeting her on Monday, in two days' time.

'If you hadn't witnessed it firsthand, you'd be sceptical,' I said. 'On Wednesday she didn't even know if she could get on a bike and then yesterday, there she is doing nearly sixty miles with barely a concern.'

Wesley raised his eyebrows and shook his head, clearly impressed. 'I know what you mean, Mike,' he said. 'You look rough, though. Hangover?'

I nodded weakly. 'I think it was part of a dastardly plot by ITN to wreck the ride. Dave Harrison came over with a bottle of beer for Jane on Wednesday – he bought it because it was called Fat Tyre and he liked the name. Jane was too poorly to drink it so you know what it's like, late at night, the bottle was calling out to me like a siren so I drank it.'

'That's all you had?' Wesley's smile broadened. 'One bottle of Fat Tyre?'

'Yep, and I feel like I've had twelve hours on the lash.'

Wesley smiled. 'It's funny you should say that – I went out for a beer with Dave and Phil last night and the barman laughed when Dave ordered Fat Tyre, saying no one drank it.'

'I'm not bloody surprised, it was dreadful,' I said. We returned to the living room where on the TV, England and Portugal were lining up for the national anthem. Wesley stretched out his feet on the small coffee table. 'Did Becca arrive okay?'

'Yeah, Becks and Jodie came. Jodie's got a suitcase that needs a forklift truck to move it.'

I rubbed my temples and looked out of the window into the hazy morning light. The school opposite, affiliated to the church, was eerily quiet. It was quite a contrast to last night when queues of minibuses had been lining the road and I had been unceremoniously awakened in the early hours by a crescendo of impromptu gospel singing on the pavement outside the house. Fortunately, after an hour of happy clappy chants and exaggerated farewells between the assembled singers, peace had been restored. But it hadn't done my hangover much good.

The ref's whistle blew and Wesley and I were captivated by the game. I could imagine the crowds watching the big screen in Millennium Square in Leeds, a Saturday afternoon and an electric atmosphere. The flags of St George flying on the cars, the sense of national pride yet knowing that at some point the usual disappointment would inevitably follow. It was odd listening to American commentators and their detached involvement with my own country. I so wanted to be at home enjoying the communal national hysteria.

'Do you get nervous when Jane's doing something like this?' asked Wesley, taking a sip of tea as Lampard tried to get on to a cross from Beckham.

I thought for a second. When Jane and her brother Luke had been cycling from John o'Groats to Land's End in 2003 and then Rome to Leeds a year later, there had been occasions when they had been incommunicado and my stomach had churned at the thought of what *might* have happened to them. 'Not nervous exactly,' I said. 'More concerned. It's not like constant butterflies. Probably no worse than waiting for a teenager returning from a night out on the town.'

Wesley reached for his cup before putting it down when he realised that he had already emptied its contents. 'You don't worry that Jane's risking serious injury then?'

'She's dying. What could be worse? Her oncologist says at this stage in her life she should do what she likes. If it's running, she should run. If she liked shopping, then she'd shop. The point of having chemotherapy is to allow her to live her life with maximum enjoyment.'

Wesley took off his jacket. Although the sun had risen a couple of hours ago, it was only just beginning to be high enough to light up the living room.

'Were they okay about her coming to the States? The doctors I mean,' Wesley asked.

'When we first mentioned what we were planning in December, we'd just been told that the cancer had spread to her liver. Her oncologist said there was no chance of us getting here. It's only very recently that it became anything other than a pipe dream but he still didn't want us to come. But he realised that Jane is not easily put off.' We turned our attention back to the match which if England hadn't have been playing would have lost our attention some time ago.

'Fancy a refill?' I said, as the referee blew the half-time whistle. I reached over for Wesley's cup but he pre-empted and handed it to me.

'It would be rude to say no, thanks Mike.'

I got up and went back into the kitchen area and flicked the kettle on. 'Was this Ironman the first time the doctors had said that she shouldn't do an event?' Wesley asked.

'No. He advised her not to do the Ironman too but Jane was determined. Nothing was going to stop her, she'd been working towards it for two years. She had this burning desire to do the Ironman – it's the ultimate one-day sporting challenge, even to those fully able. This trip is different though. It isn't a passion for Jane, it is just an opportunity to raise money for charity.'

'Yes, it's all his fault,' Becky arrived in the kitchen area fresh from waking, her blonde hair stuck up in wisps. 'What's the score?'

'Nil-nil,' I said.

'Hiya, I'm Wes,' Wesley said, outstretching his hand.

'Becky,' she said, completing the greeting.

'Have you and Jodie got any plans for today?' I asked.

'We're going to San Francisco to do some shopping. We'll get some dinner in town. What time do you want us back tonight?'

'Six thirty. Then we can all go out to a restaurant for tea. Make the most of the shops, though – you'll not see any more all the time you are here in the States.'

'Yeah right,' she said dismissively, her eyes scanning the unfamiliar surroundings.

'We'll be in the middle of nowhere for the rest of the four weeks you'll be with us,' I said. 'You'll be lucky to see people, never mind shops. No TV or internet till you get home.'

'Oh, very funny,' said Rebecca, searching through the cupboards. 'My sides are bursting. Is there any food in?' she asked, as the kettle began to emit a loud shriek. 'Tea, please.'

'Sadly your dad's right, Rebecca,' said Wesley. 'You're heading out into the desert.'

Rebecca looked at me, suddenly serious. 'Great. A holiday in the wilderness. You could have told us.'

'We did,' I said.

'Whatever,' she shrugged, then turned her back on me and continued to search through the cupboards.

I poured two more cups of tea and Wesley and I went back through to the living room. 'Where will you watch the match if England get to the final?' asked Wesley.

'We'll be in Ely which is in the middle of the Nevada Desert. It's about three hundred miles from Las Vegas so we thought we'd head down there as it would be quite a laugh. We'd have to suspend the ride for a couple of days but it won't matter. Some things are more important than a bike ride.' I gave Wesley a knowing smile.

As the second half proceeded, the conversation died along with England's hopes. Wayne Rooney was dismissed and then another penalty shoot-out resulted in an England defeat. There was a sad inevitability about the match and I was momentarily glad not to be in England where I knew the sense of disappointment would be acute. Watching on another continent seemed to lend a remoteness to that disappointment. 'At least you don't have to worry about going to Vegas,' Wesley said. 'So what's the plan now?'

'There's no set schedule, Wesley. We need to be in Cedar City in a couple of weeks because Michael flies home from there. A couple of weeks after that we're having a rest day in Pueblo as Becca and Jodie fly out from Denver and Jane wants to see them off. But apart from that we'll see how it goes. I'm not trying to think too far ahead. If I'm honest, Jane was in such a bad way earlier in the week we didn't think she'd even set off, so anything from here on in is a bonus.

'We had a big discussion on Wednesday night about whether she should start as we both realised she was in no fit state. Not for the papers but she had to take some morphine to control the pain and we always agreed that once that point was reached then we'd call a halt to any event, but Jane didn't want to not give it a go.'

'How much of her illness are you happy with us reporting, Mike?'

'Nothing that isn't already out there. Jane doesn't want anyone to know the extent of her disease. It's fair to say she's not well but she's adamant that her liver disease is kept secret and no one is aware of the type of medication and amount of bone disease.'

'I can't believe she set off, Mike, I really can't. She's got some guts,' said Wesley.

'Indeed.'

Day 3 – Saturday, 1 July
Winters, Calif. to Rescue, Calif.
80.5 miles – 8 hrs 20 mins
Total covered – 151.2 miles

JANE

Cycling through West Sacramento, we couldn't see any signs for Old Sacramento but ahead of us we spied the familiar green and black Starbucks sign and Ryan, Martyn and I headed towards it. We stopped and chained our bikes together, ordered coffee and sat outside in the shade. The sun was moving higher in the sky and the day was becoming hot.

'What's the time?' asked Martyn.

'It's just after nine thirty, so we've been cycling just over three hours,' I said.

'How many miles have we done?' Ryan asked.

'Just over thirty,' I said, consulting the map from my pannier.

'That's not too bad,' he said. 'We should be finished a bit earlier than yesterday.'

'I don't know,' I said. 'We've got nearly fifty miles left, we'd better not hang around too long.'

We finished our drinks and headed off. The route took us straight into Old Sacramento and the three of us couldn't resist walking down the street to explore a little of the log township. It reminded me of the tales I'd read of the Mississippi River and the paddle steamers of years gone by. The houses and restaurants had wooden verandas, an old railway line ran alongside the river and there was even a magnificent old steamer on the Sacramento River.

Martyn, always keen to get the best footage for the documentary, asked if he could film me mounting my bike and crossing the railway line. I obliged, making my way tentatively across the tracks.

After a few seconds negotiating the tracks, the front wheel of my bike got caught and immediately I knew I was going to fall but still couldn't manage to do it gracefully. I lay on the floor with my bike beneath my right leg, laughing out loud.

Martyn rushed over. 'Are you all right?'

'Yes, I'm fine,' I said, sitting up and dusting myself off. 'I could just envisage this happening to me.'

'I'm really sorry,' Martyn said. 'That could've ended our bike trip.'

'I'm all right. Just a bit bruised and my pride is a little bit battered.'

I recovered myself, righted the bike and pushed it the rest of the way across the railway line until we found the bike trail which ran alongside the Sacramento River for a short while before crossing the American River.

We were following the Jedediah Smith National Recreational Trail – also known as the American River Bike Trail – a well-maintained trail with a smooth tarmac surface that runs from Old Sacramento to Folsom Lake.

By now, it was eleven and the shade of the trees was welcome, as any effort we put in to crest the small hills caused sweat to pour from our bodies. My arms glistened with water and I stopped more than once to reapply sun cream that had slicked from my body with sweat.

Martyn, still intent on making sure he got great camera angles, would occasionally drop behind, film some footage and then tail us once more as we hurried on through the miles. He stopped to film Ryan cycling through arcs of water as they danced through an intricate set of movements determined by some sort of computer program. A few minutes afterwards, I glanced behind, confident that I would catch a glimpse of his white shirt following us. There was no sign.

'Its ages since I saw Martyn,' I said to Ryan, who was pedalling right beside me. 'Do you think he's all right?'

Ryan glanced behind also. 'Should we stop and wait?'

We both slowed our pace. The large trees that had shaded us earlier had become small tortured thorn bushes and we travelled over a mile before we came to some shade and stopped to wait for Martyn.

Peering anxiously into the distance, there was still no sign of his white shirt in the crowds of cyclists whizzing by. The cycle track was busy with weekenders enjoying the freedom of no work and we watched as many coloured shirts sped past, wondering where their own journey was taking them.

It was hard to believe that we had only arrived last Sunday, already so much had happened in just six days.

After fifteen more minutes, I began to worry.

'Excuse me,' I stopped one of the slower cyclists. 'Have you seen a bloke back on the track with one of these shirts on?'

The bearded man looked at my own white shirt.

'I'm not sure, man,' he said. 'I think there was some guy back there. He looked like he was having some problems with his chain. I don't know if he had one of those shirts on, though. What is it?'

'This is Jane and we're cycling across America,' Ryan said.

'Wow, that's awesome. You must be going over Carson Pass. That's one hard hill to climb,' he said, wheeling his bike back on to the track and saying his goodbyes.

Ryan was just climbing on his bike to head back to find Martyn, when he appeared in the distance. He stopped at our side and took a long drink from his bottle, his face red with the sun and the effort of trying to catch up with us. His shirt clung to his back.

'I'm so hot,' he said, blowing out his cheeks. He took his glasses off and dried the rims where the sweat had collected. 'Thanks for waiting. I only stopped for a few moments to change my flat tyre but I can't believe the heat from the tarmac.' He took another drink.

'We were starting to get really worried,' I said.

We let Martyn cool down and then set off slowly to Folsom, twenty miles away, where we met up briefly with Phil and Dave from Yorkshire Television, who supplied us with bananas and water.

It was well past midday now and my legs were feeling distinctly shaky. The sun became even fiercer as we set off up a seemingly endless hill leading out from Folsom, which seemed to be the footings of a huge ridge we would need to climb to reach Nevada.

It was Green Bay Road, which had little shelter and so our meagre water supplies quickly ran out. Our pace slowed and slowed as sweat poured from us, it dripped down my sun-creamed arms and off my knuckles on to the tarmac, and still the hill rose steadily upwards.

'I'm just going to nip on ahead to get a shot,' Martyn said and I nodded without lifting my head much but watched as he headed off. He normally pedalled away from us with ease, his rear lifting from the saddle as he moved lightly on the bike. This time, it seemed to take an age for him to create any distance between us.

At the crest of the hill he laid down with his camera on the road and, from where we were approaching, his body was indistinct and hazy, rippling with the heatwaves that rose from the hot surface. At last we reached him and he turned to shoot us on our way upwards.

'I'll catch up with you!' he called and Ryan and I slowly cycled onwards.

We passed green gardens on our right. The cool blue pool of Folsom Lake seemed to mock our efforts. One house, with a terraced garden, had a waterfall dropping down in tiers. I could hear the murmur of voices and tinny strains of music above the rush of water cascading down the garden. Above that, the chink of ice against the side of a glass.

I could just imagine holding that frosted glass and cooling myself with it. I longed to stand in the cool water but the hill just led on, upwards and upwards.

We came to a garden where a small tree overhung the road, the first shade we had seen for a long while. I stopped beside Ryan.

'Where's Martyn?' I asked. Peering into the distance I could just make out a hazy figure moving slowly. 'I think we should wait for him. I could do with the rest and its awful chasing down people when you can never seem to catch them.'

We sat and drank juice, watching an army of ants moving busily across the pavement. I let a few drops of the sugary drink fall on to it and watched as one ant then several more came to taste the sweet liquid.

Martyn finally appeared.

'Do you need a rest or do you want to carry on?' I called to him as he approached. As he cycled nearer I could see him properly. His face was white, the colour had left him, and he was bluey grey around the mouth.

'I need to stop,' he said, his body shaking slightly as he climbed from his bike and sat next to us on the kerb, drinking slowly from his bottle. His head hung low as he tried to recover.

Ryan and I looked at each other.

'Are you okay?' I asked.

'I got up from the road after those shots and I just felt dreadful,' he said. 'I've been moving really slowly so I don't get any worse.'

'We don't need you to suffer from heatstroke,' I said. 'We've not got much further to go. We're stopping at Rescue, another five miles at the most.'

We waited until Martyn's colour had returned and set off again at a much slower pace. Ryan stayed by Martyn's side until we passed into the shade of taller trees and the climbing became easier out of the heat. I could see a twisting section of road falling away from us down a deep-blue wooded valley. The cooler air made goose pimples rise on my arms as the two miles sped beneath me and I passed a sign announcing the town of Rescue.

'Seventy-nine miles today,' I said to Ryan as we all climbed off our bikes.

'That last bit was the killer,' Ryan said. Martyn came over to us, his spirit undeterred by the difficulties he'd overcome that day.

'There's a thermometer in that window that reads forty-two degrees centigrade,' he said. 'It's no wonder I found it tough.'

'I can't believe that, that's just madness, it can't be that hot,' I said and Martyn strode away.

'Come on, I'll show you,' he said and I followed him, shaking my head in disbelief even when the proof was there for me to see.

Day 4 – Sunday, 2 July
Rescue, Calif. to Caples Lake, Calif.
57.3 miles – 9 hrs 02 mins including climbs of 8486 ft
Total covered – 208.5 miles

JANE

The fourth day was the one I had dreaded most at the start of our journey. We knew that whichever route we took from San Francisco to New York, the huge ridge that led from California to Nevada – the Sierra Nevada – would have to be traversed before we could ease our passage over the Rockies.

We started out from the fire station in Rescue, setting off as early as we dared at 6.30 a.m., to allow us to get some serious climbing out of the way. After only eight and a half miles we entered Placerville, and I watched helplessly as Ryan and Martyn cycled with ease up the small incline leading out of town. I called out to them, but they were too far ahead to hear me, so I followed as fast as I could trying all the while to catch them to let them know they'd taken the wrong route.

By the time I had caught them, we had swept down a steep downhill. I looked back at the hill we would have to climb.

'Don't worry,' said Martyn. 'If we continue down here we can cycle along this way.' He pointed at the map as I followed his finger along Pleasant Valley Road. 'We can rejoin the route here.' We set off once more.

Pleasant Valley Road was an aptly named route dipping and climbing through a lush green vale. At one point, we passed a homestead high above the road and heard the baying of dogs before we saw them.

My heart pounded. I've never liked dogs. Standing on my pedals I sped down the road hoping to outrun them but the incline was against me. I glanced back and a huge hound was making its way down a snaking drive towards us. We would never outrun it.

Then, it skidded to a stop, colliding with the boundary fence, and stood flanked on either side by two smaller dogs raising their heads and howling at us. When I realised they weren't going to go any further I slowed down, but could feel my heart pounding and adrenalin coursing through my limbs.

'That was a lucky escape,' Ryan said. Martyn and I smiled, relieved.

We left the green valley behind us, having covered nearly twenty miles, and stopped at a road junction where a large shining supermarket stood out sparkling against the hillside.

'More water,' I said and pointed at the building.

'Yeah, great idea.'

I stepped into the cool interior and returned with water, energy drinks and iced lattes. The glass bottles were cool.

'That's outstanding, an iced Starbucks, you're a saviour,' Martyn said as he uncapped his drink. We sat at the roadside and finished our drinks. Ryan was the first to wheel his bike out back on to the road and I followed reluctantly, happy to sit in the sunshine longer and not keen to face the climbs that lay ahead.

We followed Sly Park Road up to Jenkinson Lake, which shone in the bright sunlight. We dismounted, stopping to take in the view of this sparkling mass of water stretching out to our left.

'That's beautiful,' Martyn said, grabbing his camera to film us dwarfed against the landscape. A cool breeze fanned us as we watched small boats bob up and down in the distance. But we could not stay long. Our way was up and out and away from the lake.

As soon as we left the lake, the climb started in earnest, the sun rising in the sky making the effort that much more physical, and I started to dread each corner which always unveiled the next steep incline.

The route we were following had first been travelled in the opposite direction by a man called John Fremont in the winter snows of the 1840s. It must have been a hostile and frightening path to take.

The muscles in my leg had become less defined during the two weeks of illness before the trip when I'd been forced to rest. The steep slopes put pressure through my back as I gripped the handlebars grimly. My body leant forward with the effort. I stopped at the roadside often, mostly hanging over my bike to catch my breath, sometimes climbing from my black steed to sit in the shade along the roadside to drink and cool myself before the next onslaught.

I was shaking. I looked at the altimeter on my GPS unit. We had climbed 4000 feet and my body was unused to such effort. This wasn't from lack of training, it wasn't from being under-prepared. I'd pushed myself harder for the last few months, but nothing can ready you for these conditions. The sun was high and hot, out on the road the trees that surrounded us gave us no shelter.

'You're doing great,' Ryan said. 'How yer feeling?'

'Crap,' I said and my lips quivered as I fought back the childish tears that I could feel hot on my cheeks. I pushed my glasses hard against my face to stop them coursing down. 'I'm sorry, this is just so hard. I can't go any faster. We're only halfway through the climbs and I don't know how I'm going to get up the next half.'

'Honestly, you're doing great,' Ryan said. 'Stop beating yourself up. You're expecting too much of yourself.'

'But we're going so slowly we're barely moving,' I said.

'It doesn't matter how slow we go, we just have to get up this. It was always gonna be one of the toughest days.'

I took my glasses off as the tears started to fall. I felt defeated. The heat was unrelenting and I was shaking with fatigue.

'I don't think I can do what we have already done today all over again,' I said, my body shaking with tiredness.

Ryan looked into his pack. 'Here, have some of this.' He forced half a banana into my hand.

'Well, that's gonna make everything fine then,' I said, forcing myself to smile. 'That's going to make this hill feel much smaller.'

Ryan smiled back. 'I'm finding it tough as well,' he said. 'I don't think I've ever cycled sustained climbs like this. You really are doing okay. We'll stop as often as we have to. The most important thing is to get up here safely.'

'Yeah, I know,' I said. 'I'll give it another go.'

Progress was slow and the heat so stifling that each time we came across a small pool of shade we stopped for a few moments' respite. In front, Ryan coaxed me on, stopping ahead when he saw me slow. Each time we stopped, the effort required mentally and physically to restart was enormous.

The paved trail led on and up with little relief from the climbs and only small puddles of shade tight against the roadside. I shook my bottle which was light in my hand, only a few drops of liquid remaining.

'Here have some of mine,' Martyn said and passed me his drink. I raised it up to my mouth and took two small mouthfuls and passed it back.

'Rob should be with us soon,' Martyn said as we stopped for a breather. 'I got a text back there which said he's on this road. He's got plenty of water in the truck.'

I sat on a large rock and massaged my calves, smoothing the

muscle upwards, placing my finger tip in the tightest knots, and pictured the stripes of muscles relaxing and smoothing.

'I hope so, my mouth is so dry and I've stopped being able to pee. I won't get much further without some more fluids.' Being outside in extreme heat after 6000 feet of climbing without fluid was dangerous. We'd left the satellite phone behind so our support vehicle was out of contact and without the hope that Rob would find us again, we were at risk of severe dehydration.

Martyn lifted his phone out and looked at it. 'No signal.' Ryan's phone was the same. Despite the road being open to the sun's rays the hill was deeply wooded and reception was poor.

We continued on our way. It was a lonely road. We had seen very few cars over the last hours and as the climbing continued and still Rob didn't appear we were starting to think we should stop the next vehicle that went by. There was a roar of a car engine and I could hear the steady grind as the gear lowered and the motor continued on its way.

I laboured on and a gold car passed me. Rob leant out of the car.

'Howdee, folks,' he chuckled, as he swept past us and then pulled in at the roadside.

'You're a saviour,' I said. 'I'm glad to see you.'

Martyn leant his bike against the car. Rob was already opening the door and Martyn reached in for the drinks, passing them out to us. I sat inside the car, enjoying the comfort of the upholstered seats, swigging water slowly and steadily, while the blokes chatted among themselves. Martyn placed the map into my lap. 'This is where we are,' he pointed his finger on the map, 'and this is Carson Pass here.'

'What's the scale?' I asked.

'It's about twenty-five miles to Carson Pass,' Martyn said. I looked at the map to see where would be the most sensible place to stop. Crossing the pass today seemed too much of an effort and would spoil the enjoyment of the achievement.

'What about finishing at Caples Lake?' I said. It was the only signed services between here and Carson Pass. 'It's eleven miles to the pass after that. It would make more sense to do that climb tomorrow with fresh legs than carry on today.'

Ryan had come over to listen. 'I think you're right. We could make it but it'll take another three hours.'

'And the rest,' I said, my whole body was tired and each mile we'd climbed had been tortuous. 'Let's leave it until tomorrow then, agreed?' I said.

The boys nodded. 'Agreed.'

Day 5 – Monday, 3 July
Caples Lake, Calif. to Carson City, Nevada (Nev.)
55.7 miles – 5 hrs 34 mins
Total covered – 264.2 miles

MIKE

The advertisement for the RV had stated that it slept seven people but at only thirty feet long, space was always going be at a premium. Every conceivable area of spare floor was used. Even the toilet was built over a wheel arch which meant it was impossible to sit on it without having your knees higher than your ears.

The RV was in three clear sections: at the back was a double bed with a window behind your head, while above and to the sides at the back were cupboard units. There was minimal floor space to navigate round and this was already covered with bags. The middle section had the toilet with a shower opposite. There was a fridge by the door across from a sink, microwave and cooker. The remaining space of the middle section was a table with two two-seater chairs. The table would dismantle and the seats would convert into a double bed. At the end, longwise, was another couch which also converted to a bed.

At the front, was the driver's cab with two seats, above which was another bed reached by a step ladder. This was meant to be a double bed.

'Yeah right,' I thought. The overwhelming impression was that personal space would be difficult to obtain and to sleep four adults would be a Big Brotherish test of endurance. How seven would manage as advertised was beyond my imagination. We'd have five in our RV and that would be sufficient.

'Are you sure you're going to be able to drive this thing?' was Rebecca's first question when we climbed on board and the truth was, I didn't know.

In the driver's seat I felt lost among the number of levers and buttons. I glanced in the rear view mirror and all I could see was the double bed in the back of the vehicle. The driver's wing mirror reflected the RV's length stretching out like a grotesque cartoon.

The automatic gear control was pointed at neutral but turning the ignition, nothing happened. I kept trying, but the only mumbling was from the kids.

'What's up, Dad, why aren't we moving?' asked Steven.

'Pass me the instructions will you, Becca?' I asked.

'Why?'

'Because I said.'

'Where is it?'

'In there.' I pointed to a magazine holder positioned above some of the lounge seats which would metamorphose into a bed at night time.

'Where's *there*?'

Frustrated, I climbed out of my seat and into the back of the van to get it myself, smacking my head against the cab roof. Thumbing through the pages of the book, I checked the index for starting the engine or the ignition but it wasn't included – too basic a task?

I got back into the driver's seat and repeated the same sequence of events that had failed minutes before; again without success.

'We're never gonna get there,' Steven said to Rebecca.

'I imagine it's very confusing driving one of these for the first time,' said Jodie. 'I wouldn't like to do it.'

'But we've got to get to Carson City which is two hundred and fifty miles away,' said Steven. 'And we haven't moved an inch yet. Dad can't even turn the engine on.'

My humiliation clearly incomplete, I tried to attract the attention of the mechanic from the garage opposite. The windows wouldn't work so I resorted to banging on them from the inside as though we were trapped.

'Can you help?' I asked, realising how stupid I looked and opening the door. The mechanic had a T-shirt hanging loose over some blue overall trousers.

'You got a problem, bud?' he said.

'I can't get the RV started,' I explained, feeling my face redden. 'Sorry, I've not driven an automatic, they're not popular in England.'

He smiled. 'No, it's just fat lazy Americans that can't be bothered with changing gears.'

He leant into the RV and went through the rudiments with me. After five minutes we leapfrogged across the forecourt as I practised stopping, starting and using the park function.

'Dad, Dad!' Steven yelled. 'Rebecca's embarrassed.'

I looked at the instruments and saw that there was no fuel in the tank. I wasn't even sure if it was petrol or diesel. My hands were sweating on the wheel. I called out to the mechanic again and he directed me to a filling station 200 yards up the road. 'I can't believe this,' muttered Rebecca. 'People are laughing at us. Dad, can we just go?'

We pulled out of the open metal gate and I edged very slowly right, giving a wide circle to ensure the RV didn't clip the side. Concentrating on the wing mirror, I heard the blowing horn of an oncoming vehicle before I saw it and slammed on the brakes, my nerves shredded. With my confidence at an all-time low, I edged forward on to the road and headed slowly to the filling station at no more than 5 mph.

The pump's canopy said it could take fourteen and a half feet of vehicle but unsure, I stopped and asked Jodie to check the height of the RV in the manual. There was no mention of it so she stepped outside and checked. 'You're fine!' she called and I inched forward before stopping and slumping my head down on the wheel when I realised I didn't even know which side the fuel tank was on. I decided to take the line between the middle pumps equidistant from both sides to ensure that I would be at least near one set of pumps.

As a teenager, I'd spent three years selling petrol at a garage in my home town of Settle but these pumps were a mystery. After minutes studying them, we realised we had to pay in advance.

'Are we ever gonna go, Dad?' Steven said from the passenger seat.

I looked at my watch. It was 12.45, three hours since we'd left Richmond and we'd only travelled 200 yards. It was a relief when we finally got on to the freeway, even though initially I was unsure whether we were heading in the right direction.

Inevitably, after less than five miles, a portable neon hazard sign indicated there was an accident ten miles ahead and it was another ninety minutes before we cleared the ensuing jam. At least it allowed me to fiddle about with the controls.

Once through the accident, Interstate 80 helped us make short work of the distance to Carson City. Through plains of wild vegetation and passed aqua lakes and snow covered peaks, we climbed the Sierra Nevada. The views of the mountains were stunning.

Driving through Reno, we were greeted by a vista of billboards with photographs of slimy middle-aged men selling real estate. Signs for newly built casinos with bulging jackpots littered the roadsides.

Nevada is a grown-ups' playground where casinos and legalised brothels are major contributors to the state income. These industries, although legal, come with tat, cheapness and a sense of the grubby and it seemed to me that if you scratched away the surface, it would reveal a cesspit of seedy human behaviour.

While Reno attempts to be a smaller version of Las Vegas, Carson City is like Reno's little brother. Surprisingly, it is the state capital. Its location makes it the perfect gateway to the desert from the rich man's paradises of Lake Tahoe and California to the west. Named after Kit Carson, a trapper, scout, Indian agent and early explorer of the West, the city has the look and feel of the modern Wild West town. It was first inhabited in the mid-nineteenth century and like many towns in the state, it boomed from silver mining after the precious metal was found by prospectors in 1859. The Comstock Lode was the largest silver find in the world at that time.

Our location for the night was Comstock RV Park which was just through the town. The cyclists and the other RV had arrived well before us so as soon as we'd parked, we sat at a table already set and dinner was about to be served. The park was clean and tidy with plenty of shade from trees but it still felt like a car park.

I'd not seen Jane since first thing Friday morning and she already seemed to be into the cycling groove. Organised, efficient and in control she was a completely different person from the one who'd arrived in California a week ago. Yesterday had been a struggle. I'd tried to keep a track of her progress but communication had been difficult and by the time we spoke I'd allowed my anxiety to come out in a sharp conversation to which Jane had responded feistily after a day in the saddle. All the time I'd known Jane our telephone conversations had never been great, so it was a relief to be able to hold her again.

Bowls of spaghetti and bolognaise sauce sat on the table together with bread. Immediately the conversation turned to Sunday, the rest day, which was six days and several hundred miles' cycle ride away.

'What shall we do?' asked Ryan who, wearing a pristine black T-shirt and with his sunglasses perched fashionably on his head, looked like he was on holiday rather than cycling across the continent.

Steven shrugged.

'We'll have a boys' night,' Ryan prompted, then quickly added, 'No, no, boys' night can be Saturday then we can stay up really really late.' He winked at Steven.

'Yes!' Steven smiled.

'And have a beer,' Jane said.

'Beer?' Rebecca piped up, trying to hear herself above the clatter of plates.

'You're a minor in this country,' teased Ryan. 'You can have a root beer.'

Rebecca smirked at Ryan then passed her plate over for a dollop of bolognaise sauce.

'What have you been doing today?' Jane said to Michael.

'We went to the Wal-Mart to do some shopping this afternoon,' he said.

She turned to Ryan. 'And what have you been doing today?'

'Cycling,' said Ryan seriously. 'And what are you doing tomorrow, Jane?'

'Cycling,' she said. 'And the day after that, cycling. And the day after that, cycling.'

'And what are you doing the next day?' Steven said to his mum excitedly.

'Probably cycling,' she said and Steven grinned.

'What am *I* doing the next day?' he said.

'Not cycling,' Ryan said and everyone laughed.

'You can cycle if you like,' Jane said.

'No!' Steven said with mock horror.

I was pleased at how relaxed everyone appeared. I'd been worried how I'd find Jane after the toils of yesterday but she looked remarkably buoyant. I'd avoided asking her about their hellish day but felt comfortable now.

'How was it?' I said.

'Very hilly. I've never been on such a horrible day's cycling ever in my life. It was very, very hard. There was actually one part when we got to four thousand feet and we had cycled only twenty-eight and a half miles and I actually wept at the thought of climbing another four thousand feet.'

'Physically wept?' I said, surprised.

'Physically wept for miles and miles. I couldn't get it out of my head that we had over twenty miles to do. The scenery was absolutely stupendous but halfway up I didn't care any more.'

For a second, she looked as though she was going to cry again just recounting yesterday's climbing. Then Rebecca dropped some cutlery which clattered and broke the flow.

Jane gathered herself. 'Ryan kept counting the road kill at the side of the road.' She rolled her eyes.

'Yeah, we're up to thirty-two road kill,' he said.

'No way!' Michael said.

'Yeah, from the tiny little bitty things to a massive great big deer.'

'A deer?' I said.

'Yeah.'

'Well, why the hell have we eaten spaghetti bolognaise tonight?'

Jane laughed. There was light-heartedness to her and a confidence from knowing that she'd climbed 8000 feet in a day. Where she found the strength of character I couldn't guess but it was, even as her husband, inspiring to be in her presence.

I looked at Jane. She'd come alive with the event and my heart swelled with pride. We were already at 4730 feet above sea level, the Nevada Desert swept out in front of us to the edge of the horizon. Only 4000 miles to go.

Day 6 – Tuesday, 4 July
Carson City, Nev. to Fallon, Nev.
66.2 miles – 5 hrs 9 mins
Total covered – 330.4 miles

JANE

Stretching myself in the tiny double bed in the back of the RV, my foot caught on Mike's leg. He rolled over.

'Morning,' I said, as I struggled to push myself upright.

'What time is it?' he asked.

I squinted at my small black travel clock but couldn't make out the figures in the near darkness. I switched on the overhead light. 'Five a.m.'

'What time are you getting up?' asked Mike. Before I could answer the alarm clock started to bleat.

'Now, I guess,' but I pushed the snooze button and lowered myself down into the crook of Mike's arm. 'I've missed you,' I said and Mike muttered something. 'It's really weird sleeping here in the same bed I've been sleeping in for the last four days, but it's much better now you're here.'

I stretched my leg and Mike mumbled again. 'Even if it means I've got less room,' I said.

The alarm clock sounded again and I swung myself out of bed into the nearest space. I'd emptied my suitcase the night before. I'd been looking forward to putting my clothes in order in the small cupboard space I'd been allotted but in the end I'd picked up my belongings and dumped them in one of the cupboards over our heads.

'Damn,' I said, reaching into the cupboard trying to find a clean vest top to put on under my cycling shirt.

'What are you doing?' Mike said.

'Looking for my clothes. I can't find anything in here.'

'What about in the other cupboard?'

'Oh yeah, you're right.' I crept round the side of the bed, cursing as I stubbed my toe against another part of the van that stuck out unexpectedly.

Dressed at last, I picked up my shoes and bent to push my feet into them. I was too stiff to crouch low enough so I opened the RV door and sat on the step to ease my feet into the tight shoes. I stepped back through into our bedroom and leant to give Mike a kiss.

'See you later,' I said.

'Will you close the curtain when you're done.'

I picked up my helmet which contained my medicines, my saddlebag, sunglasses and headscarf and pulled the long curtain that separated the bed area from the rest of the RV.

Jodie, who was asleep in the main section of the RV on a converted couch, sat up suddenly.

'What time is it?' she said, her eyes still closed.

'It's early yet so go back to sleep.' Her head slumped back down and she mumbled something unintelligible as she turned over.

My back was still too stiff to bend down and tie the laces of my shoes so I made my way carefully across the gravelled parking lot to the other RV. The sky was only just starting to show the first glimmer of the day.

The white RV with its jolly family motif mocking us from its side was just across from ours and already there was evidence of movement. Ryan stepped from the van. 'Good morning,' he called cheerily and disappeared towards the back of the van. 'I'm just going to lube the chains.' He lifted up the tube of oil. 'How did you sleep?'

'Not bad. My back's a bit sore but I'm not too bad.' He nodded and carried with his small jobs.

I opened the RV door and stepped up into the small living quarters. Cindy stood in her nightclothes by the cooker waiting for the kettle to boil.

'Morning,' she said. 'Isn't it a glorious day?'

'Yeah, looks all right,' I said and slung myself into the seat by the table. On a paper plate were two small pieces of bread and next to it a jar of peanut butter. I spread some on the bread.

'You want any cereal or anything?' She lifted the milk carton to her nose and recoiled. 'Oh no, I think the milk's off.'

The thought of cereal and sour milk turned my stomach. 'Would you ask Mike if he's got any milk?' Cindy asked.

'Yeah sure,' I said, standing up and making my way back to our RV and returning with a carton of milk.

I sat opposite Ryan as he proceeded to munch his way through a bowl of multicoloured cereal hoops. I cut away the stale crusts from the bread and then sliced the small pieces into four bite-size squares. I bit into one and chewed slowly.

'We'd better make sure we've got enough peanut butter then, hey?' Cindy said.

I lifted my head from the map I was studying. 'Yeah, that would be good. And some bread – this is a bit stale.'

'Yeah, but it's still okay,' Cindy said, pushing a cup of coffee in front of me.

'What's the address of the next RV park?' I asked Michael, who had just entered the RV.

'I dunno. What's the address tonight, Cindy?'

Cindy, standing by the cooker, put her cup down quickly. 'Oh gosh, I can't remember. All I know is that it's on the main road into the town of Fallon. It's an RV park though, you won't be able to miss it.' She turned to place the kettle back onto the hob to boil as a gold-coloured car pulled to a halt by our RV.

'Morning folks,' Rob said as he stood in the doorway, his face alight with a huge smile. 'How are you all?'

'Fine thanks,' I said. 'You?'

'Yeah, great. It's a busy town, though. Which road are you heading out on today?'

I showed him on the map. 'I'll just get my atlas and mark it down,' he said.

Mike joined us a few minutes later and as he and Rob chatted, I carried on munching my way through my measly breakfast, anxious to swallow enough food to be able to take my various tablets.

I shuddered as I swallowed each pill down. At least, I reflected, the longer I was awake, the looser my back became. I rose from the table and stepped outside to finish the preparations for the day's riding. Placing the map bag over the handlebars, I slid the Sat Nav system and the GPS system in place. I fastened the saddlebag to the rack below the narrow leather saddle and then bent down to tie my laces.

'You don't have to get down on your knees for me,' Mike laughed.

'Bugger off,' I said.

He laughed. 'What time do you reckon you'll get to Fallon?'

'Half twelvish, maybe later.'

'Cindy and Michael will meet you there. I'm going to send off the articles for the *Yorkshire Post* and then go to the shops. So I'll get there a bit later than that. Is there anything you need?'

'Something nice to eat like biscuits or cake. And if they've got a map of Utah, that would be good. I've got one of Nevada.'

'I can't wait to be out there on the road with you. It'll be fantastic,' said Mike.

I smiled at him. 'Yeah, I'm glad you're here. I've missed you.'

'Right folks,' Ryan called, clapping his hands to rally forth the troops. 'We'd better hit the road before it gets too warm.'

I pulled my bike from the side of the RV and wheeled it to the tarmac surface.

'See you all later!' I called.

'Be safe,' Cindy called and we headed for the large white gate posts at the exit of the RV park.

We headed across the road that yesterday had been a constant column of traffic. Today the hour was early, still only 6 a.m. and there were few cars around. The city flashed with neon lights, enticing people to come and try their luck at the casino tables. Our route lay parallel to Route 295 and as we approached the Nevada State Prison, a huge enclave surrounded by barbed wire, we caught glimpses of the freeway as we headed off to the pass.

After a few minutes of cycling, we at last turned right to follow Highway 50, which would take us all the way across Nevada into Utah. This was dubbed the loneliest road in America by *Life* magazine in 1986. The stretch running through to Ely was 287 miles long and would take us through central Nevada. We'd be on this stretch of road for the next five days until the rest day in Ely.

We crested our only hill of the day – a slight bump on the map but a 400-foot climb nevertheless. At the top, we stopped for a second and looked back. Below us lay Carson City, cradled by the Carson Range which hid Lake Tahoe from sight. It was still early, a little before 7 a.m. and the sun was starting to show. It glittered orange off the mountain range behind us and made the white snow of the higher Sierra Nevada glint at its peaks. We headed onwards, the headlights of oncoming cars blinding us with their brightness.

The road narrowed to one lane and we hugged the hard shoulder chugging along at 22 to 23 mph. I tucked my bike behind Ryan's, cringing when I heard a car revving behind us. A stretch of roadworks lay ahead of us in an unending line of cones and barriers. I circled my legs faster and faster, keeping carefully in line with Ryan's back wheel hoping we could come to the end of the works before some fast moving car edged us into the scrub at the side of the road.

The orange soil had darkened and dulled to a silvery yellow, the shrubs were meaner and narrower with long spine-like leaves and blue green in colour. We pedalled onwards towards the tall towers of yet another prison. Signs on the roadside warned motorists not to stop and pick up hitchhikers for the next fifteen miles and we looked around warily as we pulled up to quench our thirst.

The roadworks ended and the road opened out.

As I'd predicted, the small squares of peanut butter on dry bread had not been enough to fuel me for the whole day. I chewed on an energy bar but longed to stop and eat something more substantial, to feel I had some nutrition in my body. I kept my hands firmly on the handlebars and let Martyn and Ryan drift ahead of me, still rolling the bike along at 19 mph, cruising smoothly down a newly laid road. Ryan slowed and I soon caught him and we cycled along together side by side making steady progress onwards through the vast countryside.

The cars of the city were behind us and the few vehicles that did pass us were now bigger and higher from the ground. There were no houses close to the road, but occasionally we passed groups of trailers set back and clustered together.

As we neared the next main junction we could make out more of these clusters of trailers and decided to cycle into Silver Springs and find a café. I really needed a few minutes off the bike.

We turned right and headed down the highway towards the town. Although the map showed that Silver Springs had a population of over 4000 people, I was puzzled as to where they could all possibly be. The town seemed so temporary, there were few real buildings and it seemed that most of the people resided in narrow trailers set on bricks in dry parcels of land with mean fencing strung between haphazardly placed posts.

We came to a small all-purpose shop. There were many battered vans outside and, as we approached, another pulled in with two dogs yawning lazily in the passenger seat, their long tongues pointing down through their lower canines.

The two men in the truck started a conversation with a young woman standing on the forecourt, whose grimy T-shirt stretched taut over her large belly and gaped where her stomach overran the top of her jeans. Wide hips filled them and her feet were rusty red from the dust and in flip-flops thin with wear.

Their drawl was hard to understand but their familiarity with each other made me think they must be related quite closely.

'What do you think?' I said quietly.

Ryan shook his head. 'I'll go and check if you like, but I don't think we'll be stopping.'

I stepped from my bike and held on to Ryan's handlebars while he made his way into the ramshackle building. The eyes of the drivers were now firmly on us and we were being examined closely, although no one spoke a word. Minutes later, Ryan appeared, his face still, expressionless.

'I think we should head back the way we came,' he said and we didn't discuss this any further but stepped astride our bikes and made our way back to the crossroads.

Once a safe distance away, we slowed down. 'I think most of the people were related to each other,' said Ryan. 'I felt a bit out of place.'

'I didn't like the way they looked at us,' I said.

Martyn was cycling alongside. 'Hats off to you, Ryan. I'd have been a bit scared to go in there.'

We sat on the gravel of a nearby garage and drank down cold bottles of iced coffee, chewed on Mars bars and watched the traffic moving. Dusty flat-backed trucks and rusty cars lurched down the ill-paved road. The drivers craned their necks for a better view of us.

'What do you think of this then?' Martyn asked.

'I'm feeling a little uncomfortable,' I said. 'We're not in a Chevy, we're dressed in Lycra and we're riding bikes that are worth more than the cars we've seen. I'd quite like to get the hell out of here.'

They both agreed and we set off again.

The day was warming up as we headed into the outskirts of Fallon. It felt good cycling along a clean surface on a still day and it was still only just after 11 a.m. when we started to come across more permanent buildings. Narrow houses, some with a tall tree for shelter, whose long branches pointed out over dry red earth, began to appear.

My GPS showed the sign for a campsite just ahead and a brown wooden building with a white tin roof painted with black letters spelling out Fallon RV Park appeared. On the forecourt was a gas station with two pumps under a canopy advertising Country, Market and Gas. We stopped and Ryan went into the building while I sat on a rock that served as the divider of the RV park from the road.

'Nope, she's not got any bookings under any of our names,' Ryan said when he rejoined us. 'But she says that there's another RV park nearer the town on the right.'

A little disappointed, I pulled myself up and we cycled on for another five minutes until we came to the next park, but it seemed to be a trailer park full of permanent residents. A group of children were running around the grounds and rushed over as we cycled nearer, pressing their faces against the fence and staring at us as we got off our bikes.

'We can't possibly be staying here,' I said, horrified at the thought of my family stopping in what looked like a permanent gypsy settlement. 'It makes that first stop look picturesque.'

My stomach tightened with anxiety. I hadn't imagined the trip would involve such privations for our small group. This was not a camp I would have stopped at with my children under any circumstances.

Martyn checked his phone. 'Rob's just texted me,' he said. 'He's booked in at the Best Western hotel downtown. Come down and you can wait for your lot to turn up there.'

I nodded, there was no way I was settling in this campsite so it seemed the most sensible thing to do.

It was about three miles into town and as I sat on a bench in the shade waiting for Mike's arrival, I knew I would have to have words with Cindy.

'I'm going to tell Cindy I need the address and directions for the RV parks, because this is about the third time we've had to find our way like this, and it's frustrating when we could have finished earlier for the day,' I said to Ryan and he nodded.

We'd been in town for about an hour when an RV pulled in at the side of the road and Michael and Cindy stepped out from the cab.

'Good day, folks!' She grinned at us as she placed her sunglasses on the top of her head, pulling the hair from her face. 'Hey Jane, we've got some more peanut butter for you. We won't be running out of that in a hurry.'

'Great,' I replied with little enthusiasm. 'What about bread?'

'Oh tush,' she said, slapping playfully at my arm, 'we'll get some of that tomorrow.'

We headed back out of town with the bikes chained to the bars at the rear of the RV. Before long, we were pulling into an RV park with a wooden building with the faded letters of Fallon painted on its tin roof in white.

'See!' said Cindy. 'I told you you couldn't miss it.'

MIKE

The RV park was adjacent to a gas station and was little more than an extension of the forecourt without the benefit of tarmac. It was Independence Day and the road from Fallon to Carson City was very quiet, no cars had pulled in to the station forecourt for at least fifteen minutes.

I was grateful for the early finish. I had three blogs to write, for the *Sun*, the BBC and our own website, as well as a newspaper article and some emails to send so I wanted to find an internet connection in town. I'd also secretly hoped that an early arrival would mean we could investigate the Independence Day festivities that this flat desert outpost had to offer.

As I stood chatting to Jane outside the RV, Steven came bounding across.

'Dad, can we play pool?' he beamed, his face almost pleading.

It's not a game I'm particularly fond of but it felt churlish to say no. Facilities at the RV park were basic and an energetic nine-year-old would find little else to occupy him.

'You go on,' Jane said to me, pre-empting my question.

We wandered across the deserted forecourt to the shop opposite. It too was basic – there was clearly not much need for many supplies since it hardly attracted any customers.

'Steven, let's have a quick look for a water hose,' I said.

'Hokey dokey,' Steven said and he headed left up the first aisle while I headed right.

The hose supplied with the RV had been about as much use as a paper tent in a gale, dribbling more water on the floor outside than into the RV. We'd woken up that morning surrounded by a moat. In fact, the standard of equipment in the Cruise America RV as a whole was pretty poor. Most of the metal fittings seemed to have been manhandled by Uri Geller and the wood needed little more than a penknife to saw it in half.

At one end of the shop sat a pool table circa 1950, a broken television and piles of furniture. On the wall was a banner expressing the hope that all the service men returned home safely from Iraq.

A good-looking girl in her late teens with long auburn hair falling loose came out from behind the kiosk counter and stood propped against the wall. 'Where are you all from?'

'England.' Steven said.

'Oh wow. What brings you to Fallon, the parade or the racing?'

'There's a parade? Is it for Independence Day?' I asked.

'Yes, but it was this morning,' she said, moving around the table watching Steven as he tried to line up a shot, his cue hand wafting around like a flag pole in a gale. 'But there's the dirt racing tonight, that should be cool, there's lot of people on the site here for it.'

'What's the town like?' I asked.

'Oh you know, very quiet, nothing much happens here.' There was boredom in her voice. It must have been difficult for late adolescents living in a town right on the fringe of the desert. 'There's not much entertainment here, but the people are friendly,' she said.

'How long have you lived here?' I asked.

'Not long. My boyfriend's in the Navy. I met him in Florida

where I lived, but he was transferred up here. As soon as I arrived he was posted out, so I'm on my own now.'

A heavy silence hung in the atmosphere. It seemed inappropriate to ask where he was posted. My eyes drifted back to the poster decorated with a couple of yellow ribbons. It seemed surreal to me that a girl younger than my eldest daughter had a partner serving in another desert several thousand miles away.

Fallon is the home of the US Navy's premier air base, the real 'Top Gun' as the brochures describe it, and to peruse a map of Nevada is to understand the impact it has on the environment. Vast ranges of land measuring hundreds of square miles are used as bombing ranges and air defence restraints mean much of the surrounding area is uninhabitable.

The base was established in 1942 as part of a defensive network to repel a hypothetical Japanese invasion of the West. It was closed down after the war only to open up again in the early fifties as the result of the Korean conflict.

Since 1996 it has been home to the Naval Fighter Weapons School – 'Top Gun' – although to look at this woeful little kiosk in the middle of nowhere, it seemed a million miles away from the slinky bars depicted in the film.

This western desert outpost is reliant upon the Navy for the local economy and population growth, which bucks the trends of the other communities on Highway 50, whose population and wealth are in decline.

Established after rancher Mike Fallon built a crossroads store on his land in 1896, the town was soon boosted by a renovated telegraph line. Indeed, the Churchill County Telephone System they have in Fallon is the only publicly run one in the United States.

But although it was the Navy's construction of the air base that lifted Fallon out of two decades of depression, it has come at a significant price. As well as the uninhabitable land there is significant environmental damage from bombs and air pollution as well as oil and fuel spills.

The big question, however, is whether the enormous military

activity has caused a cancer cluster in the town among its children. The facts are startling: there were eleven cases of childhood leukaemia in rural Churchill County, Nevada, over three years and five other cases in children who had previously lived in the area. What are the chances of this happening? Apparently such a geographical cluster would only occur in the USA once every 22 000 years. Leukaemia, although the most common type of childhood cancer, occurs statistically only three times in 100 000 – so sixteen cases in such a sparsely populated area of the Nevada Desert, which just happens to have the major US naval air base, is bound to raise questions.

Several investigative journalists have tried to prove a link, but as yet, there's no proof that Fallon air base is responsible for the cancer cluster. Other suggestions for the anomaly include the fact that the town's tight water supply has high levels of arsenic – but that's always been the case. And of course there is an abundance of agricultural pesticides in the area.

But in 1963, in the Sand Springs mountain range only thirty miles away, a 13 kilotonne nuclear bomb was exploded underground. Surely this had to have some impact?

Coincidentally, there is a second town in the USA – Sierra Vista, Arizona – with a population of 40 000, which saw nine cases of leukaemia in seven years. The US military has an air base nearby.

Of course, the truth about these matters can be concealed in any number of 'expert' reports. In the years since Jane was diagnosed with breast cancer, inevitably we have taken more note of any research which has looked into why people are predisposed to the disease.

Being overweight is a factor in some research. Being underweight is another. Having children too early, children too late, smoking, drinking, not eating the right food, being healthy, regular exercise – the fact is, no one can really tell why some women are more susceptible to breast cancer. Jane doesn't fit any of the patterns and her early diagnosis at twenty-six is still without explanation. Sometimes life can provide just a cruel twist of fate.

It occurred to me that it was poignant for the ride to stop overnight in Fallon. The journey's point was to raise money for children and cancer charities.

'Hey little dude, you're a good player,' the young girl said to Steven as the cue ball bounced off the yellow spot.

'No, I'm not. I'm rubbish.' Steven looked across. 'I'm rubbish at most sports. I just like having a go.'

She moved away slightly to behind Steven's back, a little shocked by his frankness. 'Are you with the cyclists then, a Canadian guy was in here earlier.'

'Yes.'

'Oh wow. Is it your mum, the lady's who is cycling?'

'It is,' Steven said.

'Isn't that something?'

A rickety rattle of the door signalled a second customer, a middle-aged gentleman who wandered in to pick up some groceries. By the time we left, thirty minutes later, the young shop assistant was still speaking to the same customer.

Rob and Martyn were not sharing in the RV experience. Each night, after the ride, they would seek out an oasis – a comfortable, spacious, air-conditioned hotel room with modern communication devices.

The mobile phone network in the USA didn't seem to cover the area between the Pacific Coast and Missouri, apart from in major conurbations, so communication not only between ourselves but with home was always going to be an issue.

Primarily, we were relying on wireless hotspots, a Verizon card – which provided a connection where there was a mobile signal – and, as a last resort, a beacon unit which connected via a satellite. This was a feature of the Best Western hotel chain, so it was always Rob's primary choice of hotel if there was one in town. He'd found one in Fallon, only a few miles from the RV site, and had offered to drive me there so I could fire off some emails.

The weather had drawn in when he arrived promptly at 4 p.m., the blue sky had disappeared and the wind had picked up to the extent that it was impossible to keep a baseball cap on your head.

The Independence Day activities seemed to have ended and so we had spent the afternoon inside the RV catching up on mundane administration while Steven watched *Return of the Jedi*.

'Is there much to Fallon?' I asked, as I scouted round the RV collecting my laptop for the hotel room.

Rob shrugged. 'This road goes on for about four miles and there's the usual fast food diners, billboards, gas stations and real estate offices, then halfway down there's Main Street and that's the extent of Fallon.'

I gave Jane a quick kiss.

'Love you,' I said, and made a quick exit, not wishing to keep Rob waiting.

Once we were in the car, Rob said: 'I'll drive you around, you won't believe the poverty.'

'Really?'

'Yeah, you'll see, Mike. Honestly, it'll shock you. This isn't the America you see portrayed on TV series. I've never seen anything like it.'

As we drove down the flat road on either side I could see single storey wooden dwellings that looked temporary. Occasionally, a lawned area with some shrubs and sometimes a tree would crop up, usually by a hotel, but otherwise all I could see were traffic lights, advertising billboards or business signs.

Rob swung down Main Street. Apart from a solitary old man sporting a Neil Young checked shirt and denim dungarees, it was completely deserted.

'Just look at this, Mike,' Rob said, as the car began to crawl. 'Have you ever seen anything like it?'

Rows of poorly maintained prefab houses stretched out on both sides of the road, many littered with battered pickups, kids' toys and junk outside.

'Can you believe people have to live like this?' he said, turning into a different street but with the same view. 'Where are the swimming pools and manicured lawns?' He pointed to a dilapidated house where the bushes had grown through an abandoned car. 'Look at that!' he pointed.

It was a truly desperate sight. Here was an isolated town in the Nevada Desert, forgotten about and neglected by the great and the powerful in Washington, yet within only a few miles was a naval air base leading the way in cutting-edge military technology.

'Let's get out of here,' I said.

After sending the emails and writing up the blogs at the hotel, I decided that it would be sensible to remain at home and get an early night so that Jane could be refreshed for an early 5 a.m. start. Fallon only gets five inches of rainfall a year and it looked like most of it would arrive very shortly.

CHAPTER 3

Day 7 – Wednesday, 5 July
Fallon, Nev. to Cold Springs, Nev.
62.3 miles – 5 hrs 59 mins
Total covered – 392.7 miles

JANE

There was little need for the small GPS device to aid us on our way out of Fallon next morning. There was one main road running through the town and as we reached the outskirts we could see it stretching out in front of us.

'We need to stop and wait for Real Radio to phone,' Ryan called, as he slowed the pace a little. Real Radio was a station in Yorkshire which had been a fantastic supporter for some years. Their reporter, James Webster, hoped to come to New York for the finish.

We stopped at a telegraph pole and rested our bikes against the blackened wood.

'I think I'll carry on along the road,' Martyn said. 'I want to try to find a spot so I can get some good footage of you passing on the loneliest road.'

'Okay,' I said and Martyn cycled steadily away. We watched him as he drew further and further off, till the heat from the road rose and made his distant figure waiver and hover above the surface, floating with a silver glaze, until he was out of view. A dark blue car passed us, a roar of black fumes rising from its exhaust as its occupants revved their engine. They slowed to gaze at us with hostile curiosity before giving a long burst on their horn and disappearing. We watched their progress until the distance ate them up.

Another car passed. I glanced at my watch. We'd been waiting ten minutes. The sun shone down on us making my face flush.

'How irritating is this?' I said.

'We'll give them five more minutes and then we'll be on our way,' Ryan said.

'We could be three miles down the road by now.'

'I know, I know, but we ought to give them a bit of time. We'll tie them down time wise tomorrow.'

I nodded and reached out my hand to take the SAT phone from Ryan's hand as it rung. The interview lasted for just a few minutes before the line went dead.

'Thank goodness for that,' I said, handing the black brick back to Ryan so that he could stash it away in his saddlebag.

I readied myself to cycle once more. We pushed the bikes hard and by keeping my gaze fixed on the white line at the side of the road I could put myself into a near trance-like state, only aware of the bike, the road, the white line.

I rested low down on the bike, pleased to see my speed was a constant 19.5 mph. On and on we sped, the tarmac passing under our wheels as the dark grey of the road and the dashes of white fused into a constant line. The ridges in the hard shoulder were not visible as individual dents but became just darker and darker lines in the space before the desert floor.

'We should have caught him by now,' I called to Ryan, broken out of my reverie by the sudden thought that we hadn't seen Martyn.

'I was just thinking that,' he said. 'I know he had about four miles on us but he'd have stopped by now.'

We increased our pace till we were covering over a mile in just three minutes but still there was no figure before us.

Then, before one of the plastic road markers at the edge of the road, I could see a bike. Above that, a figure stood on the edge of a large stone. We kept going, aware of Martyn's camera lens.

The shimmering on the road started to become more solid. In front, I could just about make out the headlights and windscreen of a car approaching. As it neared, it slowed down, its passengers craning their necks out of the window to get a better view of us. We turned to catch a backwards glimpse of them and then they sped up and were soon racing back towards Fallon.

After passing Martyn, we waited a little further along and heard the sound of rocks clattering down the cliffside as he nimbly clambered back and lifted his bike on to the road.

'Damn!' he said when he'd caught up with us. 'I've been stood there for ages to get that shot, no cars have been past for at least ten minutes. Just my bloody luck.'

'Oh, well,' I said. 'I'm just glad to see you. We were beginning to think that somebody must have stopped and ordered you into their van. I was imagining something like *Deliverance*.'

Martyn raised his eyebrows. 'That hadn't really occurred to me, but yeah, I suppose they could shove my bike in the back and I couldn't really do anything about it.'

We pushed onwards, heading towards a gap in the Sand Springs mountain range. Around us lay mud flats, unfenced from the road. Messages written in pebbles like eco-friendly graffiti spelt out the names of couples. Some lay just by the roadside, others were further into the flats.

We passed large aluminium beer cans and brown plastic bottles discarded from drinking sprees. Large signs warned of quicksand. I had visions of getting sucked under this barren landscape as it relentlessly tugged at my body till I disappeared from view, leaving only my Gatorade bottle resting on the top.

'You wouldn't catch me wandering off the road,' said Martyn, echoing my own thoughts.

We carried on along Highway 50. Over the next week we would be dropping down into many basins only to climb up to the next range.

As we neared the base of the Sand Springs range we could feel a brisk wind forcing against us. We had been cycling freely with a breeze pushing us on at comfortably high speeds. Now the peculiar geography of the landscape was creating its own wind patterns. It slowed us down and the first pass seemed to be no nearer than fifteen minutes ago.

'Have you seen that?' Martyn pointed off the road to the left. A large sandcastle rose from the desert floor two miles long and 600 feet high. Tracks through the plain and the evaporated salt marshes led to a small series of sand dunes, above which stood this enormous peaked mound of sand. It looked as if a large bulldozer had moved some builder's aggregate into the middle of nowhere.

'Why would they bring that sand all the way out here?' I asked.

'They haven't,' Martyn replied. 'That's Sand Mountain.'

I looked at my map which did indeed show this phenomenon.

'That's a natural dune, created by years of erosion,' Martyn said.

We pushed on and up the growing incline. It was a climb of less than 1000 feet but the resisting wind made the gradient seem much greater.

As I rounded a slight bend, pedalling slowly and steadily, I swerved to avoid several large insects on the road.

'Urgh,' I exclaimed, narrowly avoiding crushing some under my wheels. They were about one to two inches long with black, glistening shells and long antennae. Their creepy hind legs bent up above the fattened rear section. Several minutes later I came across a larger mass of these crickets scuttling across my path.

Under the sun my arms were slick with sweat but even so, my skin prickled. I shivered with horror at the black crustaceous things as they spread out across the road. There was an odd stench that caught at the back of my throat and made my stomach push upwards, heaving the precious water and sports drink I'd managed to slowly swallow.

'Can I go on ahead to get some shots of you freewheeling down into this next valley?' Martyn asked as we stopped at the summit of the hill.

'I wouldn't stop too long down there though.' I nodded my

head towards the fenced-off area below. 'That's the US Naval End and I don't think they'd be too pleased if you start filming.'

'Oh yeah,' Martyn said. '"Charity bike rider arrested for spy filming." Not a brilliant idea. I'll film you somewhere else on a descent.'

'Probably very wise.'

It was a narrow valley with a straight road that allowed us to view our next climb up to Drumm Summit ten miles in the distance. The descent was perfect. The road, newly surfaced, passed under my wheels with a sweet hiss, broken only by the odd crunch as I put paid to another cricket.

I watched one large critter as he tugged at a body segment of another glued to the road by its gooey soft belly innards. I kept this one in sight and watched in disgust as its fellow species proceeded to rasp away the fleshy part, eating it off the road surface and then dragging the segment a little further towards the hard shoulder.

'Urrgghh,' I shuddered, causing the bike to wobble wildly.

'Watch out,' Ryan called, riding on before me, his strong legs and younger body moving the bike easily up the straight slope. He stood ahead of me, waiting for me once more. I reached his rear wheel and looked round at the mass moving across the road.

'So you don't fancy cycling over Carroll Summit then?' Martyn said, when we joined him further on. He was standing at the side of the road, pointing to the sign over Route 722 which directed us towards the alternative route to Austin.

'If you think I'm going to put my body through a two thousand five hundred feet ascent then you're even more mad than I thought,' I said, taking off my helmet for a second.

Martyn laughed. 'It was worth asking just to see your reaction. You looked so horrified your hair's standing on end.'

I smiled and lifted my hand to my hair. Small spiky tufts stuck out from my skull and I smoothed them down with my palm.

'Do you think we should chance it?' Martyn asked, flicking his head towards the small wooden building opposite that claimed to be a bar in the centre of Middlegate.

Ryan shook his head, mindful of our past experience. 'No way. I'm staying on the bike in case the natives aren't friendly.'

The wooden building had a large pitted gravel area, filled with stagnant water. Ryan cycled slowly on the unkempt road as Martyn and I pushed the bikes along through the rusting vehicles. The square roof shaded the dark wooden veranda and against a window was an old wagon wheel and a sign 'Welcome to Middlegate – the middle of nowhere. Elevation 4600 feet, population 17.'

Next to the 17 a number 18 had been crossed out.

'Somebody must have died,' I said.

As we neared the bar we could hear country music. A door opened and a bearded man walked through, placing his hat on his head and forcing it down over his brow.

'Well howdee!' he said – I think – his thick facial growth made the sound indistinct.

'Will we get a cold drink here, sir?' Ryan asked.

'You sure will.' The man's hand rose to the hat brim and he flicked it a little higher so that it lifted free from his busy eyebrows. He squinted at us, turning to look at Martyn. 'You're not from around hereabouts?'

'No, sir,' Martyn said. 'We're just travelling through.'

'Where's you all from then? That's no American accent. Are you Australian?'

'No, we're from England, sir,' Ryan said.

'You're not from England.' He looked at Ryan.

'No, no, I'm from Calgary in Canada but I live in England.'

'That's near Ireland,' he said. 'My people came from Ireland oh back in . . .' His eyebrows moved up and down as if to add momentum to his thoughts. 'Nope can't remember that far back. Anyways, you might know my cousins the McAndrews. They're still living there.'

'No, I'm sorry I don't think we do,' I said.

He stood looking at us, his eyebrows furrowing in towards one another, shading his eyes. He forced his hat down with a slight anti-clockwise twist of his hand and he shuffled his feet forward.

'Shep!' he whistled and a large dog came leaping out from under the veranda, making me jump. The pair walked towards a battered old pickup and drove away.

Ryan held the door for me. The place was gloomy, the dark mood from outside filtered into the interior. The ceiling was festooned with one dollar bills which fluttered as the ceiling fan made its way slowly round and round.

'Are those your bikes?' a woman asked, as Ryan made his way towards the bar. She was sitting at a table nearby and was watching a large screen opposite. She turned her head towards us.

'Yes,' Martyn replied.

'My lot are headed for Austin tonight,' she said.

'Are those cyclists we saw earlier?' said Martyn.

'Yeah, that'll be Steve, my husband, and Matt, my son. We're spending the vacation cycling across the States.'

'Are you their support?' I asked.

'Yeah. I'll hang on here a little while yet and then catch them on the road and see how they're doing.'

'Where did you set off from today?' Martyn asked.

'Fallon.'

'Wow and they're going to make it to Austin today? That's impressive,' I said.

'Oh most people do that,' she said, looking a little surprised. 'Where are you headed?'

'We've nearly finished for the day,' I said. 'We're stopping at Cold Springs. We figure we've got a long journey ahead of us and we need to take it steady. This is just the start.'

'How long have you got?'

'We're planning on finishing in New York on the first of September,' I said. 'How long will it take Steve and Matt to get to Austin?'

'They might not make it all the way,' she shrugged. 'They just cycle as long as they can and when they've had enough, I pick 'em up.'

I must have looked surprised.

'Steve's done this route twice before like you, cycling every mile, but it's hard work and he's doing this with Matt just to enjoy it, so they do as many miles as they can and then we drive on to the next stop. He doesn't feel he has to cycle every mile 'cos he's done that all before.'

'I don't think we'd get away with that,' I smiled, 'although it's a great idea. I could just call Mike and get him to pick us up now.'

'No way,' laughed Martyn. He glanced out of the window towards the bikes. 'Nice idea, though.'

The darkness of the building had cooled us as we'd supped water and Ryan had treated me to a Mars Bar. But as we set off again, the sun warmed us quickly. Against the peculiar local wind which pushed us from in front, making our wheels seem to drag against the forward motion, we passed what appeared to be stone ruins of the overland mail station. We then came to the old telegraph station, two outposts from the long since defunct Pony Express.

We laid our bikes by the roadside and strode through the sharp short grass that rustled against our legs and scratched the bare flesh to get a better glimpse of the rock walls that nature was reclaiming. I studied the ruins where riders would have changed horses as they rode through the states, laden with mail. It was a dangerous service as the riders rode through empty desert, sometimes encountering hostile Indians. It existed for only eighteen months before the cross-country telegraph caused its demise.

As we pulled into the drive that ran up to Cold Springs Station, Mike was already there, and he waved at us. I climbed from my bike.

'The bloke here says don't wander off the road too far, there's loads of rattlers this year.'

'Rattlers?'

'Rattlesnakes,' Mike replied.

'Yikes,' I said, recalling our footsteps in the long grass earlier.

Cold Springs Station, which was a bar, café, gas station with RV hook-up facilities, had the silhouette of a Pony Express rider and a horse at the entrance. A wagon and the American flag fluttered by the chain-sawed remains of a skeletal tree that stood beside the two self-serve petrol pumps.

On the station veranda I could see Rebecca and Jodie rocking steadily back and forth on an old swing seat, sipping bottles of Coke.

'Hi, Mum,' Rebecca called, leaning forward to wave. 'Do you need anything?'

I wheeled my bike to the edge of the veranda and rested against a wooden tub with a small tree in it.

'It's just good to be finished for the day,' I said. 'But I could drink one of those.' I unzipped my bag and scrambled for my purse, cursing my clumsy and sore fingers.

'It's okay, I'll get you this one,' Rebecca said and disappeared through the door that led into the shop cum café. I rocked on the swing and closed my eyes for a moment. No more cycling for the day. The sun, which had been ferocious while we were on the bike, now had a dull edge to it. Clouds were gathered on the ridges that surrounded us on all sides. Fluffy white clouds started to darken and blacken, thickening and sinking lower so that they seemed to hang from the peaks. A flash split the darkened cumulus, and the explosive noise a few seconds later made me jump.

'I wouldn't have wanted to cycle through that,' I said.

That first flash was the beginning of a stormy afternoon. Jodie and Rebecca sat in the beautifully appointed barroom in front of a Schrader wood-burning stove. There was a warming throw in United States colours draped across a settee. Jodie's head was bowed as she read and Rebecca was fidgeting, listening to her iPod, her hands and feet moving restlessly.

'What are the showers like?' I asked.

'They're okay,' said Rebecca. 'But we had to get Cindy to chase the cricket out because Michael couldn't manage to move it.'

'You should have heard Becca scream when it moved,' Jodie said.

'I did not,' Rebecca said, indignantly.

The shower was powerful and hot and I let the jets of water pummel my back to try to ease some of the pain that persisted in the lower part of my spine. I dressed slowly and when I got back to the RV I prepared my kit for the following day. I lay on the bed but I was too fatigued to sleep and too uncomfortable to lie so I pulled my sheet off and shuffled back towards the café, meeting Jodie and Rebecca coming the other way.

'I don't believe it,' exclaimed Rebecca. 'We've been sat there for hours waiting for *Friends* to come on and that last thunderstorm has taken the power out so there's no TV.' She was shaking her head furiously.

'How long will the power be out?'

'I asked that and the dumb thing said it could be twenty minutes or it could be two days.' She threw her hands up and snorted through her nose. 'I can't believe you brought me to a place like this. They haven't even got a TV that works. The woman said they'll start the generator if they need to later on but hopefully the power should come back on.'

A large thunder crack made us jump.

'I'm not standing about in the open like this while that's going on,' I said and we hurried back to the RVs as large rain drops darkened the sandy lot.

Day 8 – Thursday, 6 July
Cold Springs, Nev. to Austin, Nev.
50.1 miles – 4 hrs 43 mins
Total covered – 442.8 miles

JANE

The next morning, the air was fresh and clear after the storms, but it promised to be another scorching day.

We, the sad trio, were up early again, trying to get as many miles under our belts as possible before the temperature hit treble figures. We were following the overland stage route rather than the more scenic but challenging rail road pass as none of us felt any great need to cycle up the 7452 feet at Carroll Summit – although the road was supposed to be pretty and there would be shade from some trees.

An hour into the day, I had an urgent need to empty my bladder. The road was long and straight, skirting the ridges of the Desatoya Mountains, and there would be nowhere to 'go' for miles.

Martyn and Ryan cycled on a little way ahead as I got off the bike and walked a few steps away from the road, mindful of the rattlers that might still be lurking in the grass. The two men gallantly faced the other away while I removed my top, tugged my shorts down and squatted as low from the road as I could – but not so low that a rattler could bite my bum.

The road had been empty for at least five minutes when I'd decided to take my 'convenience break' but naturally, as soon as I'd started to pee, a cloud of churned-up dust appeared down the road and I could soon hear – then see – a red Chevy coming towards me, revving its engine.

I tried to hurry, to finish my business, but there's no rushing my bladder. So I stayed crouched as low as possible. The truck engine roared as it neared and three faces peered out at me, the horn blaring loudly as they passed me and still blaring as they passed Ryan and Martyn. Red-cheeked with embarrassment, I pulled up my shorts and struggled back into my top.

'I'm not wearing this bibbed top with these shorts again,' I said, as I rejoined Martyn and Ryan. 'It's impossible to pee with any dignity in this gear.'

'Well, you'll have made some mindless morons' day by giving them a cheap thrill,' Ryan said.

'No skin off my nose, there's not much to see and nothing to get excited about.'

'Oh believe me, that was exciting for them,' Ryan said.

We had been cycling at a steady speed of about 20 mph when the road seemed to get heavier against the tyres of the bike. I watched as Ryan and Martyn kept cycling away from me with ease as my speed fell and kept falling till I felt like I was pushing a huge weight along the road.

I looked at the altimeter and was relieved to see that the reason for the slower pace was that we were cycling up a very gradual incline.

I stopped at the roadside, my legs astride the bike, and pulled my water bottle from its cage, resting my stinging thighs and aching calves. I twisted my back first one way, then the other and stretched my neck and upper torso to try to ease my body out of the bent-over cycling position.

Setting off once more I soon had an incentive to keep pedalling. The crickets we had encountered the day before were back and each time I felt too weary to continue I counted another mass of black creatures that scurried out of the way of Ryan's wheels and back directly towards me.

As we neared the top of the pass, the stench from the insects was so bad that I pulled my bandana up over my mouth. But that didn't seem to stop the smell and the taste in my mouth, just impeded my breathing. I pulled the cloth away from my face. Big mistake. A car came hurtling over the top of New Pass, roared past us at some speed and sent the dried body parts and dust from dead crickets swirling into our path. I shook my head and spluttered to try to stop myself from swallowing the awful dust, using the back of my hand to clear dead creatures from my face.

I was just grateful I was wearing sunglasses.

All too soon we reached the foothills of our second and final pass, Mount Airey Summit. It was not a long and arduous climb – only 1000 feet – but it was a relief when we finally dropped down on to the short plain that would lead us to the final climb of the day into Austin.

The road was thick now with the insects that seemed to be crossing the plains, moving relentlessly on their eastward travel to who knows where. The crunch of the wheels as I crushed yet another large armoured creature made me cringe.

'You're nearly there now, not much further,' I heard Mike shouting at me as we neared a sandy coloured building in the town of Austin. I turned my face towards him, only wishing I could step off the bike right now. 'Smile, you'll be finished soon.'

I looked away, my face stern, my legs tired. All I could focus on was the thought that just a few minutes away was a hot shower where the grime of the road and dead creatures against my skin would be rinsed clean away.

MIKE

It was barely noticeable to the others but to me, the cumulative effect of the ride had already begun to tell on Jane. Her eyes were not opening as much, she'd lost some weight and was slumping just a little more as she sat. This had been the eighth consecutive day in the saddle and the fact that she had been barely able to walk ten days ago was long forgotten. She had become an invincible cycling machine but I knew she was in an immense amount of pain.

With the cyclists finishing just after midday, it gave me and Steven the whole afternoon to explore Austin, Nevada, while on our daily search for yet another internet connection.

It seemed inappropriate to call it a town – it was more like a small hamlet. With a population of only 400, the nearest other 'town' which had a similar-sized number of inhabitants was over seventy miles away. And if you needed a city, with the infrastructure of hospitals, government and offices of law, you would have to drive for over three hours to Reno, more than 200 miles away.

Built in the western foothills of the Toiyabe mountain range, Austin was founded out of a silver rush in 1862. Within a year, it had a booming population of 10 000 but now, it felt like a ghost town.

It had a distinct Wild West feel to it, but today there were no horses – just an occasional pickup truck and four-wheeled drive vehicle parked on either side of the four-lane road.

None of the businesses looked particularly affluent. The rather grandly titled International Hotel is said to be the oldest in Nevada. Built in Virginia City in 1859, it was moved to Austin four years later. No longer a hotel but a bar, it has a rustic dilapidated charm about it.

The RV park was located at the eastern end of town, next to the twelve-seat Baptist church. The park had an honesty box for payment by campers, which, judging by the amount of times that afternoon it was checked by random visitors, was frequently misused.

Within a couple of hours we were back in the RV park where the air-conditioning units were humming. A constant stream of cars came into the park, where the drivers would study us for a while before leaving. We wondered whether we should leave the vehicles unattended.

Jane was resting at the rear of the RV, lying on her side in the double bed, and Steven was soon playing on his Nintendo DS. The others had decided to check out the town's outdoor swimming pool. It seemed appropriate that I should begin fulfilling my pre-ride resolution of taking up running again.

Taking the rear exit out of the car park, I was soon pounding the pavement off Main Street, running down a hill and picking a route which would hopefully avoid the considerable number of yappy dogs in the area.

But within minutes, my heart was pounding, my mouth hung open as I tried to drag in gulps of air. Austin's high altitude of 6 600 feet was making even my laborious pace difficult.

I slowed even further and my thoughts turned to Jane. How were the altitude, heat and unsheltered roads affecting her?

Swinging further downhill, the tarmac darkened in the shade and bizarrely, the surface seemed to be moving. I came to a halt, my poor eyesight just able to pick out the hundreds of crickets which were inching across the surface, their shiny black shells standing out from the tarmac.

It was impossible to go forward – there was no space to even tread around them – so I cut back, turned left and headed on to Main Street and towards what was described as the town's premier tourist attraction – Stokes Castle.

After half a mile, I found it – a stone-built relic of a building which looked more like a dilapidated barn. It occupied the edge of a rise and had incredible views over the plains below that stretched out some thirty to forty miles.

Abandoned silver mines punctured the plains, their shaft openings rusting in the exposed air. It was beautiful. I sat on the ground, the sunlight on my face, and enjoyed thirty minutes of pure solitude.

That night, once Steven was asleep and Jane was busy working on the laptop, Michael and I decided to head in to Austin for a beer. I fancied the idea of entering an old-fashioned bar through the two swing saloon doors, asking for a whisky and waiting for the bar tender to slide it across the bar.

I was to be disappointed.

The only customers were three middle-aged men whose butt cheeks overhung the bar stools. Two slot machines blinked in the corner. The TV above the bar was tuned to a twenty-four-hour news channel and bar tender looked like a member of ZZ Top. Our entrance couldn't have been more inconspicuous. We took two stools adjacent to the three other customers and waited, waited and waited until almost as an afterthought the bartender, who had been wiping a glass, turned to us.

'What can I get you?' he asked.

'Two Buds please,' Michael said. The bartender disappeared and Michael turned to me: 'They're not as strong in the USA as the UK.'

Although I'd only been out of San Francisco for four nights it felt like we'd entered a separate universe. The TV screen showed world events unfolding and seemed plain wrong in this environment. Austin didn't seem like a town which should have any interest in ballistic missiles being tested in North Korea.

Michael and I sat chatting quietly for a good thirty minutes. We had nearly completed our second bottles of beer when the guy next to us suddenly turned to me.

'Were they good to you at the County Depot?'

Surprised by the sudden question I could only come up with, 'I'm sorry?'

'You're with the cyclists staying at the Baptist church, right? You went into the Depot to use the internet.' There was a pause. 'Oh, don't look so surprised. You can't come to Austin and not be noticed – it's a small town. I'm Dave by the way.'

'Mike and Michael.'

'Yeah, I know,' Dave said. 'Brits eh?' Dave turned his attention back to the TV screen showing library pictures of the North Korean leader overseeing a military parade. 'What do you make of that?' he asked.

'Not sure what's it about,' I said. 'We don't get any news in the RV not without the internet.'

'North Korea fired some test missiles on Independence Day. Would you believe that? It's just aimed at provoking us, it's like an act of war really.'

It was difficult to judge the underlying mood in the bar and a Nevada saloon didn't seem the place to share my own political views. 'What do you think the USA should do?' I said.

'Well, if they're firing missiles, we should get stuck in now. Sort them out before they build missiles that can hit the West Coast.' The bartender and the other customers listened. 'Maybe nuke 'em,' said Dave.

I looked at Michael, whose mouth was agape. 'You don't think that that might be a touch unnecessary?' I ventured. The two beers may have had a lot to answer for.

'They fired them on Independence Day!' said Dave. 'They need to be shown who's boss. We should kick their asses.'

'That's right, Dave,' nodded one of the other men, who was busily munching on a sandwich.

Changing tone slightly, Dave asked me: 'Do the rest of the world hate Americans?'

'Well . . .' I wanted to pick my response carefully. 'I think it's probably fair to say that they evoke a lot of strong opinions.'

'We know the slimy French can't stand us. But what about the Brits? You're with us, aren't you?'

'Most people support the troops, but opinion's divided. It's very difficult to say.' I was desperate to change tack. 'Have you lived in Austin long?'

'No. I come from Idaho. I only came here eighteen months ago. I like the quiet but I'll move on at some point. It's a good job you're not French. We hate the French. They wouldn't be welcome in Austin.'

'That's right, man,' the bartender nodded.

Michael shuffled off his bar stool. 'We'd better go anyway, we've an early start,' he said. 'We have to be off by five.'

Dave paused. 'Watch out for the crickets, man, especially up on the hill, it will be like driving on oil in the morning.'

Day 9 – Friday, 7 July
Austin, Nev. to Eureka, Nev.
69.7 miles – 6 hrs 29 mins
Total covered – 512.5 miles

MIKE

Waking next morning, it was still pitch black outside although at our sister RV, parked right next door, there was a hive of activity, Ryan was preparing the bikes while Michael was making breakfast.

Lying in bed, I was surprised to have my second hangover of the week. I'd only had the two Buds, but my head thumped and I groaned as Jane flitted around our cramped 'bedroom' with some dexterity. Under normal circumstances she'd be slow to move and it took some time to regain mobility first thing from the crippling bone pains, but there was so little space and so much clutter there was a need to exit the room as soon as possible.

Jodie, Rebecca and Steven were still asleep, the girls in the living area and Steven above the driver's cab. Officially, the vehicle catered for five adults and two children though we were struggling to fit in two adults, two teenagers and a junior. All of us are somewhat under average size but even so, space was at a premium. I imagined that the three adults in the other RV – none of whom knew each other well – were finding personal space something of an issue.

'How's the head?' Jane asked as she bent down to give me a morning peck.

'It's thumping, but hopefully it'll go soon.'

'Not blessed with a great deal of common sense are you?' she said, grabbing her bike bag and helmet.

'What do you mean?'

'We're at well over six thousand feet, Mike. You go out for a run in the middle of the afternoon then have a couple of beers. Figure that one out.' She shook her head and was off.

A couple of hours later, the RVs set off from Austin for Eureka on Highway 50. I was surprised that it had been billed as the loneliest road in America as there always seemed to be headlights coming towards us from another car on the long narrow road, even if it did take us ten minutes to pass each other.

We reached Eureka five hours later and a little sooner than the cyclists. Slightly bigger than Austin, it was everything you'd imagine a cowboy town to be – wide streets, saloons, wooden posts you could tie your horse to, balconies, verandas and heat.

But what really got my pulse racing with excitement was the sight of our first launderette.

I never thought I'd consider a launderette as a luxury but after five days cooped up in an RV in the Nevada Desert, you'd be surprised. There were a number of loads to do – Jane's cycling kit, sheets, towels and other items. But they would have to wait: before we knew it, Cindy had commandeered all the machines with her own clothes. I made a mental note to be quicker off the mark next time.

I left Rebecca and Jodie to bag the washing machines while Steven and I decided to explore Eureka's delights. Before we'd had a chance even to cross the road, however, a car pulled up adjacent to us and the electric windows were wound down. An attractive middle-aged lady wearing sunglasses called over to us.

'You're not wanting directions, surely?' I asked.

'What?' she said, scowling as though she could smell something offensive. A young girl, presumably her daughter, sat in the passenger seat, her hand shielding her forehead as if to disassociate herself from whatever was about to be said. 'Are you with those cyclists?'

'Which cyclists?' I said. 'There are three groups of cyclists.'

'The ones wearing white tops.' I sensed a slight frustration in her voice.

'Yes.'

She tutted and her eyes closed and I sensed a tirade coming my way.

'Well, they are a danger, riding in the middle of the road, they'll get themselves killed.'

'Thanks for letting me know,' I said, adding a little sarcasm to my tone.

'Hey, hey,' she shouted, as I started to move away. 'I want to know what you're going to do about it.' Her daughter was now looking into her lap for a hole to swallow her.

'Nothing.'

'What?' she barked. 'They're going to get killed.' She waited before adding, 'Oh . . . it's their lives.'

'Exactly. They're mature adults – well, they're meant to be – and I'm not going to tell them what to do. Anyway, it's not like you couldn't see them. You must have known for ten miles they were there before reaching them. And another thing,' I said, pointing to the front of her car. 'You need to have your headlights on.'

With that Steven and I crossed over the road.

Day 10 – Saturday, 8 July
Eureka, Nev. to Ely, Nev.
80.1 miles – 7 hrs 54 mins
Total covered – 592.6 miles

JANE

I rinsed my toothbrush under the tap and turned the shower head off using my towel so I didn't have to touch the grime that covered the sink. I had chosen the least foul smelling of the bathrooms but even so, the stench of mould was overwhelming. It was a relief when I stepped out on to the veranda and headed across Eureka RV Park back to the RVs.

As I walked across the site, I could hear raised voices coming from inside one of them, but couldn't quite make out what was being said.

Stepping into my RV, I placed my toilet bag on the cupboard and hung my towel from the cupboard handle. My pyjamas, which hopefully were dry enough from my night sweats to enable me to wear them for another night, were hanging alongside them. I was looking forward to having clean clothes. My expectations of RV sites and what sort of facilities they had had narrowed. Hot showers and washing machines were rare.

Rob was outside the RV by the time I poked my head out to see what was going on.

'I'm not happy about you setting off this early,' he said forcefully. His face was red and he was chewing his lip, still fraught from his heated exchange with Ryan.

'That's fine,' I said, calmly.

'It's too dark and the drivers won't see you until it's too late.'

'Honestly, that's fine, Rob,' I said. 'I'm happy to wait for a few more moments to set off today. I'll put the time on a little for the next few days until we go through the next time zone.'

'It's just that I don't want to be the one who has to ring someone with bad news if a car hits one of you. I nearly ran over a deer this morning.'

The experience had obviously shaken him.

'Look, I'm not going to fall out with you about what time we set off. If you feel strongly about it then I'm not going to argue. It's the right thing to do to set off a little later. We just want to make the most of the cooler part of the day,' I said.

Rob's complexion was fading from the red and his breathing was calmer. 'That's okay then. It's just that I feel kind of responsible out here looking after Martyn.'

'I understand,' I said. 'I just want this trip to be a happy trip and it's not worth doing something if it's going to upset you so much. We'll delay the start by thirty minutes and it should be light enough by then. I don't want to put anyone at risk either. It's only a minor point and it's not worth getting riled over.'

We had a long day ahead of us. Eighty miles. The edges of the clouds that had been illuminated pink as the sun rose had disappeared as the sun had gone behind them, leaving a grey dimness. Our white shirts would make us visible and we would cycle in single file, staying close to the road edge.

We had four summits to climb before we would reach our destination of Ely and the very first one was immediately after leaving the RV park.

My legs and back were stiff as I pushed the bike in a low gear slowly up the ridge. Set back from the road, I could see two low single tents nestled away from the scrubby growth. The discomfort and cramped space of the RV looked luxurious compared with camping in the middle of nowhere. At least we didn't have to shake our sleeping bags to check for rattlesnakes before we slept at night. I couldn't imagine not showering after a hot day on the bike.

We would cycle past Diamond Mountain and Battle Mountain, part of tall ranges to the left of us that crept northward away from Route 50, the loneliest road.

The first summit, Pinto, was hard on the legs but it was cooler and fresher than yesterday. We had seen the last of the crickets just outside of Austin so although the climbs were arduous I didn't have to shriek my way to the top.

Ryan would cycle on ahead to the green marker at the top of each climb and turn in his saddle to give me the thumbs up as I gritted my teeth and crept up the tarmac towards him.

At the top of Little Antelope Summit, the third summit and thirty-five miles into the day, we were greeted by the familiar sight of the RV.

Mike stepped out from it to greet us. 'Have I got something for you,' he said. I could hear clinking and he appeared with three iced coffees.

'Oh wow,' Martyn said. 'That's just heaven.'

'Wait, wait,' Mike said. 'That's not all.' He disappeared back into the RV and this time appeared with a cardboard box. Opening it, he revealed a collection of pastries.

'I just don't know what to have,' said Martyn, poring over the contents. We all dived in.

'What's it like today?' asked Mike.

'The wind's much kinder,' said Ryan, biting into a cinnamon swirl. 'It's just a little cooler. The cycling's been much more enjoyable.'

'What about you, Jane?' asked Mike. 'How are you feeling?'

I swallowed a mouthful of sweet pastry.

'I can feel the ten days of cycling in my legs,' I said. 'I'm looking forward to the rest day. At least there's only one climb left.'

Robinson Summit was the highest of the climbs that day, but from there, it would be a glorious coast into Ely and our first rest day.

We arrived in Ely in good time. The campsite was a real luxury – a Kampground of America or KOA, with laundry facilities, a shop that sold iced Starbucks and chocolate. It doesn't sound a lot but expectations weren't high.

Day 11 – Sunday, 9 July
Ely, Nev.
Rest day

JANE

We'd eaten as a team, Steven had enjoyed his 'boys' night' and as we woke up on the Sunday morning I was so relieved to have a day without getting into the saddle.

'Cindy and I will stay here. We've got loads to do,' said Michael. He stretched his arms above his head and his T-shirt rose, exposing his midriff.

'Stop showing us your body!' Ryan said.

'Oh, I don't mind,' Cindy cooed, watching Michael as he gathered up the campsite directions.

'We'll try to book some accommodation ahead,' he said. 'You lot go with Rob and enjoy the train ride.'

We were looking forward to our steam train experience. It was advertised as a step back in time, the sole survivor of a grand era in the silver state.

'Howdy, yawl.' Rob stepped from his four-wheel drive. The campsite was several miles from the town and he'd kindly agreed to pick us up to take us to the railway. 'Is you ready for your train ride, young man?' he asked Steven.

'Sure am, partner,' Steven said.

I watched Rebecca and Jodie sloping back to us, chatting away. 'Come on, Becca,' I called. 'We'll miss the steam train if you don't move now.'

'Okay, we're coming.'

'You're supposed to be ready. We're going to have to go without you if you're not ready now.'

She muttered something under her breath as she turned away but grabbed her bag and climbed into the car.

We waited in the queue for the Nevada Northern Railway and came away with our light blue tickets, with a picture of a steam train on them. It was advertised as 'The ghost train of old Ely'. Martyn fidgeted, anxious for the train to draw into the station. A black-painted engine glided up towards us, smoke billowing from its chimney. We climbed aboard and sat in the open carriage just behind the engine. The driver made the engine whistle 'toot toot' and Martyn stared open-eyed ahead.

'It's great not to be cycling,' he said. 'I've got so much work to do but I wouldn't miss this for the world.' He took out his camera. 'You don't mind if I film us, do you?'

'Of course not,' Mike replied. We sat back on the hard bench seats and as the train pulled out of the station, a woman's voice came over a speaker and started to tell us the history of the ghost train.

'Built in 1905–6 the Nevada Northern Railway is the best preserved standard gauge short line and complete rail facility left in America. If you're sitting in the open carriage you'd better watch out for the ember – it can get mighty dusty and dirty up there.'

At each turn, the engine driver blew his whistle. We headed towards the mountainside and into a black hole shored up by metal supports. As darkness descended on the open carriage, the embers, which had previously flown up into the air, streamed down on us, hot and greasy.

Steven and I shrunk into the carriage, where he held my hand tightly in the darkness which dim lights only just held at bay. Soon we were back in the daylight and Monica, the guide, continued her chatter.

'Oh look, we're real lucky today,' she said. 'There's a digger making a trench in the side of that slag heap.'

I burst out laughing. Martyn turned to me.

'What's so funny?'

'I can't believe we're spending our day off visiting what is described as the biggest slag heap in the world. It's fantastic.'

As we headed into town, Monica pointed out the various points of interest, including the pink-roofed brothel. Before we knew it, we were back at the station ready to disembark.

'I don't want to hear another train whistle again,' Martyn said, as the driver let out a familiar 'toot toot' as the engine rumbled slowly down the rails into a siding.

The boys were looking at their watches. On the other side of the world, the World Cup Final between France and Italy was about to start and, despite the rival attraction of the biggest slag heap in America, it was to be the highlight of Mike and Steven's day.

'I'm sure there will be somewhere we can see it,' said Rob. 'We'll have a look and see.'

We found the casino, which was lined with gaming machines occupied by ill-dressed men and women, who sat before them inserting coins and watching the wheels spin. Sure enough there was a restaurant with a television showing the final. We ordered food and had a good view of the screen, eating our meals and making drinks last to watch the entire final.

We watched in astonishment as Zidane completely lost his bottle and headbutted Materazzi's chest, then we were gripped by penalties. I wanted France to win and was bitterly disappointed when Italy did.

'I'm right glad I got to watch football on my day off,' I said to Mike, as we headed back to the RV campsite.

'Oh, come on,' he said, teasing. 'You wouldn't let me miss the World Cup Final, would you?'

'Of course not. And at least I'm not cycling. I'm not looking forward to getting back on the bike tomorrow.'

'Oh, I am,' Ryan said, from the back seat.

'Yes, you would be,' I said, grinning at him. 'At least it's our last day on Route 50 tomorrow and we'll have cycled the loneliest road, all the way from Carson City.'

'I don't think it's been that lonely,' Mike said.

'Martyn would definitely not argue with you. Every time he's tried to get footage of "the loneliest road" another car goes by.' Ryan chuckled.

'You'll have another state out of the way, too,' Rob said. 'We're nearly in Utah now.'

The car bumped across the gravel road and into the campsite. I'd noticed some tents with a collection of assorted bikes surrounding them.

'There's a group of lads over there cycling across America from coast to coast. They're fundraising for Cross Country for Cancer,' Mike explained.

'Oh, what are they like?' I asked.

'"Enthusiastic" would be one way to describe them,' Mike said. 'They're quite keen to swap experiences.'

'It would be good to know how they're coping. They look like fit young men.'

I wandered over to the bench outside the campsite shop and was greeted by six tall men who looked like babies in comparison to Martyn and me. 'Hi, I'm Jane,' I said.

'It's good to meet you finally,' said one of them, smiling. 'We've heard your name at some of the places we've stopped.'

'So when did you lot set off?' I asked

'Monday we cycled to West Sacramento, about ninety miles, although we had a twenty-mile detour into the countryside courtesy of Ezra's directions.'

'That's a bit harsh on top of ninety miles,' I said, knowing all too well how interminable twenty miles can feel at the end of a long day. 'So who are you all and where are you from?'

'I'm Jacob and this is my brother Ezra,' said the first one. 'We're from San Fran.'

'I'm John. I am from Ohio.'

'David, San Diego California.'

'Max and Paddy, Brits.'

'You must have put in some long days to get here now,' I said.

'Yea,' John said. 'Fallon to Austin was a long hard day. One hundred and forty miles. Max pulled a muscle and he's used some muscle rub which has helped a little.'

'Oh, magic muscle cream! You'll have to share some of that with us,' I said laughing, but knowing how cramped my legs were each day after seventy or eighty miles. 'So, what did you make of the crickets – I've been cycling and squealing all the way.'

'I thought they would jump up and attack us.'

'Crickets can't jump too high. Ryan's been entertaining me with tales of grasshoppers the size of tennis balls in Kansas that really can jump high enough to hit you in the chest with a bang.' I shuddered just thinking about any evil-looking creatures we might meet in the future.

'So how are you coping?' asked Jacob.

'I think the first ten days of any long ride are the best,' I said. 'After that you just want to go home. It's fun but after that amount of time, the group dynamics begins to change and can cause friction. It takes some time for your backside to get used to the daily assault on your buttocks, but that goes off after a while. You seem a very together bunch of lads, I'm sure you'll enjoy the journey.'

We chatted a little longer, exchanging tales of the previous day. Ezra had been the instigator behind the ride and he was also responsible for the routing. I sympathised with him as that was my territory too and I couldn't help feeling responsible for the tiredness in our legs on some of the harder days. I knew I'd planned for some high mileage days in the future, hoping that by then we'd be fitter and 100 miles wouldn't feel too bad. Now, I wasn't so sure.

'So who's on your team?' John asked.

'Mike and Steven are here to support me. Rebecca and Jodie are along for a few weeks and then there's Cindy and Michael in the other RV for support. That's where Ryan sleeps. Ryan's foolishly agreed to come along to help me get through the tough days and he's doing a great job at motivating us – sometimes too much of a great job.' I rolled my eyes. 'And the other guy is Martyn. He's someone we know from our other two tours. He's a freelance cameraman who's working for Sky. He's quite amazing. It's hard enough just cycling but Martyn cycles on ahead, leaps off his bike, climbs the hills, films us then leaps back on his bike, catches us up and he's got to carry all his gear on his bike as well. We don't know how he manages but he's got some fantastic footage.'

We exchanged hugs and I stood in the middle of the group for a photo. I was truly dwarfed by six men all under the age of twenty-five and at least six foot tall. I barely came to the shoulder of any of them.

The group had been unable to find anyone to drive support for them so they were taking it in turns to drive the station wagon that was packed to its very roof with camping kit, bike spares and food. It stooped at the back, its suspension groaning under the weight.

JACOB

We took our sweet time waking up this morning and getting our day started. I personally managed to sleep from 10 pm until 7 am and I was the last one up. Plus, we're at the most remote KOA in America and it has great people and great facilities. It's our own personal oasis after so many miles of nothingness in the desert. This is our first rest day . . . and it's truly glorious.

We did laundry, updated the website a bit, fixed lunch, and read some books. Not much to speak of, but everything a rest day should be.

Then came Jane.

Jane is a name we had heard from time to time at places we'd stopped along the road. Occasionally we'd be prompted with 'Oh, are you riding with Jane?' by shop owners and locals. A bit confused, I finally looked Jane up on the internet last night and found out she is a tremendously strong athlete and human being first and terminally ill cancer patient second. She's the only terminal case to ever complete the Ironman, in fact. Right now she's on her third of three tours: a ride across America to raise donations for cancer research. And she was a few days ahead of us on the same route, but at a slightly slower pace (only on account of the media attention weighing her group down, I assume).

Well, we ran into her today staying at the KOA in Ely, Nevada when an English man asked if we wanted to do an interview with her for the BBC. That's like accidentally staying over at the same monastery with Lance Armstrong in Tibet. Quite a coincidence.

So we did the BBC interview (radio podcast, really) and afterwards talked for a while about riding strategies and opinions of the people and scenery thus far on the ride. We exchanged T-shirts and photos and parted quite pleased to have found other lycra-clad warriors along the road. She is a woman of small stature but seemingly effortless inner strength. Quite awe inspiring and perhaps even a little perplexing. I'm honored to have met her, and I'm pleased to have had a slice of her personality without knowing any of the celebrity context. I can see how she manages to raise multiple millions of dollars for cancer on her tours.

Jane's Appeal are heavily sponsored by a few groups, but happened to have had far too much gear from Gatorade. So we walked away with new water bottles, energy bars and endurance powder drink packets. Speak of a massive morale booster-shot . . .

Both our groups are following a nearly identical route and pace for the next few days since there are no other ways to go or places to stop in the desert, so perhaps we'll cross paths again.

As we sat eating our evening meal, I felt rested. I had been exhausted when I arrived in Ely but actually found myself looking forward to the following day's ride as I laid my kit out in preparation for another long hot day on the bike.

Day 12 – Monday, 10 July
Ely, Nev. to Baker, Nev.
58.7 miles – 5 hrs 10 mins
Total covered – 651.3 miles

MIKE

The savageness of the climbs had taken us all by surprise and although refreshed from the rest day, Jane looked ill at ease. At the summit of Sacramento Pass, which at 7154 feet was 600 feet lower than Cannon Pass, I decided to drive on ahead, park up and cheer her on. The twenty-five miles since Cannon Pass had been a steep descent then flat road across Spring Valley. It had seemed to take the cyclists an interminable amount of time to cross the flat lands and now the weather was closing in and thunder looked imminent.

A rough track led off towards the battered remnants of a ghost village and in the well-appointed parking area Jodie and Rebecca sat at a covered table supping a can of Coke each. Surprisingly, considering the low volume of traffic, a second RV pulled in behind us and a sprightly man who looked to be in his sixties jumped out. His body was wiry and lean and his bones seemed to point at right angles from his skin. To bump into him would be akin to walking into a jabbing finger.

He and his wife were experienced RVers and had a classic Harley Davidson coupled to the rear of their vehicle.

'How do you find America?' he said.

'We've only seen Nevada and California,' I said. 'So I can't really judge.'

'Is this the most remotest place or what?' he said, looking through some powerful binoculars. 'We went to Alaska last year but didn't get past through Canada – the wife was pissed.'

'Are you going to give it another go?' I asked.

'God knows. Set of cowards those Canadians, they were all assholes, never seen so many rules. There was a huge queue to get over the border, everything got searched. It was just a nightmare.'

'We've got a Canadian travelling with us,' I said, anxious to make sure he didn't make any faux pas should Ryan arrive.

'Best of luck to you, best place for them Canada, they're meant to be our allies but you wouldn't believe it.' He looked across at his wife whose stare would stop a child dead.

'Are you carrying?' he asked.

'Pardon?'

'I said are you carrying?'

'Carrying what, we don't have a bike only an RV.'

'Carrying a gun,' he said, as though I was an imbecile.

'What?' I said. 'Why would I want to carry a gun?'

'Connie!' he shouted across to his wife who was watching for the first glimpse of the cyclists. 'They're not carrying,' he said. 'You need a gun man,' he said, turning to me. 'Where are you heading?'

'Across the country to New York.'

'Wooohh man, I wouldn't go without a gun.' He rested his binoculars down. 'I'll show you ours.'

'No, it's not necessary,' I said. The man had a natural enthusiasm and exuberance and there was no sense of menace but I was keen his firearms remained in his vehicle.

'We have a law called the right to carry, lots of states allow you to carry a concealed weapon. Those that don't, turn a blind eye. There are so many immigrants, hoodlums and criminal types you need one, especially in remote places.' He looked across at his wife. 'Connie, tell him he needs a gun.'

'Oh, for sure he does,' she said, nodding.

'We'll be all right without one, we haven't got anything worth taking,' I said, hoping I sounded forceful without being rude.

The man shrugged. 'Your funeral,' he said. 'The druggies in this damn country will have you. Are you going to Chicago?'

'No.'

'That's a good thing. That's one mean city, you need to stay away from there.'

As a child my dad had always had guns stored in the alcove of the attic. He'd used them for hunting pheasants and rabbits mainly. It was a lovely feeling as a child taking the weight of a twelve bore, the fine wooden handle smooth to the touch. I used to hold it in position against my shoulder, seeing how long I could hold it steady without my arms beginning to tremble. I didn't feel intimidated by guns but likewise didn't feel the need to own one.

And certainly, on this trip, it seemed absurd to consider whether to carry a gun, especially with children in the vehicles. We'd take our chances.

Baker in Nevada was our next overnight stop. By now, we were accustomed to small towns but even by the standards of this trip, it was tiny. You could stand in the centre of the main street and lob a cricket ball in any direction out of the town. The new RV park was closed and the only gas station was an unmanned one. The blue road sign displayed the message 'Next service is 83 miles'.

In the near distance abandoned vehicles and discarded oil drums, car parts, tyres and general waste were scattered around. Accommodation was low grade static caravans in a poor state of repair.

We were booked into the Whispering Elms Camp Ground but it occurred to me that if the elms could talk they would have been screaming 'This place stinks!' It was smelly, dirty and a haven for varied insect life.

Our original thought had been to park up and head into the Great Basin National Park and specifically the Lehman Caves. Practically, though, it was becoming impossible to move the RVs once the cyclists had arrived. They needed to rest and our transport was their home.

Baker had been founded in the 1890s to serve ranchers, miners and visitors to the caves. It now has a permanent population of sixty-five and most of these appear to be 'artists', as many of the fence posts each side of town are various sculptures. As we'd parked up, Rebecca and Jodie had skidaddled to explore the town. It left Steven and me needing to await Jane's arrival before we could do the same.

It was ninety minutes later that Jane, Steven and I met

Rebecca, Jodie, Cindy and Michael sitting outside the Silver Jack Inn, a café which, from the décor, looked like it had been transported from the bohemian districts of San Francisco. Opposite was an antique shop flying a gay rights' flag. I suspected this was as near as liberated people could get to the border of Utah, the Mormon State. One local advertisement read 'Work in Utah, play in Nevada', although it did look like it would be a forlorn hope in Baker.

'What's the café like?' I asked.

'Really nice,' Rebecca said. 'There's some really nice home-made cakes. The owner's really miserable though. He won't serve us any more as he's shutting for the afternoon. You're wasting your time trying to get in.'

It seemed commercial suicide to me, especially as the traffic was coming through at one vehicle an hour.

'Best of luck anyway,' Rebecca said, as I wandered into the café. She had that smug air of someone who'd just been well fed and watered.

Three of the Cross Country for Cancer lads were stretched out across the veranda on wooden chairs reading, dozing and writing. They started their rides earlier in the morning, which meant they were generally finishing two or three hours in front of Jane so that once they'd erected their tents, they chilled out in the early afternoon. We joined them, sitting on the porch, Jane tugging up her trousers which were already hanging a lot looser than they had been two weeks ago.

A lone cyclist pulled up, his panniers trebling the width of his bike. It was such an extraordinary sight, a lone cyclist crossing a desert hundreds of miles from any major habitation. He dismounted, propping his steed against the wooden veranda like a twenty-first century cowboy. His bike was not the gleaming metallic finish of others, his helmet, a yellow pudding-basin BMX type. He opened a rear pannier, took out a half-empty gallon container of water, its brown discoloured plastic making the contents look unappetising. There was a collective nod of heads and hiyas. He ambled round to the front of the bike and ran his fingers through his hair before wiping the sweat from his brow with his right hand then dragging it dry across the cycle top.

'Hi,' he said. 'I'm Dave. Is it open?'

'No,' I said.

'Have you come far today?' Jane asked.

'About eighty miles. Are you all cycling as well?'

'Yes, but we're in two separate groups. We're going from San Francisco to New York,' Jane said, 'these guys are going from San Francisco to Baltimore. Are you on your own?'

'Yes.'

'I couldn't do that, it's incredibly brave,' Jane said.

'Brave or foolhardy, I haven't figured it out yet,' he said.

'So where's your journey taking you from?' I asked.

'I set off a few weeks ago from Oregon. I'm heading to Kansas to catch up with some friends and family then maybe reaching Boston by mid-September.' He delivered it in such a matter-of-fact way it was as if he was out for a day trip – not a three-month cycle ride across a continent. His demeanour indicated someone who was truly comfortable in his own skin, although he seemed to be finding conversation difficult.

'Have you finished for the day?' Max asked, raising his head from his book.

'No. I'll see how far I can get before that storm breaks.'

'Where will you stay? There's nothing until Milford.'

'I'll just pitch up at the side of the road in the desert.'

'That'd freak me out,' Jane said. 'What about the snakes and the scorpions etcetera.'

'I won't deny that it gets a little scary when the sun goes down and all you can hear are the surroundings coming to life. You'd be surprised how many creatures there are and how much noise there is.'

By now Dave had an unintentionally captive audience. We watched in silence as he checked his bike, secured his belongings, climbed on the saddle and pedalled away into the wilderness while the skies began to darken.

By early evening, the day's heat had vanished, the sun had begun to set and the heavens let go a mighty roar throughout the surrounding Nevada Desert and by a trick of light we were treated to pink and purple rain.

Throughout the night the rain battered the RV. Baker's average rainfall in a year was only four inches so we felt blessed. We wondered how Dave was getting on in his tent.

Day 13 – Tuesday, 11 July
Baker, Nev. to Milford, Utah (Ut.)
83.6 miles – 8 hrs 29 mins
Total covered – 734.9 miles

MIKE

It was a relief when next morning, we came across Dave twenty-five miles east from Baker. We blasted the horn once past him so he didn't feel buzzed and we all waved. He acknowledged us by raising his right arm.

Dave was an adventurer on a shoestring. There were no people supporting him and he didn't appear to have any communication tools or shelter within this area of Nevada. It was hard not to be inspired by him but at the same time, it made us feel totally inadequate.

Half an hour and thirty miles later we passed the three amigos spread out over a mile on the road. Martyn was in the rear having just been shooting some film, Jane's position was good with Ryan some 400 yards ahead barely turning his legs over. They'd been cycling for five hours and realistically they still had another three to go. We passed the Cross Country for Cancer lads just as they were entering Milford.

Earlier, almost as soon as we'd left Baker we crossed the state boundary from Nevada to Utah. I was surprised at the immediate contrast between the states. The tarmac changed colour, road signs changed focus from warnings about gambling to warnings about alcohol and it was as if the state took real pride in its cities. The most significant difference, however, was that it seemed a lot wealthier. Milford's houses were more substantially built and it seemed to take a lot of pride in looking good.

Although the town only had a population of 1500, the facilities were the equivalent of a town twenty times that size in the UK. The school pitches were so lush that Wembley would have been jealous.

The further we travelled into the USA, the further the temperature rose. It was unusual now for it not to reach a hundred degrees and coupled with the high altitude, it was becoming intimidating.

Certainly, it was impossible to venture out in the afternoon so we decided to settle into a routine of staying inside the air-conditioned RV after lunch. But it seemed the cyclists' finishing times were becoming later, partly because of darker mornings but also because of tougher terrain and physical conditions, increasing heat and winds that would pick up soon after lunch. The late finishes meant their recovery times were reduced and, in turn, that increased the strain on the next day.

We began to notice subtle physical changes in Jane. Eating was more difficult for her as she lost her appetite and the fare being offered wouldn't reinvigorate that. She was beginning to sweat more profusely at night.

It didn't help that our provisions were becoming a little unimaginative. It had been ten days since we'd seen any reasonably sized supermarket and fresh food stuffs were not easily accessible. So late dinner in Milford for Jane consisted of a tuna mayonnaise sandwich on a sweet bread which, although not particularly unappetising, would not begin to write off the 6500 calories that she was burning each day.

There was also an unsettling feeling of perpetual motion, a sensation that even though we were parked up, it would only be temporary. This led to a disorientation in all of us, which was at its most acute for a couple of hours after arrival, as everyone wandered in and out of the vehicles as we became acclimatised to our new surroundings.

Ryan's distinctive rap on the door signalled his arrival at our RV. 'Hiya, you all good? Do you want to watch a DVD later, Steven?'

'Yes, please.' Ryan had become Steven's best friend on the journey and each day he seemed to arrive with a fresh memento of the day for Steven's scrapbook.

'Do you want to bring one of your Star Wars DVDs over?' he said.

'Sure,' Steven said.

Ryan was carrying a plastic plate and a sandwich. 'Can I use your microwave, I was using ours and it's fused the RV.'

'Oh,' I said.

'Don't worry, Michael's having a look at it.'

'Help yourself,' Jane said.

Within a second, Ryan was tapping in the timings into our microwave and as he hit the start button there was a little pop, then a whirr as the air conditioning stopped and then silence.

'That's what happened to ours,' he said. 'There must be a common fault.'

'Yeah, the doylem who's operating it,' I said.

'Whooahh,' Ryan said as he took out his sandwich and sat down opposite Steven.

Outside Michael was looking puzzled. 'Problems as well?' he said.

'Only Ryan.'

Michael laughed.

'Is your generator working?' I asked.

In the second RV all the curtains were drawn, emphasising the light of Cindy's laptop as she reviewed her day's photos. As Michael fired the generator, the RV shuddered into life having blown Ryan's theory. We traced the fault back to the plugs in the toilet block where both sets of sockets had blown.

'Shit,' Michael said and looked across at the sixty-seater coach that doubled as a mobile home parked adjacent to his. 'We've fused their power. Any thoughts?'

'Are they in?'

'I don't think so. Are you thinking what I am?'

As our eyes traced our cables back to their vehicle, it was clear that we had lost them their power as well as ours. Suspecting that discretion was probably called for, we unhooked both RVs and drove them to the other side of the RV park to put some distance between us and the failed power.

We appreciated that they would have lost electricity so any fridge or freezer would begin to defrost but there was little we could do and we didn't need to attract unnecessary animosity.

Day 14 – Wednesday, 12 July
Milford, Ut. to Cedar City, Ut.
55.1 miles – 7 hrs 29 mins
Total covered – 790.0 miles

JANE

We left Route 50 just after Baker and before long entered our third state – Utah. It felt good to tick off our second state, we had covered over 700 miles in just twelve days but cycling without a break for ten days had been tough.

Yesterday, we'd been on the road for eight and a half hours and covered eighty-three and a half miles. Today was a baby in comparison – just fifty-five miles. We'd be finished in time for lunch and be able to rest properly before the big climb up to Cedar Breaks the day after.

The map showed that our route for the next few days would lead southwards before heading eastwards through the Escalante Desert. There was a much more direct route but it wasn't cycle friendly so we were stuck with the extra miles.

The long straight road out of Milford had maize crops on either side. One large climb over the Black Mountains dominated the landscape ahead and the only town between here and Cedar City was Minersville.

It was early, we had only been cycling for half an hour when we stopped by the roadside to admire a group of deer. They looked at us from the shelter of the tall maize. A large doe continued foraging on the field floor then, as if on a signal unheard by us, they lowered their heads and disappeared back from view. I caught sight of white rumps and then they were gone.

The road was silent and few cars passed us. Locals were the only other users of Route 21 but we were glad of the lack of cars and spread out across the road, able for once to chat as we cycled alongside each other.

After ninety minutes, we turned left towards Minersville and into the wind. At the gas station, we paused and sat on the pavement outside, our bikes rested against the wall. My phone rang.

'Hi, we're just setting off from Milford,' Mike said. 'Is there anything you need?'

'No, we're fine. We've just got to Minersville and are having a break before we tackle the climb.'

'You're a bit slow, aren't you?'

'Yes. But it's quite windy. Hopefully it'll be better on the other side of the mountain.'

We finished our drinks and Ryan looked at his watch.

'We'd better get moving,' he said and I gathered up the empty bottles and wrappers and waddled over to the bin. The business part of the day was about to get underway.

We had been climbing steadily all morning but as the gradient got steeper, the two men pulled away from me unhampered by the wind and slope. I plugged away slowly up the incline all the while conscious of the pass that loomed.

I could see cars and lorries slowly travelling up through the man-made Black Mountain Pass. I dug deep to keep my tired legs moving. One two three, one two three. I sucked in more air through gritted teeth.

'How yer doing?' Mike yelled, as the RV pulled alongside from behind.

'Fine . . . thanks,' I panted.

'We'll see you at Cedar City.'

I nodded, unable to speak.

'It's not much further. You'll be finished by one at the latest.'

I nodded again, my face set, my breathing rasping, then he was gone, pulling away and eating up the slope.

I was struggling. As I rounded each corner another blast of wind slowed me more until my legs were shaking. A little further on, I stopped at the roadside to gather myself for another onslaught against the slope.

Martyn had slipped ahead and away from us and I could make out his mic by the road side much further up the slope. Cursing the ease with which he had cycled away from me, I stood panting.

'It can't be much further,' I said.

'No,' said Ryan. 'I'm sure I can see the summit not too far ahead of us.'

Heartened, I set off once again and ground my way to what we assumed was the last climb. But it was a false summit and the road continued up. What had happened to the easy day and early finish I had been counting on?

The climb was slow and so long that it was nearing midday before we reached the summit. I half expected to see Mike watching us at the top, waiting for us, but no such luck. The people in the RVs were looking forward to civilisation and showers and had taken us at our word to carry on.

Deflated, at least we could look forward to the descent into Cedar City.

After resting, I set off down the slope that led off the mountain top, lowering myself to freewheel downhill. But I didn't get very far before I was forced to sit upright and start pedalling.

'Is it an optical illusion?' I asked Ryan. 'Is it one of those bits where the road rises but looks like it's falling.'

'No, I don't think so. It's the wind. It's worse here than it was on the other side.'

We carried on down the mountainside. My speed dropped, dropped, dropped and dropped again till I was moving downhill at 8 mph – barely faster than I had made my way up the damn thing.

'Bollocks, bollocks, bollocks,' I muttered. 'Bloody, bloody wind, bugger off.'

Ryan and Martyn cycled on ahead but I just couldn't do it. I slumped over my handlebars, hot tears of frustration running down my cheeks and pain in my eyes. I had no energy to even climb from the bike and none to give it any momentum. I just stood there watching my companions diminishing as they continued their journey away from me.

Summoning what small amount of spirit I had remaining, I placed my left foot in the cradle and forced myself forward. My speed dropped to 6 mph and it was an effort to keep it even at that pace as the wind blasted me from ahead.

The two guys sat at the roadside waiting for me. As I reached them I climbed from the saddle and dropped to the floor, legs stretched akimbo, head bowed down. Even off the bike, there was no respite from the wind. It blew at us, chilling me, piercing its way through every item of clothing I wore. It eased its way to my back, my ears were chilled by it and it tore at my coat.

'Well, Jane,' Martyn said, pointing the camera at me, 'can you tell me how you feel cycling in this wind.'

'There doesn't seem to be any point in me being here at all today,' I replied through gritted teeth, trying to stop the tears of tiredness from falling down my cheeks.

Up ahead we could see a vast cloud of dust yards and yards high and wide. It looked like a localised whirly.

'Oh no,' I said, screwing up my face. 'We're going to have cycle *through* that.'

'It'll be okay,' said Ryan. 'Come on.'

As we set off again, my speed slowed and slowed as the wind tried to force me back up Black Mountain. Stubbornly, we carried on till I could bear the flurry of sand and grit against me no longer. I pushed my glasses firmly against my face and closed my mouth, breathing only through my nose.

'I need to rest guys but I want to stop out of the wind,' I said.

'The next place we can get to that looks sheltered, we'll have a rest,' Ryan said.

The road had been lonely with no buildings but as we reached Enoch some appeared, although they were still sparse. Directly in front of us, was a modern church.

'Let's rest here,' I said.

'I'm not going inside any church,' Ryan exclaimed.

'No, no,' I said, cycling through the car park to the rear of the church, where blissfully we were sheltered as the wind raced either side of the building. I climbed from my bike, sat on the steps where the wind couldn't reach me and hugged myself, glad to be free of wind's constant pulling of my clothes and my spirit.

We sat and looked at each other.

'This is bloody awful,' I said. 'We've only got six miles to cycle but at this rate we could be another one and a half hours.'

The look Ryan gave me changed as he realised the truth of my statement. I knew that Martyn and Ryan could be finished much sooner but I was not going anywhere fast.

'Look at us, grateful to be outside a church,' Martyn said and we looked at each other and burst out laughing. What a state we must have seemed in to anyone zipping past us in their huge motor vehicles, oblivious to the wind.

'Come on then,' Ryan said, mounting his bike and cycling up through the parking area back to the entrance we'd come through.

At last, we were crossing Interstate 15 and would soon make it to the campsite. Once we reached the roads that led into Cedar City, the buildings provided a little more protection from the wind and our progress quickened.

We reached the campsite in seven and half hours, a pathetic eight miles an hour for the day, and Mike was waiting, holding out a recovery drink to all three of us. I took it eagerly, gulping down the liquid. It tasted better than it had tasted on any other day.

'The guy from the local paper has been waiting for ages,' said Mike, as I was finishing the last dregs in the bottle. 'Can you come and do that interview with him when you've finished that so he can get off, he's had a long day.'

I looked at Mike and felt a deep fury welling inside me. I actually wanted to thump him on the nose but didn't have the energy.

I walked away from him, too angry to actually speak to him. 'Did no one think I might be too tired to do an interview when it started to be obvious how much we were struggling?' I muttered.

I sat on a bench outside the RV watching Martyn pack his kit into Rob's car. I was sleepy, exhausted from the seven and half arduous hours it had taken us to cycle a mere fifty-five miles. It was by far our worst day on the bikes and I wondered how many more days we would have like this.

'Do you know what the local name is for that range of mountains we just passed?' Martyn said, hauling the last of his bags into the back seat.

I shook my head wearily.

'Hurricane Cliffs,' he said.

'That explains an awful lot,' I replied.

Day 15 – Thursday, 13 July
Cedar City, Ut. to Panguitch, Ut.
58.7 miles – 7 hrs 36 mins
Total covered – 848.7 miles
Highest altitude – 10 601 ft

MIKE

By the time we awoke, Michael had already gone with Rob to the airport. Michael was heading back to the UK and would return for the penultimate week. Mentally, it was a signal that the beginning of the trip was over. During the five-week interior leg of the trip, our road crew would shrink further as Rebecca and Jodie would leave in two weeks' time.

The intensity of each day's weather had become less bearable. Unbroken blue skies would welcome each and every day as the temperatures ramped up a couple of degrees. Jane had sweated profusely again overnight, her body so damp that she needed to change her pyjamas; two towels were soaking as if they'd spent the night in a sink.

Respite from the heat, however, was at hand because we were about to climb to over 10 000 feet for the first time and we would finish the day at Panguitch – 1000 foot higher than Cedar City.

Many souvenir T-shirts in Ely had boasted that the nearest Wal-Mart was 285 miles away. That fact was worn as a badge of honour for them but for us there was no more a welcome sight than the giant supermarket that was indeed 285 miles on. We stocked up with essentials – water, bread, ice and fresh produce – and the odd treat such as poundcake before we headed out into the Utah desert and a further ten days of wilderness.

Cedar City centre was beautifully presented, had streets you could eat off, and there was a certain civic pride to the place. Pots of plants stood outside each shop and the abundance of red flowers seemed to have been deliberately designed to contrast with the sunlight beaming on the desert hills, which surrounded the eastern side of the town. There were nice touches such as the old-fashioned iron railroad clock which adorned the main street.

Unfortunately, apart from the centre, the rest of the town seemed to be just one long strip of fast food franchises, gas stations and real estate lots. Hastily built, inconsequential properties with florid design logos, they were the twenty-first century's convenience buildings at their worst. Since we'd passed Sacramento it seemed that very little had been built to last and a lot of the properties were dilapidated.

We didn't hang around too long in the morning as I wanted to join Jane to ease my anxiety as she made the long climb to Cedar Breaks. As we joined Utah 14 it was heavily shrouded with rich vegetation; there were vivid green and yellow flowers. The climb was gradual rather than steep but stretched over eighteen miles. Jane was two thirds up when we pulled over the RV and I peered out of the rear windows awaiting her arrival, laptop perched to my side as I worked on an article.

They were soon upon us and looked in good spirits. Physiologically Jane would, if only for a short time, exceed 10 000 feet and I'd been agitated at the strain this would place on her heart, but the nervous energy was wasted. Jane's heart had suffered damage as a result of taking Herceptin and her heart function test rarely got above 50 per cent. No one could explain why Jane could continue competing when, in most people with those results, climbing stairs may have proved a challenge.

There was, though, a nagging doubt that at some stage it could just go bang.

For two hours we leapfrogged them each mile and travelled on a further four, passing the pudding-basined Dave as he worked hard to get to the top. There was a romantic feel to his journey and it was a total antidote for the gas-guzzling pickups, RVs and four-by-fours the Americans seem to love.

Dave pulled in to stop by the RV and say hello and reluctantly accepted some Gatorade. It seemed almost as if it was selling his soul to accept any assistance.

'How are you doing?' I said.

'Oh fine.' As he removed his helmet his hair seemed to spring into life and he moved his hands through it twice as though locating an itch.

'How far are you hoping to get?' I asked.

'Bryce Canyon, I hope. I want to camp there for a couple of days.'

'Did you get caught in the storm outside Baker?'

'Yes. I had to stop just after I saw you. I only got about twenty miles. I felt a bit vulnerable and didn't sleep too easily. Yesterday was worse with the wind.' He took two strong gulps and half the container had gone. 'How is Jane doing?'

'Okay.'

'Before I met you, everywhere I went people were talking about her. She's sure brave.'

'I know,' I said. Rebecca left her seat in the RV and went to the loo, uncomfortable to share the conversation. She was always reluctant to listen to others praise her mum.

'Is there a reason for you cycling across the USA?' I asked. 'A long held ambition?'

'I guess it's something I've always wanted to do and I figure this is the last chance before I have to grow up. I get married at the end of September and after that, the days of adventure will have to stop.'

'Does your girlfriend mind?'

'No. It's in my system I guess, it's a rite of passage. It's a little selfish but she gets me for the rest of my life.'

I sat and contemplated his thoughts and wondered if it was really possible to sacrifice your desires for another human being. Maybe for a short time, but surely you would lose the essence of the person?

I thought of how, when we knew Jane was going to die, I'd stopped going out or to football and playing golf. It seemed perfectly natural to want to spend as much time as possible with Jane and inevitably there was guilt if we were separated. Slowly, over the years, I'd resumed going to the odd football match here and there and with Steven growing older and joining me it was only natural.

Many people had asked why Jane had continued to do the challenges when her time was so short. Some accused her of being selfish. How could she do it when she could be spending time with her family and friends?

But to me it was obvious. Since her diagnosis, I sensed that Jane needed an element of adventure and freedom in her life. It was her way of defying the disease. But at the same time, adventure and freedom were two things that I felt I'd stifled in her in our early years of marriage. I'd been selfish and so I hoped that by encouraging her in whatever way I could to take part in challenges, it would not only assuage some of my own guilt but help her along her personal journey now.

I looked at Dave, about to enter a new phase of his life, but I doubted the spirit of adventure would vanish so easily.

'Do you want some Gatorade for later?' I asked.

'I'll be fine, thank you.' It was as if by taking our hospitality, he was selling himself short. We watched him prepare to climb back aboard and with an almighty push of his right leg he started to propel the solid metal frame of the bike and panniers uphill.

One advantage, or disadvantage, of being constantly on the move is that you have little time to reflect on where you've been or where you're going. Short of knowing we were passing Cedar Breaks National Monument and finishing in Panguitch, the day was a mystery.

In the recesses of my mind I'd imagined a barren mountain

top but upon getting to 10 000 feet the vegetation was as lush as anything we'd seen since leaving the West Coast.

From the turning off the Utah 14 on to the 143 it was only a short way to the National Monument and we pulled in, closely followed by Rob. For the last two weeks, Rob had been the cyclists' best friend, unconstrained by the immobility of the RVs, he'd always been the quickest to react when food and especially drink were running short.

He would advise Jane, Ryan and Martyn of distances, hazards and road conditions. In short, he was becoming the most valuable addition to the team.

Pulling alongside, his elbow rested on the open window.

'I'll nip back, Mike. But this place is bloody magnificent. I've just had a view from the road further north. I've never seen anything like it.'

I parked across three car park spaces conscious that I didn't want to be blocked in, and looked over at Steven.

'Come on, Steven,' I said, 'let's go and have a look at the view.' He shut the lid of his Nintendo DS and got up.

'Can I take the camera?' he said, referring to the camcorder.

'If you like. Becca?'

'What?' she said not lifting her head from her book.

'Are you coming?' Jodie had already placed her book down and was putting on her flip-flops.

'No.'

I shook my head, but didn't see the point in arguing. A small wooden kiosk marked the entrance to the National Monument; the car park pavements and amenities were beautifully cared for.

It was a small inauspicious walk to where the view opened up to what can only be described as the most beautiful sight I'd ever seen. My mouth was agape as the view disappeared over tens of miles in front of us and I let out a sigh.

'Wow,' Jodie said, 'incredible.'

We walked slowly to the wall protecting the sheer drop behind it and realised that the initial view had been only a prologue to the stunning multicoloured limestone formations that dropped away several thousand feet in front of us. The sun beat down, casting shadows which increased the intensity of the coloured strata, ranging from violent orange through all the reds to white. The drop fell to 2000 feet below with formations of rocks in various stages of erosion.

Steven looked out over the wall.

'Dad, Dad, Dad, look at this. I need to film this. It's so wonderful, look at the colours.'

Jane arrived moments later. She looked at me and muttered 'Wow.' We stood together, looking out across the Utah plains, and despite all the efforts of getting to America and the pain that Jane had been through during the year's planning for the ride, it was worth it for this single moment.

'Is this the most incredible sight?' I said.

'Unbelievable. I never imagined we'd see anything like this. It's a shame Michael's gone home today.' Jane moved closer to the edge, her eyes scanning the whole vista. Martyn went and collected his high resolution camera and took some photos of Jane and me specifically for our personal benefit and then one of Jane with her bike at her side.

Within thirty minutes we were back on the road, caught in a temporary traffic jam of roadworks. The road dropped off away from Cedar Breaks, passing Panguitch Lake, a vast expanse of water surrounded by luxury homes.

The road to Panguitch dropped down in a gradual descent over a number of miles. It provided a welcome respite for Jane and despite being tired when she pulled in she wasn't as desperately weary as she had been yesterday.

Each day I'd scribbled a few notes down on a website blog for the appeal; my incoherent ramblings were rattled off quickly and I never actually considered that they might actually be read by anyone.

Yesterday I'd had a bit of an unthinking rant after watching Jane arriving totally exhausted at Cedar City and only raising £30 through online donations on the day. I'd said the ride was futile, that we weren't raising much money and that I wondered why she was doing it at all.

I'd looked at the comparison between how much had been

raised on the 'Rome to Home' and we were failing badly. The easiest way to remedy this would have been to do more media but Jane's health was declining and we needed to protect her. The article she'd done yesterday was for the front page of today's local paper and the US media were clearly keen to cover the ride but we simply hadn't the resources to cater for the demand. Since the *Today* show, we'd received a number of requests but had answered none. It was a case of catch 22 – the ride was too demanding, so media were being turned away, so the whole point of us being in the USA was being negated.

Upon arriving in Panguitch we noticed that there had been a number of calls to the satellite phone and there was one message from my work saying that various members of the UK press had been phoning all day as they couldn't contact us directly. The press had read into it that Jane might give up and wanted to find out why.

I immediately thought of Suzanne back home and the effect that this news might have on her. I decided to call her.

'Hello,' Suzanne said at the other end of the line and I felt an immediate need to be home.

'It's me.'

'Hiya.' There was a slight delay on the phone but she sounded as though she'd just woken up from a deep sleep.

'Are you in bed?'

'Yes. I'm worn out. I'm on earlies at work and so I've been up since half past five. It's half past eleven in England.'

'Oh, I'm really sorry, Suzanne. I'll phone back tomorrow.'

'Don't worry, I'd rather speak to you now. Are you okay, is Mum okay?'

'More importantly, Suzanne, are you okay?'

'I'm fine. It's been very warm in England, my stomach's getting bigger by the day, I feel very uncomfortable but I've only got a few weeks left at work.' Suzanne was due to go on maternity leave in three weeks. We weighed up the option of whether to come to America once we knew that she was pregnant but fortunately she was due four weeks after the ride was scheduled to finish.

'How's Mum?'

'She's had a good day today.' I carefully repositioned the satellite as the signal began to fade.

'It said on the telly she was fed up and tired.'

'No, she's fine. We're not raising much money so it seems pointless being here. Yesterday was a bad day but she's not too bad, you know how Mum is.'

'I thought if Mum was bad you'd give me a ring.'

'Were you worried?'

'No. I knew you'd ring if you needed to.'

'If Mum gets ill or anything we'll ring before the media say anything. You know Martyn and Rob from Sky are really good. They'd not report anything until everyone knew at home, so don't worry.'

The conversation petered out as the signal broke up, leaving me with an unbearable yearning to hold my daughter.

JANE

After the horrendous experience cycling into Cedar City, I was reluctant to even think about getting back on the bike the following day.

Arriving at Panguitch was a relief but although I was tired, I had enjoyed the cycling. Following the disastrous day before it felt good to have a rewarding day's ride.

Panguitch was a small town with an RV park within walking distance. I showered and ate a small cheese sandwich and walked down the long main street with Mike and Steven. We passed a supermarket on the left and came to the main road junction. Tomorrow we would head off right at this junction out towards Red Canyon but first there was a town to explore.

We passed a Wild West store and I wandered in with Steven. There was a tableau with a scary looking model cowboy hanging over a bed, his face slumped on one side. His clothes were shabby and moth-eaten and a cowboy hat rested precariously on his head.

From behind the counter, a rotund man with florid red cheeks above the most enormous beard and moustache greeted us.

'Howdee folks, take a look around,' he said, checking that his black hat was still firmly on his head before gesturing with his large hands for us to explore.

We looked through his collection of musty old clothes and hats and his ropes coiled into lassoes. Pictures of a long ago Wild West hung from the walls. There was nothing here we wanted to buy.

A brighter, more modern store beckoned on the other side of the street, its main attraction being the café. We sat in the café while Mike waited for the counter people to figure out how to make the fruit smoothie he'd ordered. I sipped at a coffee and took a slug out of Steven's Coke.

'Oi, get your hands off,' he said.

'Yes, siree,' I smiled and left my coffee to cool and wandered into the store. They had a selection of cowboy hats piled up on shelves. Some were ridiculously priced at $140 to $160 but others were more affordable. I wanted to buy a hat for Rob who, in a few days, would be leaving us for a while until the end of the trip. I wanted to mark his experience and thank him for the help and support on the road.

A hat would keep the heat of the day off his face and neck as he was reddening more and more as the trip went on. I selected one and tried it on. It was a little on the large side but about right for Rob's red bonce. I returned to the café.

'There's a hat in there that would be perfect for Rob,' I said to Mike.

'We'll look later,' he said, reluctant as ever to part with his money. When he'd finished his drink, I nudged him to come inside and take a look.

'Yeah, you're right, it's perfect,' he conceded. 'Are you paying, Steven?'

'No!' said Steven, wide-eyed.

'Don't worry. We'll find you a hat if that's what you want, we've got loads of time to get something for you.'

He grinned back at me, good humoured as ever.

'Okay, Mum,' he said, putting his hot hand into mine as we waited for Mike to pay for the hat.

Day 16 – Friday, 14 July
Panguitch, Ut. to Escalante, Ut.
81.9 miles – 8 hrs 07 mins
Total covered – 930.6 miles

JANE

Next day, we were up early again. With a long hot eighty-two miles to cover we needed to get as many miles as possible out of the way before the sun became too fierce. We were heading towards Escalante, which, looking at the map, meant heading southwards and then east.

We met Martyn in town and cycled onwards along the most major road we had seen for a couple of days. It soon headed southwards where we took the eastward turn through the outskirts of Panguitch. The scenery suddenly changed and we found ourselves cycling beneath a stretch of red rocks that overhung the road like an enormous natural gateway. The day was still early and the new sunlight made the rocks glow deep oxide red, a vibrancy that we might have missed had we arrived later in the day.

We headed away from the narrow road through the canyon. The steep meandering road had no hard shoulders and it was unsafe for three cyclists. Instead, we swooped along the red canyon bike trail, sometimes riding side by side, sometimes one of us stretching ahead to admire the views.

Clattering over a small wooden bridge, the three of us dodged overhanging branches as we lost sight of the road and felt the closeness of the wooded area. The problem with wooded trails became apparent after only a few miles. Leafy debris, hidden thorns and other nasties can all snare their way through a tyre and, sure enough, Ryan soon pulled up with a puncture.

I sat on the rocks and watched as he mended his bike,

expertly removing the rubber wheel and carefully feeling the inner tube to check for any offending sharp particles. It is always well worth checking that there is nothing more in the tyre as it's annoying to repair a flat, only to have it reoccur within minutes.

I could hear voices quietly passing comment just above the hum of the wheels of the tarmac. Two lads swooped past us, bare-backed, their T-shirts tucked away in the top of their black panniers.

'Aren't those the guys we saw a few days back?' I called.

In fact, they were the two lads we had encountered on the second day – the ones who had been less than chatty as they overtook us just outside San Francisco. I couldn't believe we were tracking them so closely. They whizzed by with the merest wave of their hands, mumbled a greeting and then disappeared around a bend.

With a spin of the front wheel, Ryan was once more sitting astride his bike ready to set off. We coasted down a small hill before climbing briefly away from the road and back into the shelter of the more wooded area.

After another mile and still before 8 a.m., we were back on the road travelling up along a slow hill towards Bryce Canyon National Park, named after Ebenezer Bryce who had set up business in the area in the 1870s.

We stopped at the entrance to the canyon where spectacular pink and white rocks stretched out before us. I longed to have a little more time, to be able to explore among the huge fins of jagged rock. But we had so many miles to go. Reluctantly, I set off down the slope and away from this huge natural tourist attraction, which I would probably never see again, and towards the small town of Topic.

Ryan sped past me only to come to a sliding halt a few yards ahead. I could hear him cursing and watched him upend his bike once more. No matter how carefully you check a tyre, you can't put enough pressure on it. There must have been a small thorn lodged in the inner tube which had caused another puncture.

'At least it didn't go further down the hill,' I said, as I sat on the roadside beside him. 'You could've come off at thirty miles an hour and really done yourself some damage.'

Ryan grunted and turned back to his bike, wiping the sweat from his eyes and pushing his sunglasses higher up his head.

'I'm a bit worried now,' he said. 'We have plenty of tubes but we're getting through them and I'll need to get some more.'

'Oops,' I said, knowing full well that for the next few days we were in desert country, where there would be very little in the way of civilisation, let alone bike shops. In fact, the only reason we would be cycling higher mileages for the next few days was that there were so few places to stop.

We met up with Cindy at Cannonville, which at the thirty-seven-mile mark wasn't even halfway, and we were glad to see her. It was only the second day without the company of Michael and it would take some adjustment for her to be travelling alone. As she pulled alongside us, Ryan grimaced once more. Yet another puncture.

'I'm glad that happened now,' he said. 'I'm going to change the tyre. I can't feel or see anything but it must be in there somewhere, the little bugger.'

I sat in the cool of the van, relieved to be out of the heat, even for a short while. Cindy pulled out a glass bottle of sweet brown coffee from the fridge. It was enough to lift me. She pushed a tall pack of pastries towards me.

'Sorry,' she said. 'I haven't had time to get to the shops. I've been trying to book accommodation and there's none around here.'

I shrugged my shoulders, aware by now that to pursue a point with Cindy would mean her hackles rising and it was a waste of time. She would argue that none of it was her fault and I couldn't be bothered to express my true feelings.

'Perhaps they might have something at the next stop,' I suggested. 'Or maybe the store back there.' I pointed to a sign which advertised a general market just two miles down the road.

'Nah,' Cindy said, waving her hand at me. 'I'm not driving back there, we'll be fine.'

I raised the bottle to my lips, unwilling to make any further suggestions to the woman who was providing such vital support to Ryan and me.

'Gosh, do you know I've been sat here thinking how beautiful. Thank you, Jane, it's amazing.'

'Yeah, I can't believe the scenery. It's shining. Did you see Red Canyon?' I said.

'See it? I nearly got stuck in the arch across the road. Boy, that was a tight one.'

Ryan's studded shoes clattered on the steps of the RV and he appeared carrying the box of tools and spares. 'Where can I put this?' he said.

'Oh, just throw it in the shower with the rest of the rubbish,' said Cindy.

Ryan slid back the shower door. 'There's not much room here,' he said, bending down to pick up the full litter bag. 'Is there a bin out there for this? It stinks.'

Cindy snatched it from him. 'Yeah, fine. I think that's one across the parking lot.' Her flip-flops clapped against the steps as she tossed her head and flounced out of the RV with the offending bag.

'Oops, she likes you,' I said, smiling at Ryan.

'She's a bit difficult,' Ryan said, rubbing his forehead. 'I've been dreading Michael going. But the earphones and laptop work so I just wear those and she doesn't bother talking to me. I don't even have to have the music on,' he said, breaking into a smile.

I winced and then smiled. 'Yeah, the voice can get to you,' I said. Cindy was not only vocal but a little loud as well.

'I'm hoping no more punctures.' Ryan held up his hand, fingers crossed. 'Otherwise we really are in trouble. I'll have to start patching up tubes.'

Martyn had been stalking around the parking lot and opened the door just ahead of Cindy. 'Are we nearly ready for the off or do you need a few more minutes?' he asked.

'No,' I said. 'Just have to have a pee and then I'm ready.'

The next few miles were relatively flat. It was only after

Henrieville that the road started to rise more steeply towards Powell Point. The scenery was still breathtaking – table-topped mesas with orange, silver and red strata.

We climbed to nearly 8000 feet and then the road dipped gradually, small rises and falls but more falls than rises, as we headed for Escalante.

We had done sixty-seven miles and I longed to finish in this quaint small town. But the plan was to head towards the Escalante River about fourteen miles further, because tomorrow was already a very difficult ninety-six mile journey to bridge the gap to Hanksville. The major problem was that there was no stop between Hanksville and Blanding, which were 125 miles apart, so our days were elongated anyway and it was important not to make one day completely impossible.

A small but cruel climb led us out of the town and past a very new-looking school with immaculate green playing fields.

'Look, Jane!' Martyn called, as we slowly made our way up the hillside.

'What?' I panted. The sun was beating down on our heads and the heat waves from the hot tarmac assailed us from below. I lifted my head from its wearyingly heavy position down towards the handlebars.

'An airport! Out here!' he said. 'We could sneak on a plane, get all the way back to California and be back home by tomorrow night.'

'You say that jokingly but you're messing with my head now,' I replied. 'I could go home right now, this is too much like hard work.'

Just then, the familiar SUV passed us and Rob's red face hung out of the car. 'You wanna see the view at the top of those climbs, folks,' he called. 'Talk about stunning.'

We carried on wearily, sipping more often from our water bottles as the heat took its toll. Before we knew it though, we were at the top of the head of rocks.

Martyn swung his bike from the road where Rob had set up a static camera for him to take images of the scene before us. The road slowly circled a mass of rocks, revealing a world of red and orange stretching out and down away into the distance. I carried on cycling, taking in the magnificent peaks and the deep narrow gulleys around us. The road dropped down, down and down and we swooped through the desert air which felt cool against our cheeks. It took concentration to position the bike before the next bend, first right and then left. Out of the corner of my eye I spotted a sign with a lone cow on it. I pumped on my brakes, gently on, off, on, off, slowing my bike by degrees.

Ryan was behind me. I pointed at the iron cattle grid across the road that could snatch the wheel from under you and at 45 mph cause serious injury. I clattered over it and scarcely had time to turn and check Ryan was safely over before the next corner appeared, a tight left-hand bend that took me round sharply towards another bend. This roller coaster was just the sort of cycling I loathed, the energy put in to climb to the top of one slope was not enough to carry you over to the peak of the next.

We passed some weary cyclists creeping up the slope in the opposite direction.

'Don't envy them the climb ahead,' I said to Ryan. 'It could take them ages. They already look exhausted.'

'Yeah,' nodded Ryan. 'I sure am glad we came down it rather than up. Wasn't that awesome though?'

'I've never seen anything like it,' I said.

We'd reached the bottom of the hill and were in the valley through which ran the Escalante River. We could hear the water nearby which was absorbing the still heat that we'd usually felt in such valleys.

'Boy oh boy. What a sight,' exclaimed Cindy from the roadside as we pulled over. Cindy had made sure she was at the agreed finish waiting for us.

'Let's get the bikes inside the van and see if this thing will go back up that hill, hey guys,' she said. 'Escalante looks a real pretty spot. There's a nice café there as well.'

'I think I might try that out,' I said. 'I can't face tinned soup and stale bread again,' I added under my breath.

Ryan nodded, 'I know what you mean.'

The RV groaned until it found a gear low enough for it to grind its way slowly up the slope we had just made our way down, as our accommodation was in Escalante the last town we'd past fourteen miles previously.

'Watch out for the . . .' I shouted. 'Cyclists,' I finished meekly as we squeezed past one of the group making their way up the pass.

'I was miles away, see?' Cindy said, forgetting how much the wing mirrors stick out, unable to tell how close we were to the cyclist's head. I closed my eyes not wishing to see any more of the journey.

Opening them warily as we reached the outskirts of Escalante, Mike was already there, waiting for us. It had been a long day and it was always a joy to see Mike and receive the familiar hug.

'You've got to see the view down towards Escalante River,' I said. 'I bet first thing tomorrow it's awesome with the sun.'

'I can't wait but first let's get you something to eat. There's a smart café just down the road,' he said.

'So I've just heard. Let's go,' I said.

Day 17 – Saturday, 15 July
Esacalante River, Ut. to Hanksville, Ut.
96.1 miles – 10 hrs 13 mins
Total covered – 1026.7 miles

MIKE

The sickening sound of metal crunching against rock could be heard distinctly above the water flowing in the Escalante River. At five thirty on Saturday morning the small valley car park was as cool as any place we'd been in since arriving in the USA. Although the sun was rising, the tall rocks all around were providing plenty of shade to this little enclave. It was a small oasis of vegetation, fertilised by the locality of the stream in contrast to the barren landscape which dominated all around.

Cindy climbed out of the RV, her face white contemplating

the damage to the side of her vehicle. Rob was Indiana Jones-like moving away the foliage which had disguised a large boulder.

'Oh no, that means we'll lose our deposit,' Cindy said.

'It's why we paid the supplementary premium,' I said. 'It was inevitable on a trip like this we'd suffer some damage. I'd have put odds on it happening to me first.'

Rob looked down at the RV. There was a large dint on the back. 'It's driveable,' he said. 'Just cosmetic, it could have been worse.

We'd have lost the deposit anyway as they'd have charged us for the damage already done.'

Since picking it up, Cindy's RV had systematically started to fall apart. Cupboard doors had come off their hinges, door handles flopped as screws had come out, the toilet door was permanently kept open by a piece of elasticised rope tied to the shower opposite as it would have continually banged shut while driving. Outside there wasn't one lock that worked. The water hose had more leaks than the government.

Jane, Martyn and Ryan made final preparations for the bikes, attaching water bottles, checking tyre pressures, before Jane wandered off with Martyn to film their daily blog.

In typical grandiose fashion, Highway 12 from Panguitch to Torrey some thirty miles west of today's destination was labelled the 'all American road or the National Scenic Byway'. There's no explanation for what an all American road is but the pompous sounding nationalistic title didn't quite seem to fit the tranquil surroundings.

'You'll never get a thirty-foot rig over that road,' a fellow bus passenger had said yesterday and I had immediately wondered whether his judgement of width was affected by his own girth, as he shuffled his expansive backside across two seats. Even so, it had triggered me into asking total strangers, 'Will my thirty-foot RV navigate Highway 12?'

It was like an uncontrollable tick. And despite the general consensus that a thirty-foot rig would be all right but if I was driving 'a big rig' it wouldn't, I couldn't stop asking.

When Jane had been planning the trans-America bike ride

routes, the description of the 'Hog's Back' as a three-mile stretch of narrow road along a ridge spine with no shoulders or guardrails before Boulder had excited Jane and terrified me. The guidebook had advised cyclists to ride carefully and defensively so I'd envisaged the motoring equivalent of Striding Edge. For months I'd had nightmares of meeting an oncoming vehicle, politely moving to one side before tumbling down 2000-foot cliffs and becoming engulfed in a ball of flames James Bond-style at the bottom.

After an incredible two days travelling through Cedar Breaks, Red Canyon and Bryce Canyon we could have been blasé about the road quality on Highway 12. The cyclists had ridden a few extra miles from town to the river the previous evening to clip some miles from today's marathon stage. As always with Jane, I knew there was a cocktail of motives for this decision. She wanted to ensure that I treated the road with respect. She also wanted to see me shitting myself at the thought of sheer drops down the cliff. Her incredible dry humour was difficult for me to fathom sometimes – even for me, who has over twenty years' experience.

At a café last night, the owner had said it was impossible for Jane to reach Hanksville in a day and he didn't even know about her illness. As if Jane needed motivation.

I considered turning round and retracing my steps to Cedar City, joining the interstate system and seeing the riders a couple of days later. But I had some solace knowing that Cindy had driven the road already to Escalante and quite frankly, if she could manage it, it should be a piece of piss.

Jane, like the morning in San Francisco, was alive and physically buzzing, relishing the impossible challenge. It was as if the two days of back ache from Cedar City had been banished with the merest whiff of a positive attitude.

The early morning sun cast its shadow on the rocks, playing tricks on the coloured strata. Since leaving Cedar City, we had climbed on to the Aquarian Plateau, the highest in North America, which was the summit of the grand staircase of different coloured strata.

The drive from Escalante to Boulder was astonishing. It was a beautiful Saturday morning, peaceful and barely another vehicle on the road.

The Hog's Back was a major disappointment in terms of risk and was no challenge even to our cumbersome RV. Indeed, there are much scarier journeys to be had in the Dales, though I have to admit the unencumbered views both to the left and right were stupendous. It was one of the many times I'd been envious of the cyclists – seeing the vista from outside on a bike would have been wonderful.

We dropped off the top of the Hog's Back and down the road to Boulder, a town of less than two hundred people. There, we planned to refuel the vehicles and find some fresh food.

Cindy was still rattled by her early morning adjustment to her RV's trim. But she still managed to throw the vehicle around the forecourt of the gas station in Boulder like a test driver on a skid pad.

A few minutes later, having failed to find a single shop, café or any establishment even to buy a bag of peanuts, we headed off to the edge of the village and parked at the top of a slight climb with a great view of the long stretch of road behind us. Steven held his camcorder out in front of him, filming the view. His baseball cap was protecting him from the sun and the temperature was rising to a level which I knew would soon become uncomfortable.

In the distance, I spotted Martyn and Ryan approaching like two sprinters at the end of a road race, heads down, bikes being thrown from side to side, oblivious to their surroundings.

'Yes!' shouted Martyn triumphantly, as he sped past us. There was barely a wheel's width between them. Ryan looked peeved.

'My foot slipped on the pedal,' he said, but that wasn't going to stop Martyn gloating. He had the smile of a boy who'd just defeated the school champion. Jane, still 200 yards away, chugged up the road. All three of them looked physically drained.

'Thanks for waiting, you two!' Jane said jokingly, as she pulled up and dismounted. Beads of perspiration glistened on her forehead and as soon as she swept them away with her fingerless gloved hands, new ones appeared.

At that moment, a bare-chested middle-aged jogger ran past us on the opposite side of the road. He was solidly built and clearly in some pain as he pounded the road. It was such an unusual sight that we all turned in unison to watch him.

'Madness,' Rebecca said. 'In this heat.'

'Said the idiots cycling across America,' said Jane.

As we stood in the shade of the high-sided RV, the day was getting hotter by the minute. It was almost as if the man upstairs was adjusting the central heating thermometer.

'Phew, put the air conditioning on, Dad,' Steven implored, as we resumed our seats to move on and leapfrog the cyclists. With the turn of the ignition, cold air blasted out on our faces. I scrabbled for the iPod to turn on the music, but it was hot to the touch.

'Ouch,' I said, fanning my fingers. Letting it cool, I picked it up again five minutes later to find it had frozen on one particular song: 'Keep on Running' by The Journey. It couldn't have been more apt.

We set off again, leaving the cyclists behind and it wasn't long before we started to climb Boulder Mountain, which at over 9000 feet would be the highest climb until the Rockies. As we rose steadily, the riders benefited from a drop in temperature. At various points up the road were beautifully laid out observation areas which afforded the most dramatic of views of the Nagava, Fifty Mile and Henry mountain ranges. The guidebooks said that on clear days you could see up to a hundred miles away and looking out at it, I couldn't argue with that.

Today the conditions couldn't have been better, no heat haze, a cloudless sky and more importantly, views to share with no one. We stopped at each rest area and soaked up some of the finest panoramas America has to offer. Incredibly, this thirty-mile stretch of road known as Boulder Mountain Highway was paved only in 1983.

Rebecca was singularly unimpressed.

'Why are we stopping again?' she asked when we pulled up for the fourth time. 'It all looks the same.' I didn't bother to answer. Jodie, Steven and I were more than happy taking in the inspiring views.

A Jeep pulled in and two middle-aged couples got out.

'How do?' said a small silver-haired man in a broad Yorkshire accent.

'All right,' I said.

He looked surprised. 'Bloody hell, no guessing where you're from,' he said. 'Eh Elsie, there's some Yorkshire folk 'ere.' He moved forward and shook my hand. 'Alan.'

'Mike,' I said. 'That's Steven, my daughter Rebecca is in the RV, Jodie here is my daughter's friend.'

'Hello,' Jodie said.

'That's a strong Barnsley accent,' Alan said. 'Are you on holiday?'

'No, we're supporting a charity bike ride. The cyclists should be here shortly. Are you on your holidays?'

He shook his head as his wife and the other couple came round from the other side of the car to greet us.

'No. We moved out here from Huddersfield three years ago. This is Kath and Steve, an American couple who are giving us a guided tour of the area. It's beautiful, isn't it? We're heading towards Lake Powell. Have you come far today?'

'We set off from Escalante and we're heading to Hanksville.'

'Elsie, did you hear that?' he said. She nodded. 'That's an incredible distance in this heat and these hills, you must be very fit.'

'I'm not, hence the RV, but the cyclists are. Is it always this hot?'

'No. But there's a heat wave. The weather forecasters are saying this could be the hottest summer on record. There's folks dying in California. It's intense at the moment, even for the desert. It's probably twenty degrees higher than normal. Your cyclists need to be careful.'

'Thanks for the advice,' I nodded. 'Clouds have never looked so good, eh?'

Alan studied me and then looked at my T-shirt with the charity logo. 'Jane's Ride Across America,' he said. 'That wouldn't happen to be the Jane I'm thinking of – is it Jane Tomlinson?'

'Yes.'

'Bloody hell, Elsie, Jane Tomlinson's coming, would you believe it? What an honour! Jane Tomlinson, here!' I felt a surge of pride rise in me as the other couple gathered round. He thrust a $50 note in my hand. It was the first donation we'd received on the road – a marked contrast to when Jane had cycled across Italy and France where, despite the language barrier, money had been donated daily.

Within minutes, Jane arrived with Martyn, another Huddersfield boy.

As we stood there chatting, a small part of America was claimed as Yorkshire. A fleeting sense of homesickness overwhelmed us all and we were all quiet when we set off again twenty minutes later. Suddenly home seemed such a long way away.

There was now a fifteen-mile descent into Torrey which, like most communities in this part of the world, was built at a road junction and had the obligatory filling station just on the corner. There was also a small motel, a little coffee shop and a Subway sandwich place.

Somehow, it seemed sacrilege seeing the lurid green sign of a fast food chain outlet in the middle of one of the most beautiful and lonely places on the continent. Nevertheless, desperate for carbohydrate and energy, Jane needed a mega Subway sandwich and so we settled for this and a latte at the coffee shop. Jane looked drained as she bit into her sandwich, but not half as knackered as Ben and Amos, the two American cyclists they'd met on the way and who had also stopped to refuel.

'How are you both?' Jane asked.

'Okay,' said Ben

'Tired,' said Amos.

Both men looked flushed from their exertion on the bikes. Their cycling tops covered bodies that hardened athletes would have been jealous of.

'That was a tough descent with the wind against us. Are you still aiming to get to Hanksville?' asked Ben.

Jane nodded, finishing her mouthful. 'I'm going to try,' she said and my shoulders slumped slightly. 'Though Mike thinks we should stop here. But we'll never get across to Blanding in two days.'

Steven sauntered over. 'Mum, how far have you got left to go?'

'About thirty miles.'

'Thirty miles!' Steven screeched.

Jane looked wrecked and I was concerned that pushing on for the last thirty miles would be too much, but she'd got it into her head that unless she did she'd never breach the gap to Blanding in two days.

As we left, Ben and Amos wearily nodded their heads towards Jane as if they were trying not to waste any surplus energy. Outside, the furnace had continued to be stoked and even the sweltering walk back to the RV made Steven and I puff out our cheeks. I couldn't believe Jane, Ryan and Martyn were going to cycle another thirty miles in this stifling weather.

Within minutes we were passing through Capitol Reef. It was as if one stupendous piece of scenery had to outdo the last. Still the ability to take your breath away remained undiminished.

Within minutes the landscape had changed dramatically, the colour and texture of the road resembling the surface of the moon. It was as if a huge bomb had exploded flattening the mountains, breaking the landscape. If Neil Armstrong's moon adventure really had been a hoax, this was surely where it was filmed.

It was approaching 5 p.m. when Jane arrived in Hanksville, ten hours and ninety-six miles after departing Escalante. Jane looked excellent upon dismounting the bike, tired but amazing considering today's physical feat and that she'd just past the 1000-mile mark. It was incredible, the fear of San Francisco was banished and the challenge was well and truly on.

They had been cycling in temperatures well above a hundred degrees up big climbs and at altitudes never less than 5000 feet.

It had been Jane's decision to push on and complete the

objective and seeing her I had to reluctantly agree that she'd been vindicated.

'Bloody hell, Jane, I can't believe you've managed to get here. We're knackered from driving. Are you all right?'

'No,' she said, getting off the bike.

'Is your back sore?'

'Back, pelvis, shoulder, ribs, stomach – do you want me to go on?'

'Is there anything I can do?'

'You can bloody well shut up.'

I gave it a try for fifteen seconds. 'Did you do too much today? Wouldn't it have been better to stop at Torrey?'

'No. It's a huge distance to Blanding and we'll have to do it over two days.'

Day 18 – Sunday, 16 July
Hanksville, Ut. to White Canyon, Ut.
55.6 miles – 6 hrs 44 mins
Total covered – 1082.3 miles

JANE

The Colorado River is a fast moving body of water which slices its way through the Colorado Plateau. Over a period of six million years it has created the world famous Grand Canyon.

Unfortunately, we would not be visiting the wonders of the Grand Canyon as we were a couple of hundred miles north and instead were to follow Route 95, 'The Trail of the Ancients', all the way from Hanksville to Blanding.

We rose early and from the RV park watched the dawn sky fill with hundreds of bats moving in black clouds to the caves that surrounded the town. They would be resting for the day until dusk when they would once again swoop and float through the night sky.

The two American cyclists, Ben and Amos, were still asleep in their tiny single tents, their bottles and plates from the night before lying in front of their zipped doors. Ryan was busy putting lubricant on the chains as I stumbled over to him, my back still stiff from another poor night's sleep. I sloped across, my feet half in and half out of my cycling shoes because I was unable to bend to tug them on any further. My pain relief, Coproximol, needed a little more time to kick in and ease the little hammerings along my spine and the shocking jets of pain down my leg. Most of the sensation in my left foot was lost.

'It was a long day yesterday,' I grumbled, as I hauled myself up the steps to Ryan's RV.

'Could be another one today,' Ryan replied. 'How many miles is it?'

'About seventy,' I said, sitting down on the steps and tugging on my shoes. 'But I'm not sure we'll get that far. It depends on the heat.'

Ryan stood up, wiping his blackened, oily hands with a cloth. 'Well, see how we get on. We should get on the road before it gets too hot.'

I nodded and entered the RV where Cindy was pottering about with a kettle.

'Drink?' she asked breezily, as I gently lowered myself onto a small bench.

'Yes . . . please,' I said, noticing the small array of stale pastries on the worktop. 'Is there any toast?' I asked.

'Sure is, do you want me to do you some?' Cindy asked.

'Yes, please, that would be very kind.'

She reached over and took four slices of bread from a bag and placed two of them in the toaster. I watched as she busied herself with jars of jam and a tub of butter.

'You're going through some real rough stuff today,' Cindy said.

'Yeah, it looks a bit lonely,' I replied. I held my head above the table, my elbows taking the full weight. 'Do you know what I really want to do today?' I asked.

Cindy turned to look at me. 'No, go on tell me.'

'I want to dangle my aching feet in the cool waters of the Colorado River,' I said.

'Okay,' said Cindy. 'Do we cross that today?'

I nodded, focusing my attention on spreading the smallest amount of butter on my toast as possible.

'Yeah, it's right after the Dirty Devil River,' I said. I had the map out in front of me on the table and traced my finger over the names of the valleys and rises we would be cycling through. It looked ominous. Dry Valley was followed by Skulled Knoll, Little Egypt, Poison Spring Canyon and Hell Hole Swale. It was going to be a hot and intimidating landscape.

I straightened my back all the way through the spine, feeling the pull and the stretch of the muscles. The pain seemed to be easing, so I forced my hands down towards the uppers of my shoes and tied the laces. I took a glass of water and began to swallow the vast number of tablets I needed to see me through the day.

'I'll just fill the water bottles,' I said, gulping down the last tablet.

'Already done,' Cindy said.

I was impressed. 'Thank you,' I said, easing myself up from the bench.

'Oh, it wasn't me. Ryan's been up for ages. I think he's missing his girlfriend.'

I walked out of the RV, taking the map with me. The profile of today's ride looked less testing than the day before and I was ready to be on my way. There were no huge steep climbs but there were long slow steady ascents with small drops between them. Just the sort of cycling that wears out the legs.

The road rose gradually over the first seventeen miles but it was clear that today's primary challenge would be the heat. Before eight o'clock the temperature had risen to above 100 degrees and the open desert landscape provided no respite.

Once over the high point near Lone Cedar Reservoir the road started to fall in altitude, dropping towards Lake Powell over a twenty-mile stretch. All the while as the morning progressed, so the temperature continued to rise. We cycled in ten-mile stretches at the end of which we needed to replace the fluids. I filled one of the bottles full of ice as opposed to water but after only ten minutes it was a tepid warm mess. As we cycled towards the lake the heat was becoming a real issue; radiating off the rocks, it was like being placed in a very big oven.

I was grateful that we'd eaten and rested well the night before. We knew that the 130-mile stretch between Hanksville and Blanding had no services and that at some point we'd have to stop and travel on to Blanding before returning again the next morning.

I picked up speed, freewheeling down towards the lake, slowly watching the bike speed up to 20, 30 then 35 mph. Without warning I approached a bend and noticed gravel all over the road. My heart stopped as I felt sure that I would lose the bike in a high speed crash. I feathered the brakes but couldn't exert any pressure, only managing to stop increasing velocity. I whispered a prayer, loosened my grip on the handlebars and prepared for a tumble.

I arched the bike, the front wheel slipped but not enough to throw me, and I turned the corner and faced the most wonderful sight of Hite Bridge framed by the red rocks of Glen Canyon National Recreation Area. There was a lay-by at the bottom where Mike's RV was parked. Steven and Mike stood outside capturing the moment. I freewheeled down, enjoying both the spectacular view and the knowledge that I was still in the saddle.

I dismounted. The heat in the valley bottom was like a furnace.

'How are you?' Mike asked.

'Hot and bothered.'

'At least you're used to hot flushes, it's a new experience for some of us.'

I smiled at him before screwing up my nose. I took the top off the water bottle and emptied out the dregs of water where they hit the tarmac and evaporated immediately. Within seconds there was no trace that there'd been any fluid on the surface.

Within five minutes of standing in the RV's shade the temperature had become completely unbearable.

'We'll head off,' I said, sweat dripping from my forehead while I wrung the buff out. 'Will you meet us in ten miles? We can't manage further than that without replenishing the water.'

'Can you give us a couple of minutes to take some shots of you going through that gap in the rocks,' said Steven, giving me cow eyes. 'We'll need to get a hundred yards down the road.'

'Okay, but don't be long and I'm not doing any repeat passes.'

As we set off, we soon crossed the Dirty Devil River. A bridge spanned the canyon and below the river was just a bare brown trickle of water. Within minutes we were crossing Hite Bridge and the Colorado River. I'd been so looking forward to dipping my legs in the lake beneath but the drought was so severe that even the Colorado River had nearly dried up and Lake Powell which was usually used for recreational sailing and bathing was nothing more than a brown puddle. I was bitterly disappointed.

Rising from the Colorado River the sight that met us was a continuous climb snaking around through the ravine for the next four or five miles. We stopped and looked at what faced us, the temperature was now 120 degrees. At least riding created a slight wind which helped keep us cool.

I picked the lowest gear and ground up the valley, drinking from the bottles regularly. Sweat dripped from every pore of my body and it needed replacing. I could feel a headache beginning to develop and was aware that I was feeling the symptoms of heatstroke without the dehydration. As we turned a corner, it was such a relief to see both RVs. It was an even bigger relief when I stepped inside to find that Mike was using the air conditioning. Even so, it was still stifling.

'How are you guys doing?' Cindy said.

'Struggling. I'm gutted I couldn't dip my feet in the water,' I said.

'Oh well, you'd have been more disappointed if you'd gone down the bottom. The lake is so low that it's not safe as it's completely populated by poisonous snakes.'

'Yuk.'

'It's just as well we're not camping. I spoke to a couple of guys who said they'd had to shake scorpions out of their clothing and tents.'

Cindy moved across and handed us the last remaining couple of iced coffees. We'd used so many litres of water today that there were no cold coffees left in either RV.

'I think we'll try another ten miles,' I said. 'Are you okay with that?' I asked Martyn and Ryan.

'I'm good,' Ryan said.

'Me too,' Martyn added.

'You definitely need to meet us at ten miles, Mike,' I said. 'It's dangerous out there without fluid.'

As it turned out, we had to meet Mike at the twelve-mile mark. It was impossible for either RV to park two miles before. It meant we'd only cycled fifty-six miles as opposed to the planned seventy and was the first time we'd not achieved our mileage, but we had to stay out of the furnace otherwise we'd have seriously compromised our health.

It was a relief to climb inside the RV and discard the helmet, buff and gloves. The journey to Blanding would be sixty-five miles which wasn't ideal but better than parking the RVs here.

'You won't believe what happened, just before,' Mike said.

'What?'

'It was freaky, Mum,' Steven piped up.

'We were sitting about four miles back waiting for you to come in. I was in the driver's seat and was just resting my eyes for a minute; I opened them, turned to the door window and there was this bloke's head.'

'Why? How?'

'I know. We'd not seen another human being all day, in the middle of the desert, no vehicles around. His head was heavily tanned but there were pigments of his skin that were really brown, parched as if he'd been in the desert for a week.'

'Is your dad joking, Steven?' Jane said. 'Becca?'

'No, he's not,' Rebecca said.

'Anyway this guy had been sitting behind a rock, said he'd broken down and wanted some help.'

'What did you do?'

'There's no way I'd have opened the door or windows to the guy. He had the complete look of a homicidal maniac. I called

911 on the SAT phone and gave them the exact position.' I looked in Jane's eyes, 'I felt guilty but this guy was a freak in the desert.'

'Where is he now?' I said, looking in the wing mirrors. 'I haven't seen any broken-down vehicles, although there are off-road routes going through the desert.'

'I know, maybe he was okay but better safe than sorry.'

CHAPTER 4

Day 19 – Monday, 17 July
Colorado River, Ut. to Blanding, Ut.
68.6 miles – 8 hrs 10 mins
Total covered – 1150.9 miles

MIKE

I woke to hear the crunch of bike tyres spitting out loose gravel from underneath them. Jane was departing. Seconds later, the other RV chugged into life and set off behind her. It was 4 a.m.

Resisting the urge to go back to sleep, I sat up in bed and blinked. Jane had asked me to pull the sheet back from the bed so, with eyes still unaccustomed to the darkness, I scrabbled around for the corners of the material.

My left hand smoothed over the area where Jane had been sleeping. It was damp. Further into the centre, it was as wet as a sponge. It *had* been hot in the night but even so her profuse sweating made us question whether her liver was working too hard as a result of the day's exertions.

Deciding that all the bedclothes were too wet I stripped it completely and put them in a pile to take to the laundry as soon as the time became respectable.

We'd always known that the 120-mile gap from Hanksville to Blanding was going to take two days. For Steven, Jodie, Rebecca and me it meant a welcome break from driving as we were already at today's finish. It had been psychologically difficult for Jane to be at the stage's finish and then have to drive back to the start. She'd had a sneak preview of today's road, so it was rather like dreaming the nightmare and then having to live it for real.

Blanding, with a population of 4000, was the biggest town we'd visited since leaving Cedar City a week ago. More significantly it marked the eastern edge of the Nevada and Utah deserts which had dominated our lives for the last two weeks. An irrigation system supplied by the canal from the local mountains had turned the desert scrubland into an area where livestock and agriculture could flourish. In 1952, after thirty-one years' work, a 5400-foot tunnel was completed to bring water to supplement the reservoir. Like many of the desert towns we'd visited, the town's infrastructure had benefited greatly from the booming oil and uranium industries of the 1950s. Of course, depression had followed but boom times were surely on their way again with rising oil prices and the growth of nuclear energy.

I sat on the stripped bed and worked through some emails and wrote some blogs until the hour was respectable enough to go into the RV's central area where the others were sleeping and head out to the camp amenities.

I gathered up the sheets and went across to the laundry. It was a wooden block, raised slightly off the ground, and contained the laundry, toilet and shower blocks. The site was peaceful, only a handful of vehicles were parked on the dusty strip of land.

'It's gonna be another hot one,' said the owner, as he continued with his morning routine, sweeping and cleaning. Indeed by 8 a.m., the temperature was already too high to stand outside and I made a mental note to apply some sunscreen on Steven the moment he got dressed.

'Yesterday was fierce,' I said. 'Does it always get this hot in July here?'

The owner, a short, spritely, wiry man of about sixty, leant against his brush and shook his head. 'No, this is feverishly hot.'

'Really?'

'Yep, it's a good twenty degrees hotter than normal. We're having a heat wave here in the desert, can you believe that?'

'Sadly, I can.'

'The radio's advising folks to stay indoors today. It's the hottest year on record,' he said, moving away slowly. 'Yes, indeed, the hottest year ever.'

By mid-morning, everyone was up. Rebecca and Jodie had headed off to find the town's library, presumably so they could spend hours instant messaging their mates at home. It was a good mile but for Rebecca walking was infinitely more preferable than getting a ride with her dad and younger brother in a vehicle that could only be described as a thirty-foot embarrassment to her. Naturally, when Steven and I passed them both on the road, we wound down the windows shouted out and blared the horn.

For a town with such a small population, Blanding's services were spread over a wide area. The blueprint for all American towns seemed to have two main thoroughfares – one north to south, one east to west and usually unimaginatively called Main Street.

Steven and I parked close to the centre of the town. Our task for that morning was to complete several menial tasks such as finding printer cartridges, posting a FedEx parcel, replenishing supplies and cashing some traveller's cheques. We arrived at the bank to finish our final task just before lunch.

After traipsing up and down in the dusty heat, the air conditioning in the modern bank office was a welcome relief. Steven immediately removed his cap.

'Good morning, sir,' a middle-aged lady, dressed very primly, welcomed me to her counter.

I leant over and my elbow slipped on the highly polished wood. 'Do you cash traveller's cheques?' I asked hopefully. Cashing money had been a problem from day one in America. Retail stores would accept them and give you change but if you wanted a wad of cash it proved troublesome. Drawing out cash usually meant trailing around a dozen banks until we found one that would do it.

'We do, sir,' smiled the woman.

I took off my rucksack and put it down on the counter, shaking my T-shirt to allow some air to breathe around my body. The blue folder containing our passports, driving licence and money was tucked in a pocket behind the laptop. I groped ineffectively for a minute, lazily tugging at the folder and eventually realising that sheer force would not release it. I did what I should have done initially and emptied the rucksack on the counter.

By the time I'd finished meticulously placing all the valuables on the work surface, the lady's patience was clearly wearing thin. I smiled apologetically.

'The stuff you have to carry,' I said and she flashed some brilliant white teeth and a smile that had all the sincerity of a beauty pageant queen.

'If you're ready, sir . . .' I felt a wave of pity for her husband.

'Thank you. I'd like to cash one thousand dollars please.'

'Certainly, sir. And are you a customer?'

'No, we're from England.'

'Yes, I can tell from your accent.' She smiled again. 'Are you on holiday?'

'Yes,' I said, I didn't want to get drawn into a conversation.

'I'm sorry, sir, we only cash traveller's cheques for customers.'

My forehead creased. 'Please explain the point of that,' I asked.

'It's a service we offer our customers.'

'Yes, but you are a small bank in Utah. Why would one of your own customers *from* Utah want to cash a *traveller's* cheque here?'

'I doubt they would, sir.'

'How many traveller's cheques have you ever cashed?'

She thought for a beat. 'In ten years I've never cashed any.'

'So, why didn't you say all that when we came in, it would have saved a lot of trouble.'

She flashed me that smile again. 'Thank you, sir, have a nice day.'

By five thirty, it had cooled to a manageable temperature. Jane had arrived at two, physically shattered and needing to rest in the RV. She looked unwell.

Steven and I had discovered a public swimming pool just off Main Street and we decided to go for a dip.

'Why don't you come?' I said to Jane.

We arrived at the open-shuttered concrete kiosk to the accompaniment of 'Have a Drink on Me' from ACDC's *Back in Black* album. Two highly athletic swimming attendants accompanied by a long-legged blonde-haired girl manned the desk.

'Australian, hey?' said one.

'No, Brits I'm afraid.'

'Cool.'

'Does the locker take a dollar coin?'

'Oh, we don't have any lockers, there's no need. If you just leave your belongings at the side. No one will touch them.'

'Does nothing ever get taken?'

He shook his head. 'No, there's practically no crime in Blanding.'

'It must be lovely to live in a town with no crime.'

'It is,' he said, handing me the change. 'Everyone's proud to live here.'

'What's it like growing up in a town hundreds of miles from the city?'

'Well, when you're young it's fantastic, very safe with a good sense of community. But a lot of us go to university in St George or Salt Lake City.'

ACDC's 'Hells Bells' began belting out of a ghetto blaster. It seemed oddly incongruous in a community that seemed so sheltered from the harsher world. The attendants directed us to a changing area.

The poolside staff all seemed no older than sixteen with many acting as childminders to the patrons' infants. Almost all the children of a comparable age to Steven engaged him in conversation and within minutes he'd made new friends. Our time was cut short after only twenty minutes when the pool was vacated as a storm became imminent.

As we approached the exit, the young man who'd chatted to us earlier called us over.

'Excuse me, sir,' he called.

'Yes.'

'There's your money back.'

I looked at him, bewildered. 'Why?'

'You hardly had any time in the pool, it was unfair.'

I was astonished. I held out my hand and he deposited the cash we'd paid only half an hour earlier in my palm.

'Thank you,' I said.

That night, after a day of relative relaxation, I found settling difficult. Jane had already dropped off, her breathing heavy and nasal. Her body was already generating enormous heat. It was going to be a long night.

Day 20 – Tuesday, 18 July
Blanding, Ut. to Dolores, Colorado (Colo.)
85.5 miles – 7 hrs 45 mins
Total covered – 1236.4 miles

JANE

When I arose my body felt heavy. My face was set with tiredness, my upper body turgid and my back crooked with pain. My thigh and calf muscles felt hard with fatigue. I strapped my helmet on ready for another day's cycling then tugged at the strap, which seemed to dig into my neck. No matter how I adjusted it, it still irritated me under my chin.

My waterproof was in my back pocket and chaffed my back just where it ached most of all. I felt sorry for myself and was unprepared for the long mileage into the foothills of the Rockies. Today, eighty-five miles seemed too far to achieve.

I mounted the bike and cycled across the road, my body wishing it was back in bed. The bike was moving slowly, the wheels seemed to be cycling through mud.

'Stop Jane! Your back tyre's flat!' Ryan called out. I was so weary I hadn't recognised the threading sound that meant a puncture. I climbed from the bike just yards from our RV. Ryan set his own bike back against a post and took my bike from me.

'Bad day, hey?' he asked and I nodded wearily and rested myself down on the kerb while he took my rear wheel and removed the tyre and inner tube.

Martyn met us with his hotel keys. Rob had driven to the airport to swap the job with Lia. 'You must have picked up a bit of glass from the side of the road. I've just pumped these tyres up this morning,' he said.

I nodded again and sat glumly.

'It's not a good start to the day, is it,' I said. 'I think I might need a breakfast stop this morning.'

I pulled out the map. 'Look, this town Monticello looks quite a good place. Shall we let Cindy know?' I said.

'Yeah, we can call her later,' Ryan said. 'Right, let's roll.'

He turned the bike the right way and passed it to me. I climbed on it and pushed off, cycling into town.

'At least there's no huge hills today. I couldn't face climbing today my back's too sore,' I said. The road wasn't entirely flat but it had no peaks to speak of, just some gentle hills.

We headed northwards towards Verdure and Monticello. The initial climb out of Blanding had made me slump over the handlebars and I was glad to reach Verdure. The road was narrow, too tight to cycle safely. On the outskirts of Verdure, a car pulled in front of Ryan, causing him to brake as the car made a swift right turn.

'Bloody idiot,' Ryan said, loud enough for me to hear. We carried on, my legs cycling without any real push in them. We mostly cycled single file and in silence. I was too weary to talk and toil. Ryan would pull alongside me occasionally and check on my progress, which continued to be slow.

A black car overtook us and a man craned his neck out of the window, peering at us so long that he didn't realise he had crossed the white line and was driving into oncoming traffic. As his attention was drawn back by the long shriek of a horn, he quickly swerved back into his own lane and sped away.

Ryan pulled up alongside me. 'What was that all about?' he said, his eyes narrowing and chin jutting. 'That was the same guy as before. I'm almost a hundred per cent sure that he cut me up about three miles back down there.'

A car behind hooted its horn impatiently at being held up briefly by a cyclist and Ryan quietly sped on ahead but we stayed close together, spooked by the thought that someone was deliberately cruising by us. All of us were worried as to what might happen if he pulled up and he made us stop.

We put our heads down and my legs found a short lease of life which helped speed our little group along. Cars continued to pass us, some waiting to pull over wide around us, others screeching past us making my bike wobble. I concentrated hard on the tarmac which had been resurfaced at regular intervals, making me screw up my eyes at every bump across each small fault.

A car sped past us and a red light lit up as it pulled into the narrow shoulder of the road. It was the same car we had seen twice that day already. The door of the car was opened and a man dressed in dark trousers and dark shirt stepped from the car. His belly strained against the shirt which announced him as a police trooper.

The open door and large-bellied law enforcer blocked our way and we pulled up. He continued to swagger, his legs apart, his feet facing outwards and his hat screwed on to his head, making his coarse features even redder than they might have been. His arms were held away from his body, his shoulders bulking against a neck as thick as his thighs.

He held out his hand to stop us from continuing, although the gesture was entirely unnecessary. His bulk and the car beyond him made a nearly immovable barrier.

'Who's in charge here?' he growled, no pleasantries were to be exchanged apparently. The three of us looked at each other, puzzling over who was in charge. We all had different roles on the ride but cycling wise we regarded ourselves as equals. No one took charge of the day's cycling, we agreed route changes together and cycled as a threesome but within our own space.

Our reluctance to come up with an answer was obviously irritating to Captain Porkie and he pulled out some cheap sunglasses and pushed them on to this face, hiding his little piggy eyes.

'Well then, let's see.' He squinted at our shirts. 'Is that Jane then?' he said, not talking to me directly – obviously communicating with the female sex was beyond him.

'Yes, I'm Jane, so I suppose I'm in charge,' I said, pushing myself more upright and facing Captain Porkie straight on. 'What seems to be the problem?'

'I've had lots of complaints about cyclists riding in the road and stopping the flow of traffic.' He paused, such a long sentence must have required a gargantuan level of concentration. 'It was the same yesterday. Cyclists riding three or four abreast. You need to let the rest of your team know that they'll get arrested for doing that here in Utah,' he said.

'I'm sorry, there's just the three of us cycling together, although we have bumped into a couple of other groups cycling but they're nothing to do with us.'

Captain Porkie turned his body towards Ryan. 'I've been watching you, junior, and you seem to be taking pleasure in stopping the cars passing.'

Ryan frowned. 'I don't think I have. I might have pulled alongside someone just to ask them something but the road's too narrow to cycle together.'

'Well anyways . . .' Captain Porkie glared at Ryan and pointed his stubby finger at us aggressively. 'If I see any of you on the road again I'll have to take action.'

My hackles were well and truly risen now. 'So where are you expecting us to cycle, officer?' I asked, keeping my voice as even as possible so as not to antagonise this hideous creature who seemed to be looking for an excuse to 'run us in'.

'I'll need you to keep to the right of the line there at the edge of the road.' He pointed to the litter-strewn hard shoulder. It was too narrow to cycle on safely, the debris meant we could easily be unseated at 20 mph.

'Well,' I said, 'we'll certainly try to do that as long as it's not too dangerous. We'll do as you are asking but may need to use the road occasionally.'

I faced him defiantly, willing him to confront me.

'I'll be keeping an eye on you,' he said. 'Now get into the side of the road and stay there.'

We moved our bikes slowly and waited as he swaggered back to his car, his buttocks churning against the shining cotton of his black trousers. I could hear the grunt of effort it required to push himself into his black unfriendly car.

His car door closed, he revved the engine hard and pushed grit from beneath his rear wheels, causing us to shield our faces.

'What a wanker,' I said and Martyn nodded his head in agreement.

'We're not far from the Colorado border now then he can go teach his grandmother to suck eggs,' he said.

I nodded. 'Yeah, but I think we should do as he asked else he'll have us and our bikes on the back of his car at the smallest excuse.'

I mounted my bike and we continued our journey towards Monticello and breakfast.

MIKE

Jane pulled up not a yard further than the RV park's entrance. Her hands left the handlebars and her shoulders slumped forwards as though she were carrying a hundredweight of coal. I stood ten yards from the park entrance with Steven, just far enough away to avoid any traffic. Cindy walked over to her and silently wrapped her arms around Jane's shoulders, but Jane's only response was a slow shudder as she began to weep.

I went over to her, shocked. 'Are you all right?'

She couldn't answer me.

'It's been a bad day,' Ryan said.

Martyn moved gingerly towards Jane, his camera pointing two feet from her face, capturing the moment she crumbled from exhaustion.

'This madness can't go on,' I said. 'I'm not going to permit it. There's going to be some changes, this is fucking stupidity. She's fucking dying in front of us.'

Ryan looked as though I'd held him personally responsible but my tirade was aimed at no one in particular. Everyone remained silent, conscious they were witnessing a human being on the edge of exhaustion. Martyn kept filming. He looked apologetic but he was only doing his job and we all knew that one knowing look and he would stop without being asked.

Two minutes must have passed without Jane moving, too physically exhausted to summon the energy to even dismount the bike.

'This is fucking madness, Jane,' I said softly. I put my arm around her as soon as I was sure that she would welcome it.

She gave the slightest of nods, her head still bowed from exhaustion. 'I'm not disagreeing with you,' she said, regaining her composure a little. 'But I can't do this now.'

'Some fucking rednecks threw a bottle at Jane just after we saw you,' Ryan said.

I shook my head, speechless.

Martyn put down his camera. 'Are you okay to do the video blog, Jane?' His voice was tentative.

Jane surprised me by nodding in agreement. She removed her helmet, bandana and eyewear to reveal bloodshot eyes and moist cheeks. I held her bike and waited for her to do the blog and return.

That night, Jane was adamant that she didn't want to discuss anything so the ride was put away.

Day 21 – Wednesday, 19 July
Dolores, Colo.
Rest day

MIKE

I wriggled my toes which were poking out over the edge of the bed. Jane lay next to me, intense heat radiating off her still body. I couldn't tell if she was asleep and I was trapped. My bladder felt like a tightly filled water balloon. Going to the toilet in the RV would probably wake Jane and the others and going to the toilet block outside would mean getting dressed, walking a hundred yards and sharing the facilities with other smelly hairy campers. I decided to lie still and try to doze in the half-light of dawn. Today would be a rest day in Dolores, Colorado, the first one after nine days and six hundred miles.

Eventually, however, the bladder discomfort forced the decision. I pulled back the covers, stumbled over the bags by the side of the bed and grabbing yesterday's discarded clothes from the trim over the wheel arch, I threw them on.

For the first time in weeks there was a cool dampness to the morning. The RV park was adjacent to the Dolores River and was shrouded with trees. For a change, it wasn't a gravel car park with power points, sewage and water but was set up to cater for holidaymakers visiting the Rockies.

At least a hundred pitches and log cabins were dotted around the site. Our thirty-foot RV – although a giant by UK standards – was no bigger than a Fiat Panda compared with the huge monstrosities parked nearby. They had air conditioning, washers, dryers, dishwashers and satellite TV; they were proper home from homes. Most of the RVs were parked up for the whole holiday season and many were towing four-by-fours, boats or sometimes both.

Walking across to the wooden toilet block I met Ryan, freshly showered and returning to his RV.

We sat on a wooden picnic bench and discussed yesterday and wanted a less extreme schedule to be identified. Tensions on the road had been rising and it was good to have ten minutes where a balanced conversation could be held without the frantic need to do other jobs.

Inside the toilet block there were six sinks, each of them occupied by unfeasibly hairy men removing their beards as if in a charity shaving fundraiser. There was a queue for both the cubicles and showers and as the doors to each had gaps below and above, every bodily function was clearly audible.

As if to drown out the background noise, a number of loud conversations about the size of RVs, the parks and the fishing were taking place. It was like a Monty Python sketch on one-upmanship.

'How are you?' I asked Jane, as I returned to the RV. She was swallowing a mouthful of Frosties, dabbing away a drip of milk that had escaped her mouth.

She made no attempt to answer. Steven peered down from his bed. 'Hello, Dad.'

'Hiya, little dude.'

'I'm going to have to get this tooth sorted,' Jane said.

'What tooth?'

'The one I told you about last night, you never listen. You nod as if you have but your mind's elsewhere.'

Steven pulled a smiley face and pointed a finger at me from above his mum's head as she delivered the admonishment. 'It's so sore I can't continue like this.' Her face grimaced and my tongue rolled through my mouth simultaneously checking my own teeth.

'I'll check the internet,' I said. 'Where's Becks?'

'She and Jodie have gone for a shower,' Steven said, as he slowly started to descend the ladder that led down from his bed.

'Get dressed before you get down,' I said.

'Aww,' he said and stepped back up.

I looked at Jane. She was clearly in some discomfort.

'We need to sort things out, Jane.'

She nodded. 'I know.'

'Will you be able to continue tomorrow?'

'Not now, Mike,' she said, her voice rising with frustration. 'At least let me get up and get going.'

'We need more rest days at least,' I said.

'Later, not now.'

'I'm just saying.'

'For goodness' sake, Mike, shut up.'

Steven was quickly dressed and tentatively peered outside the RV to see if his newly acquired friend Joey was around. The previous night Joey, only a couple of years older than Steven, had introduced him to fishing. Joey had travelled up from Arizona with his family, keen to take advantage of the outdoor sports in a cooler climate. For Steven, it meant he had

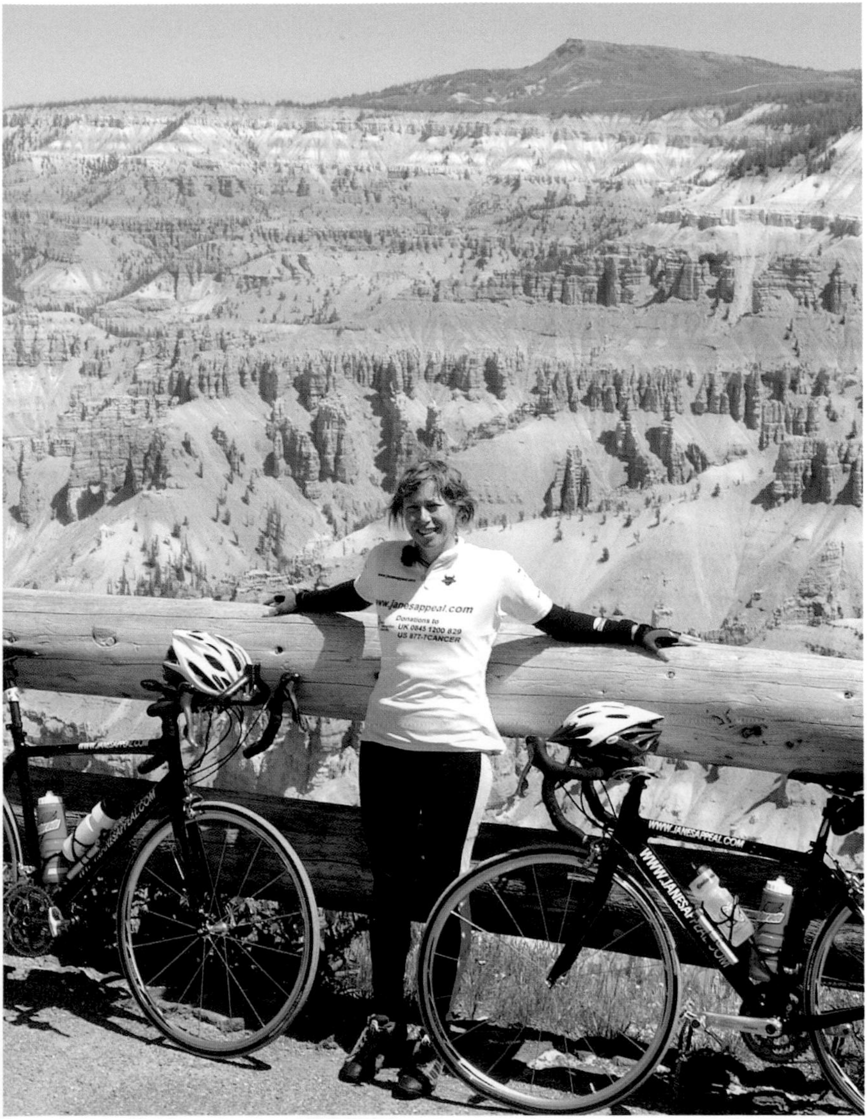

How Good is That?

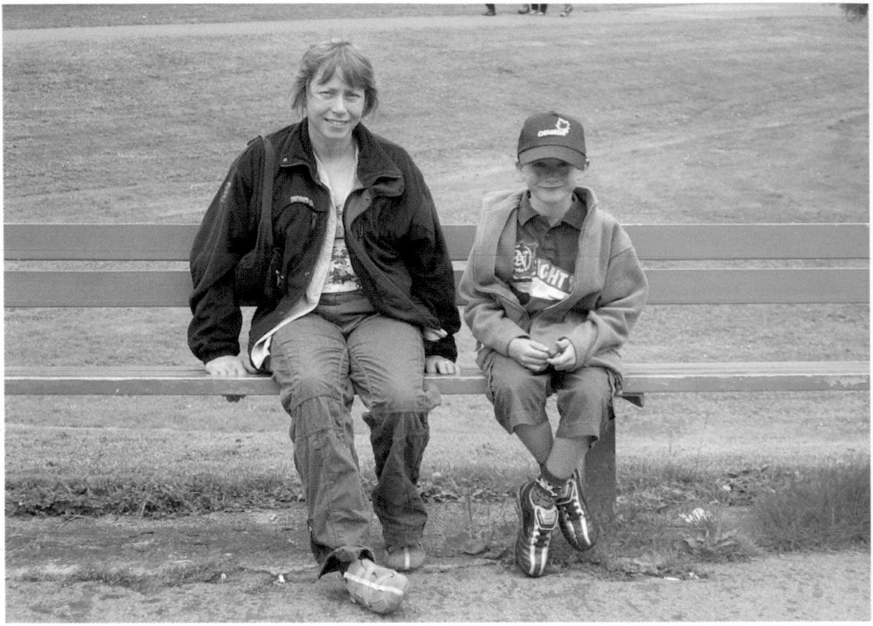

Jane, on the eve of the ride at Golden Gate Park, still unsure whether she could sit on a bike.

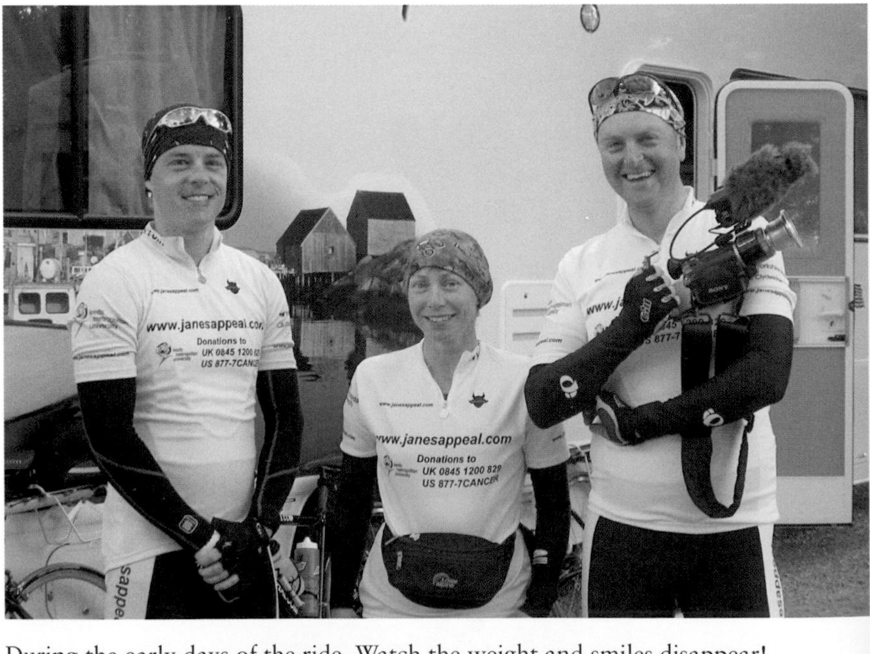

During the early days of the ride. Watch the weight and smiles disappear!

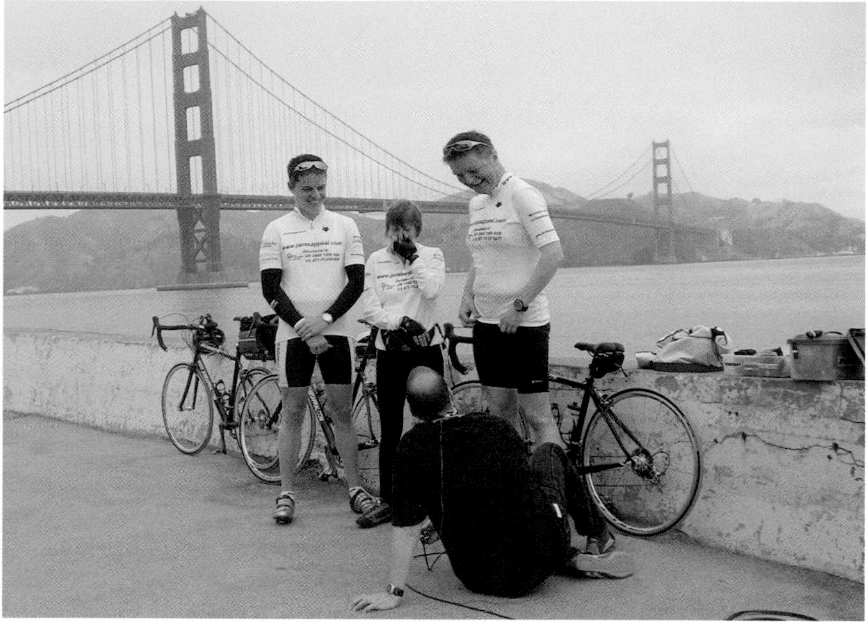

Jane being interviewed for Sky News just before the start.

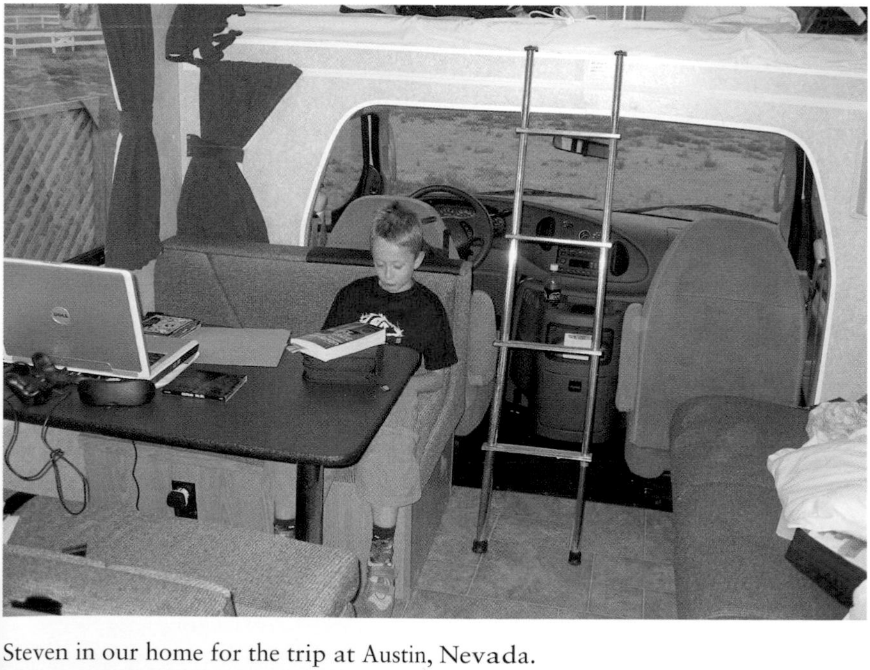

Steven in our home for the trip at Austin, Nevada.

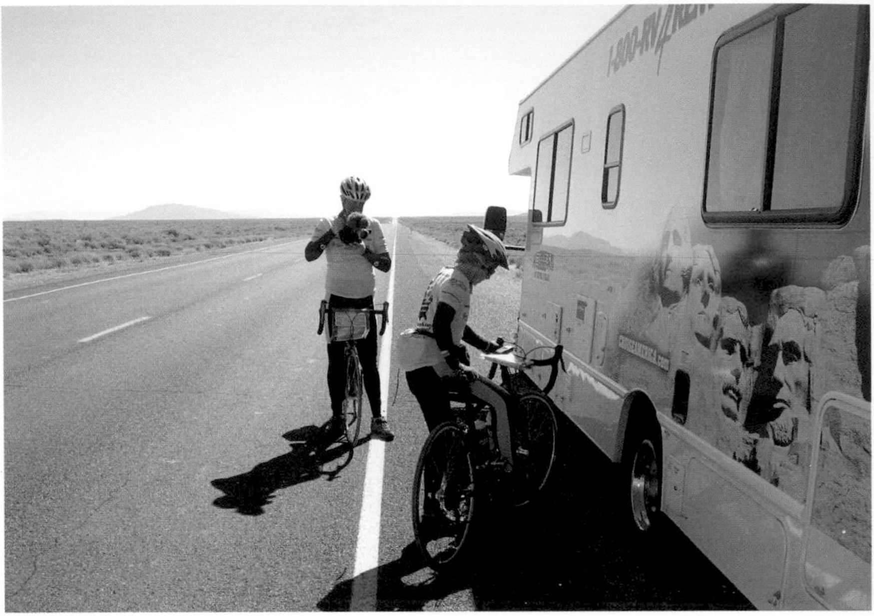

US Highway 50, Austin to Eureka – America's Loneliest Road.

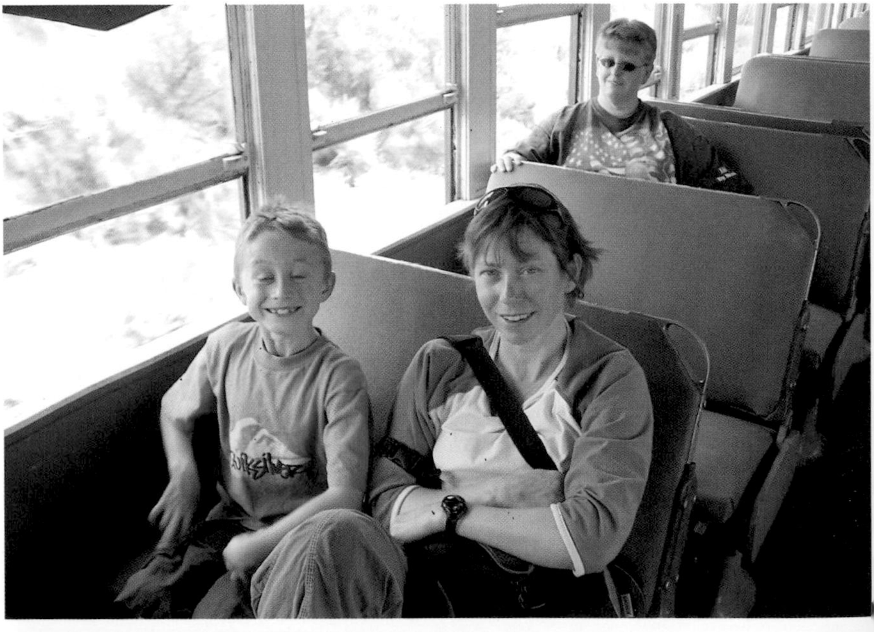

Ely, Nevada. A train journey to discover the local tourist attractions; slag heaps and brothels!

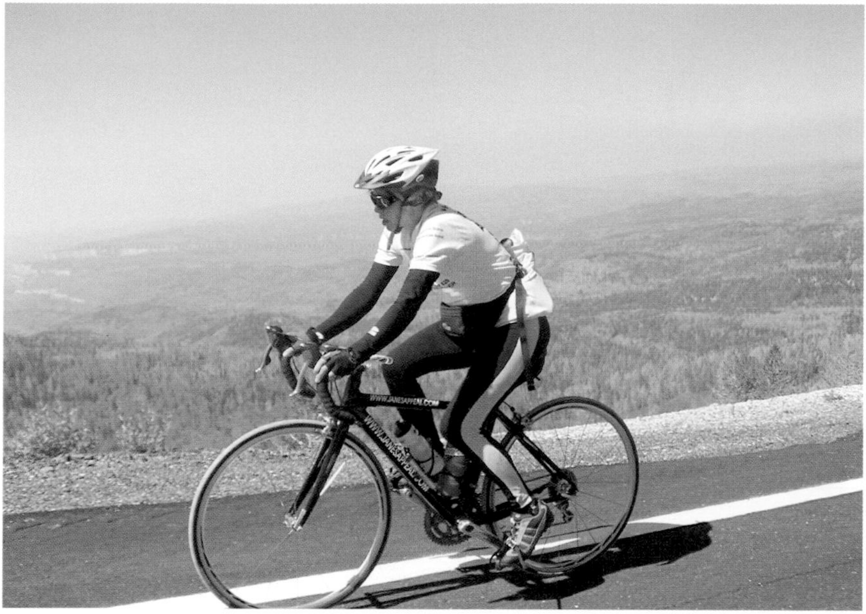

Jane climbing to Cedar Breaks Utah, the first 10,000 ft climb.

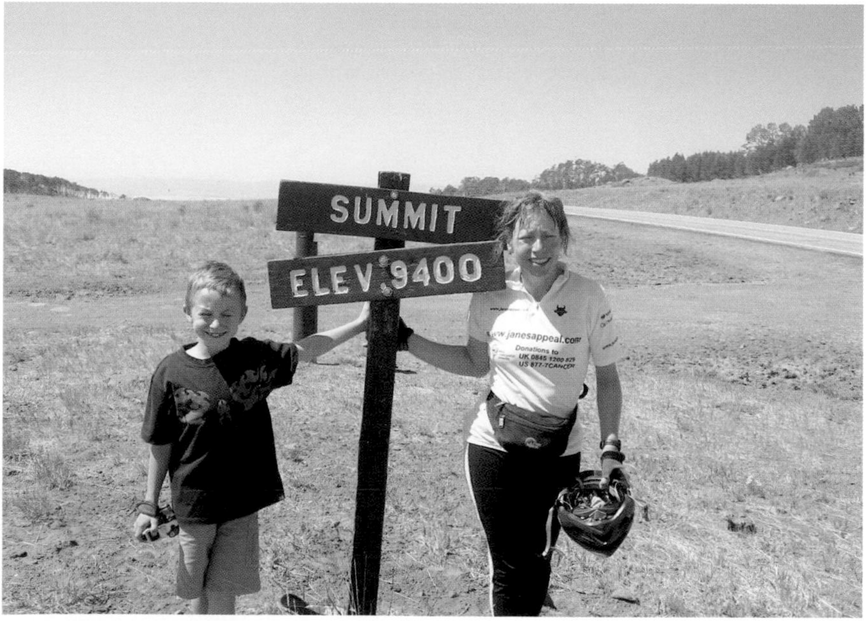

Jane thirty miles into her longest day's ride; Escalante to Hanksville. The day was already taking its toll.

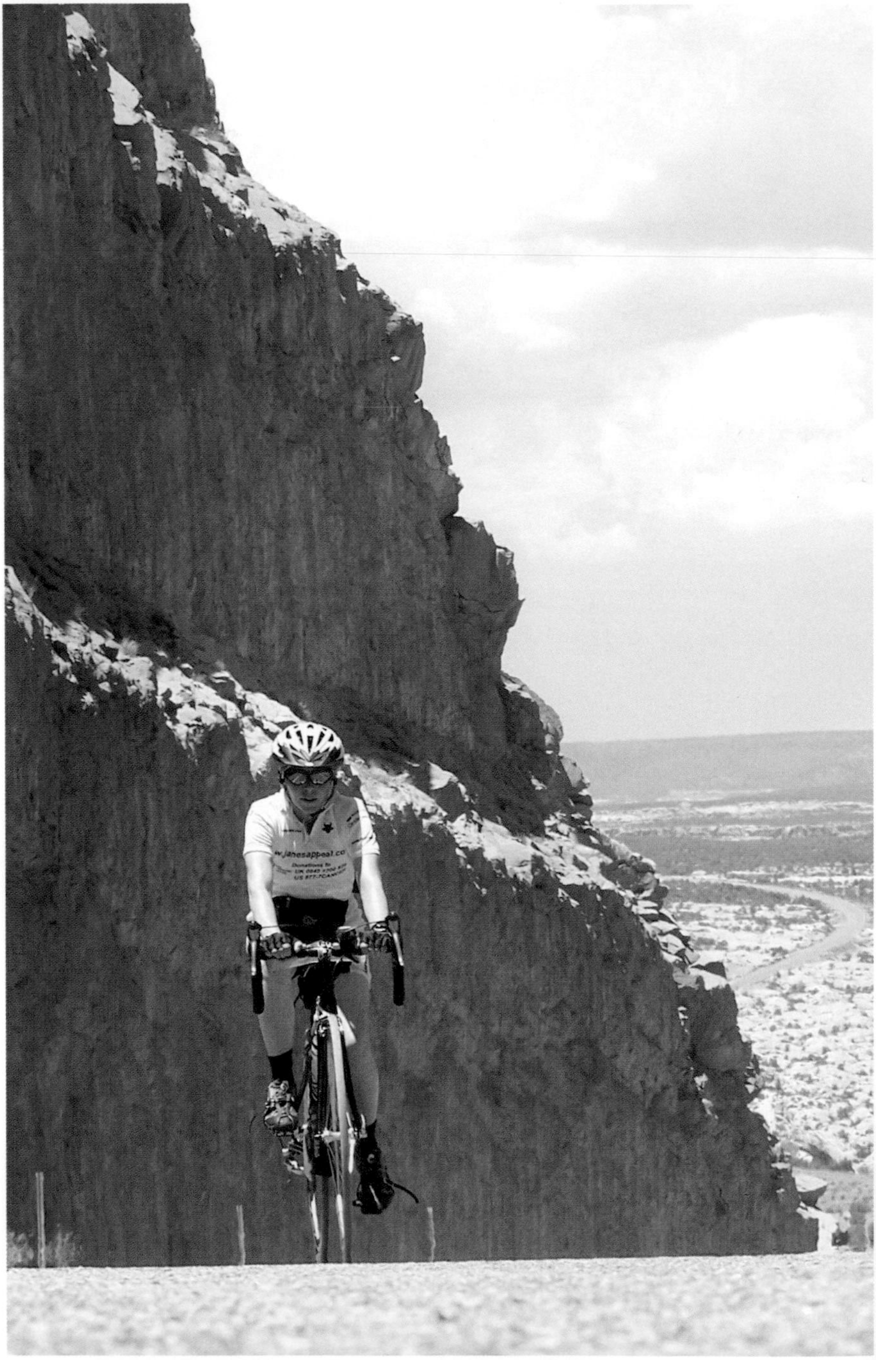

Glen Canyon, Utah. A reminder of how insignificant we all are.

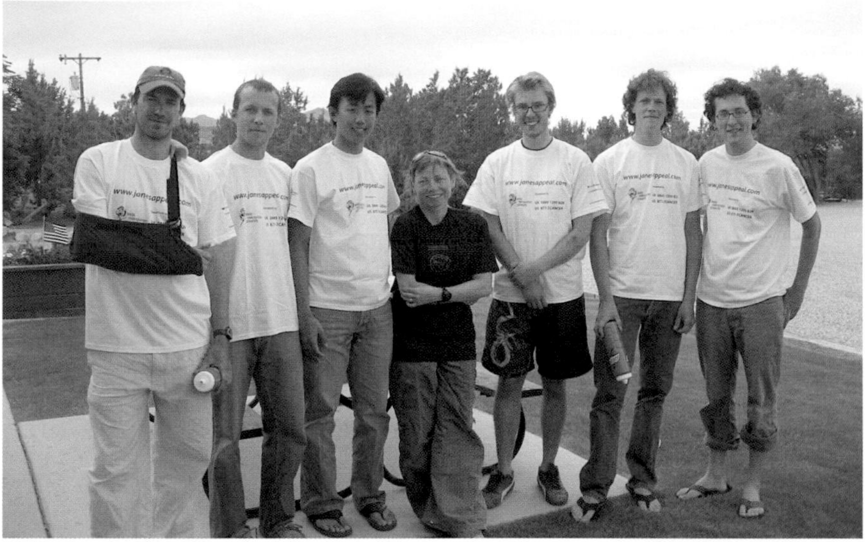

Jane with the Cross Country for Cancer lads – clearly they had some physical advantages.

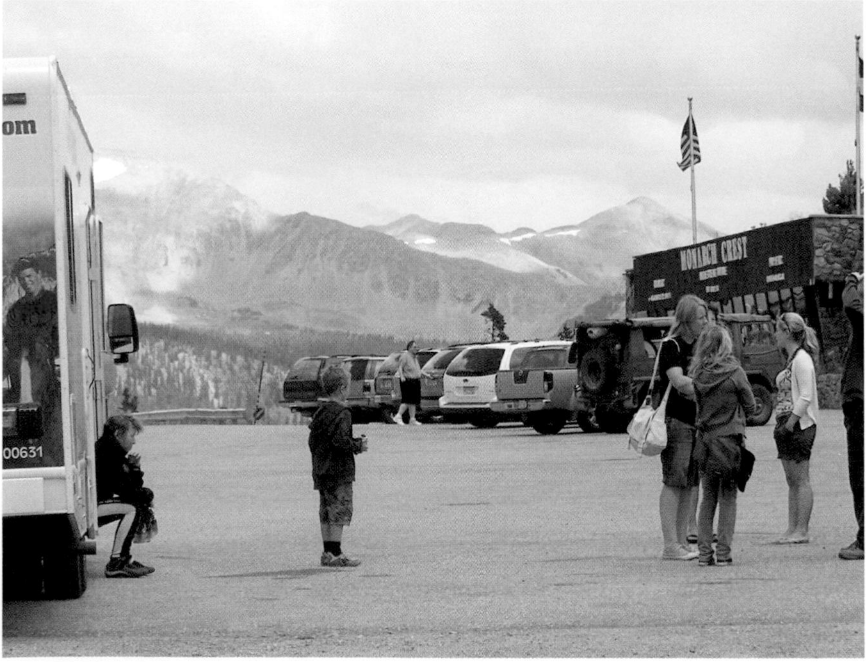

Top of Monarch Pass – Jane lost in thought.

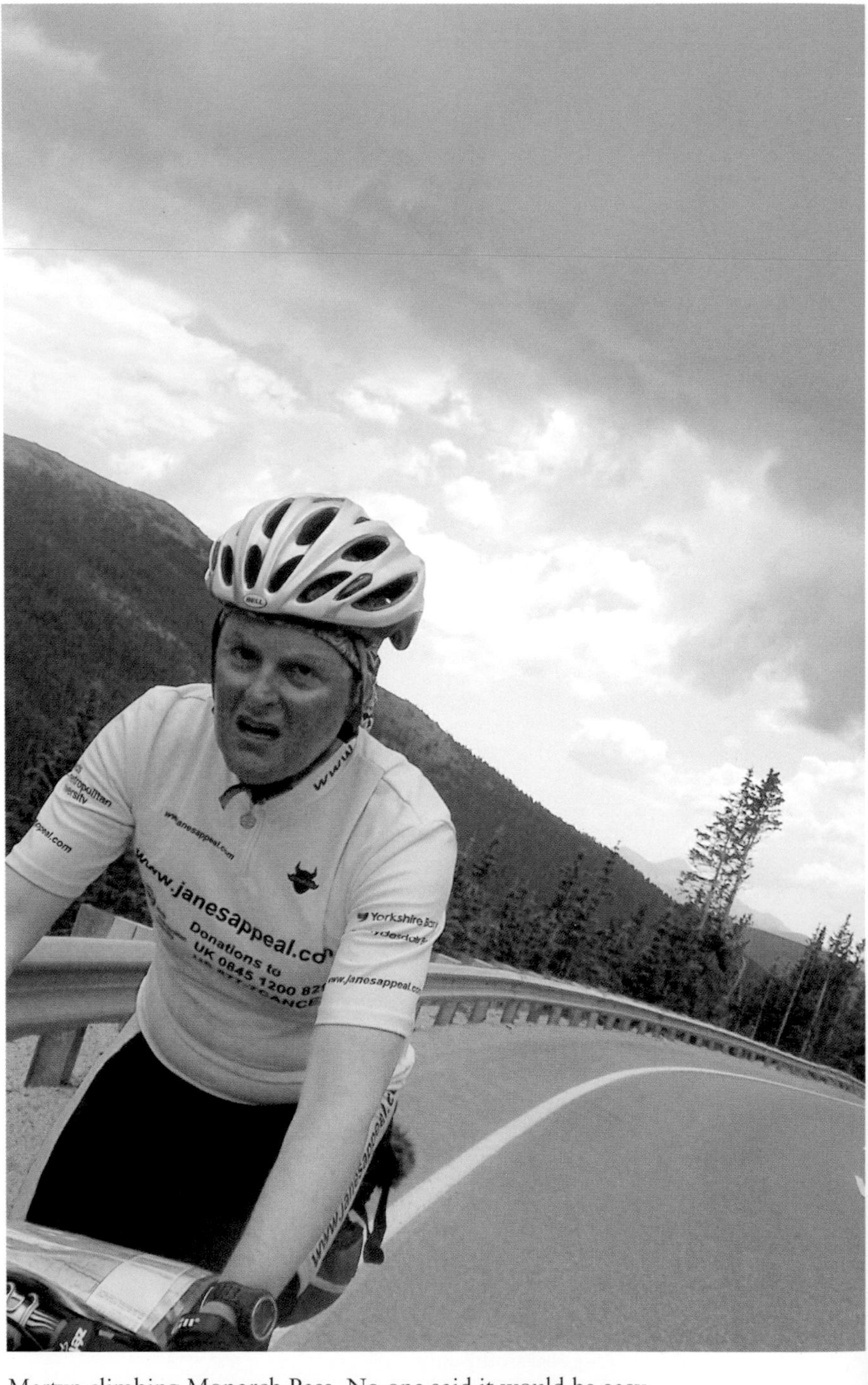

Martyn climbing Monarch Pass. No one said it would be easy.

La Crosse, barbed wire capital of the world. Only recommended for someone with a huge boredom threshold. The experience brought Jane to tears of laughter.

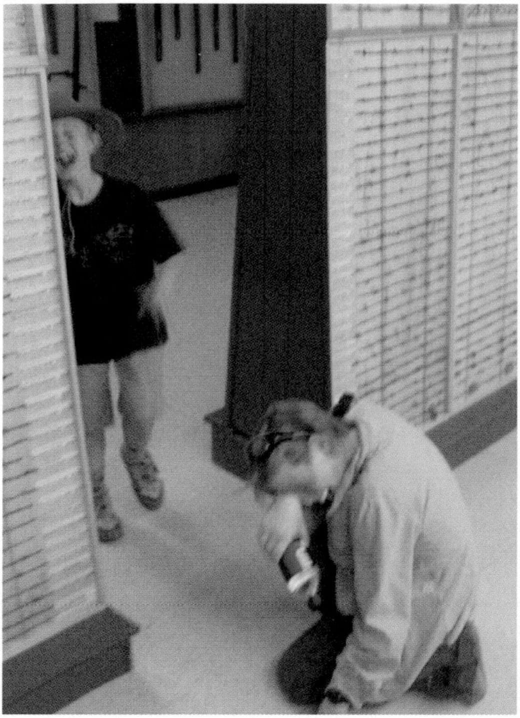

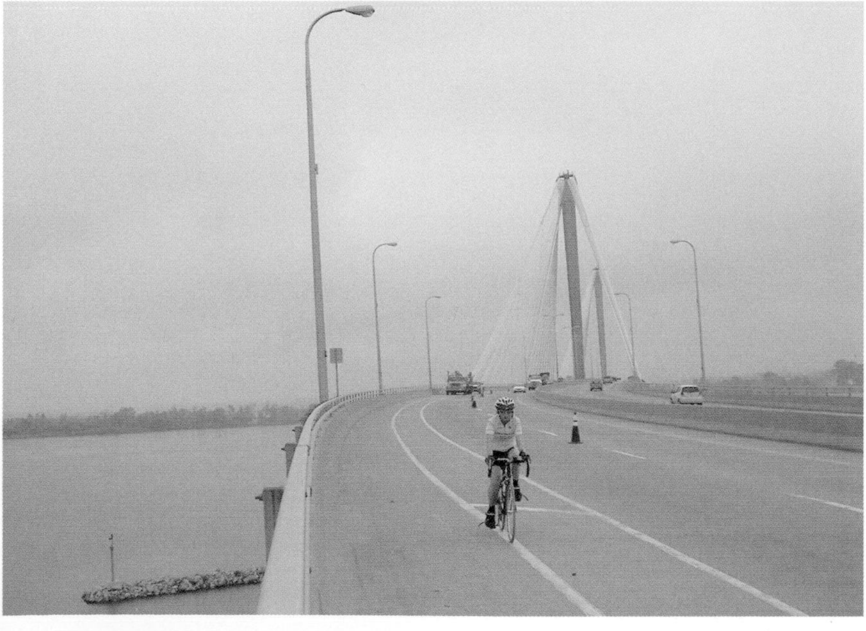

Jane crossing the Mississippi near St Louis.

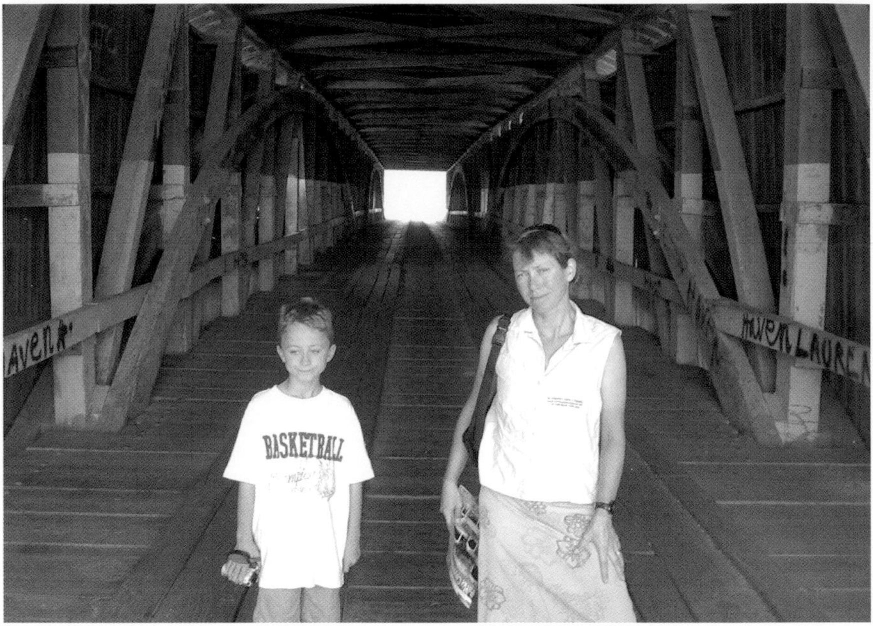

A covered bridge. Check Jane's tan lines even on her fingers.

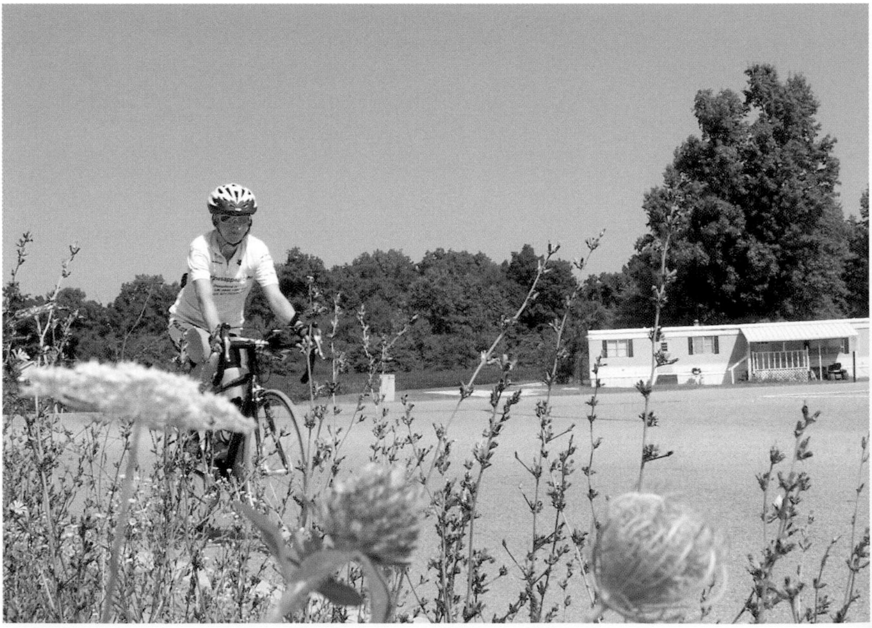

Typical Midwest US accommodation.

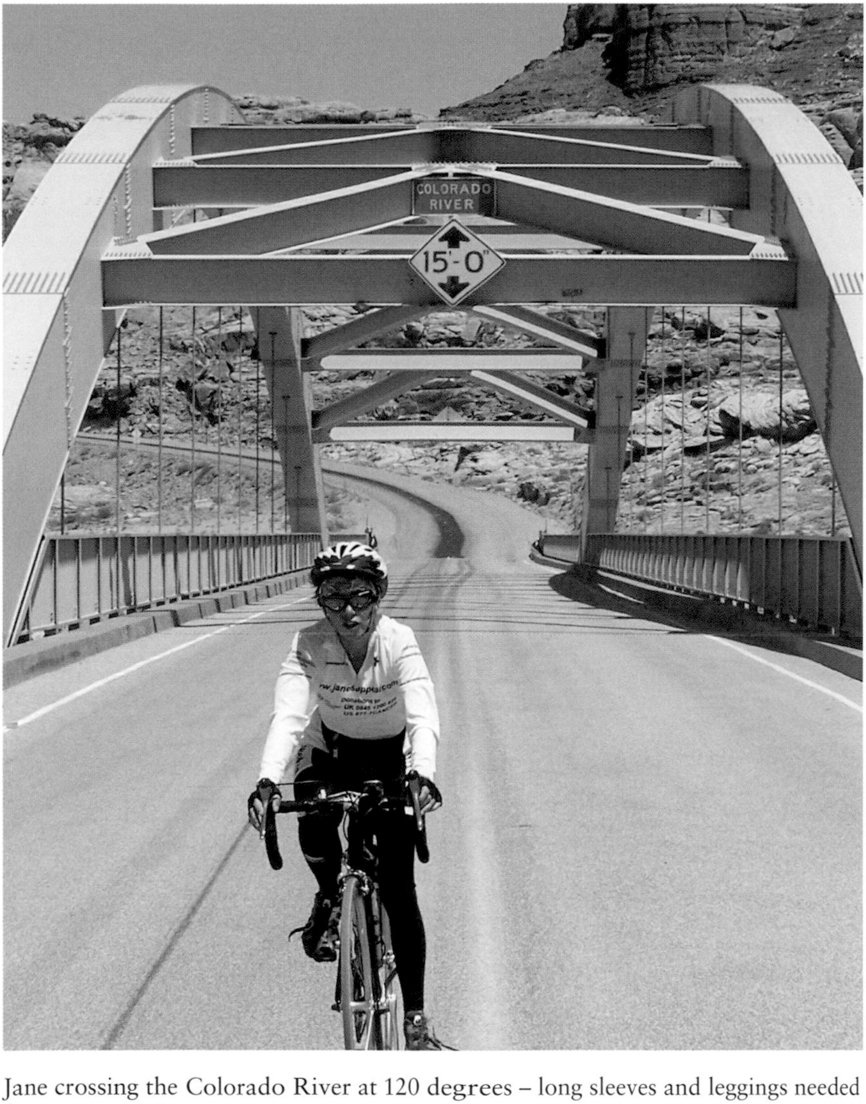

Jane crossing the Colorado River at 120 degrees – long sleeves and leggings needed for sun protection.

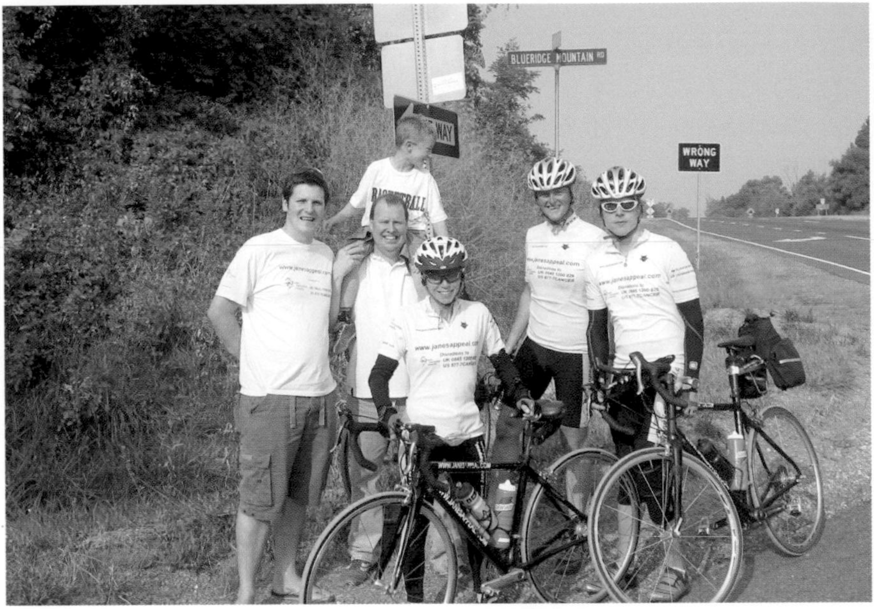

A group photo, paying homage to Laurel and Hardy at the Blue Ridge Mountains.

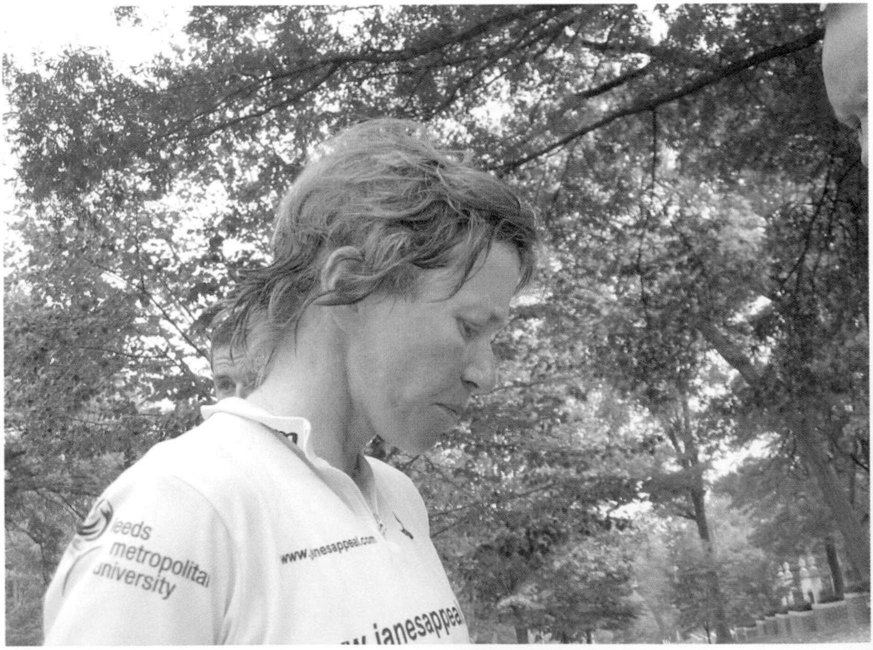

Jane showing a rare glimpse of the strain she was under.

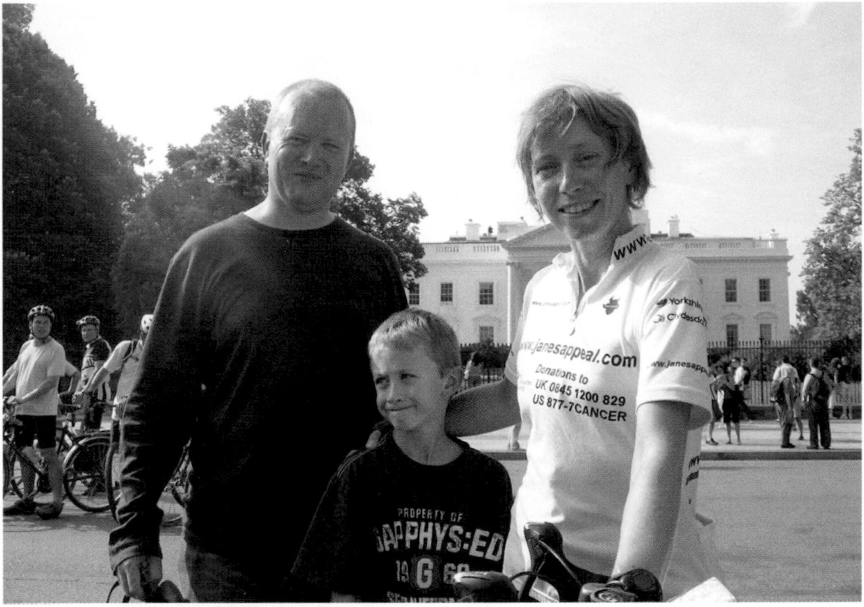

I'm not sure why Mike's the one sweating. Check the colour-coordinated embassy team!

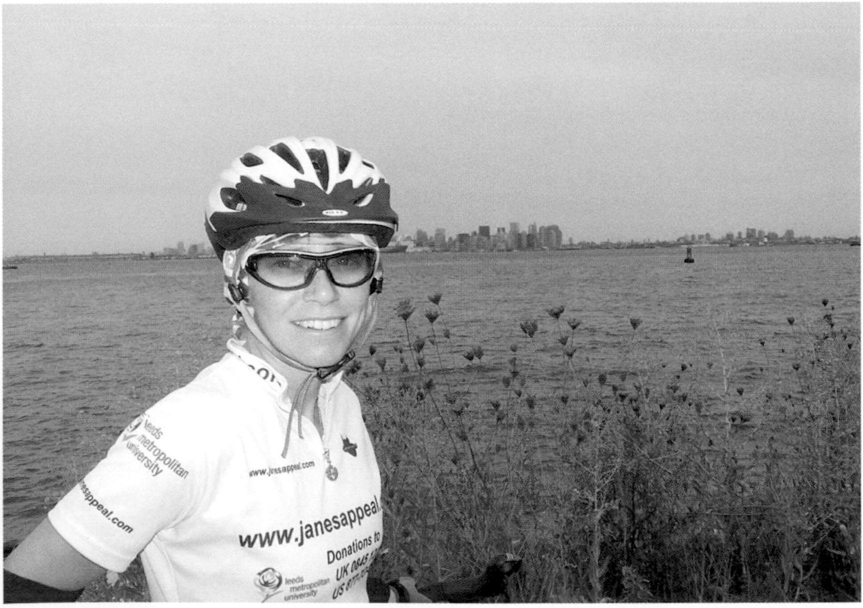

Jane on Staten Island with Manhattan in sight. Never a more welcome sight – Manhattan and the finish. How different to the previous nine weeks.

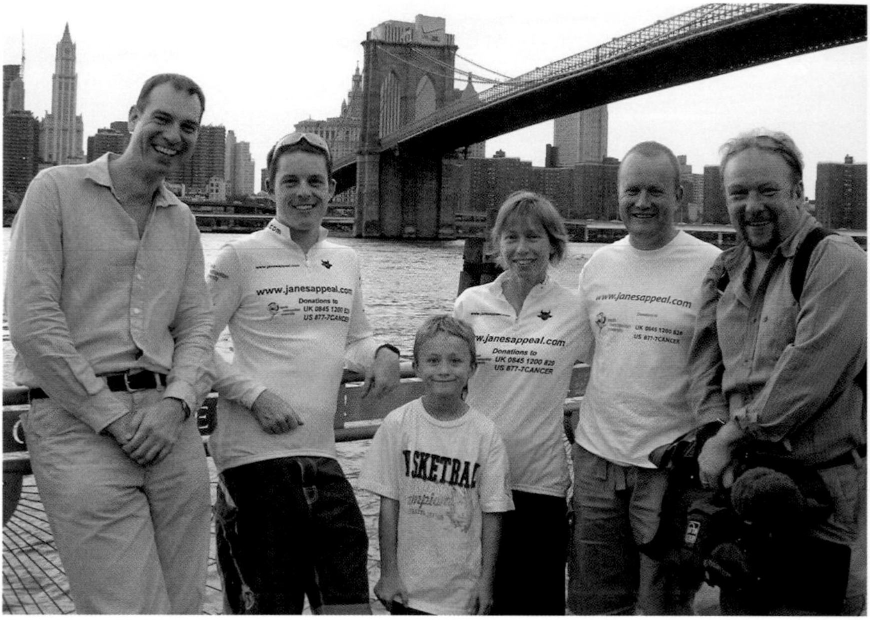

The night before the finish. Dave Harrison (YTV), Ryan, Steven, Jane, Mike and Phil Iveson (YTV).

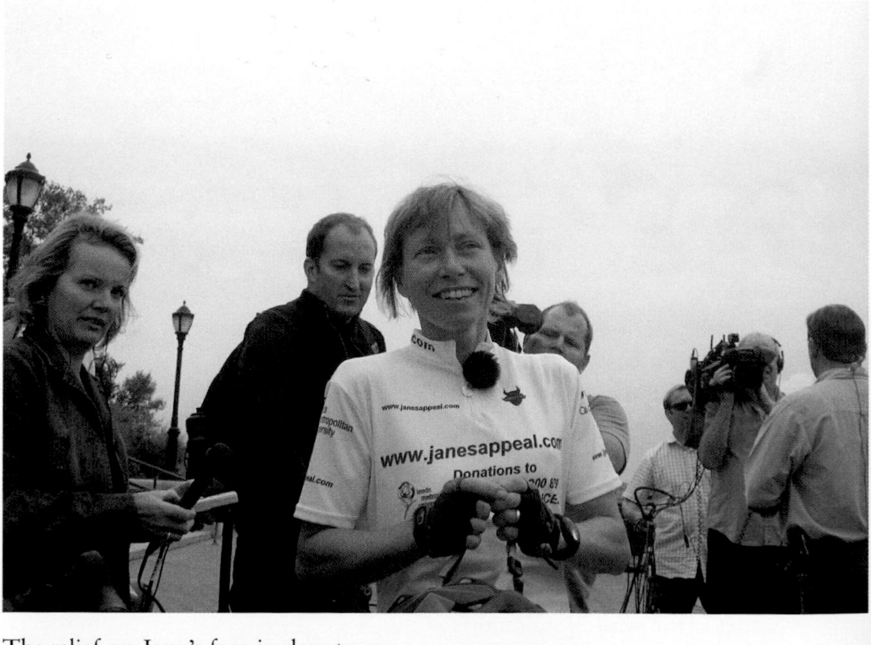

The relief on Jane's face is clear to see.

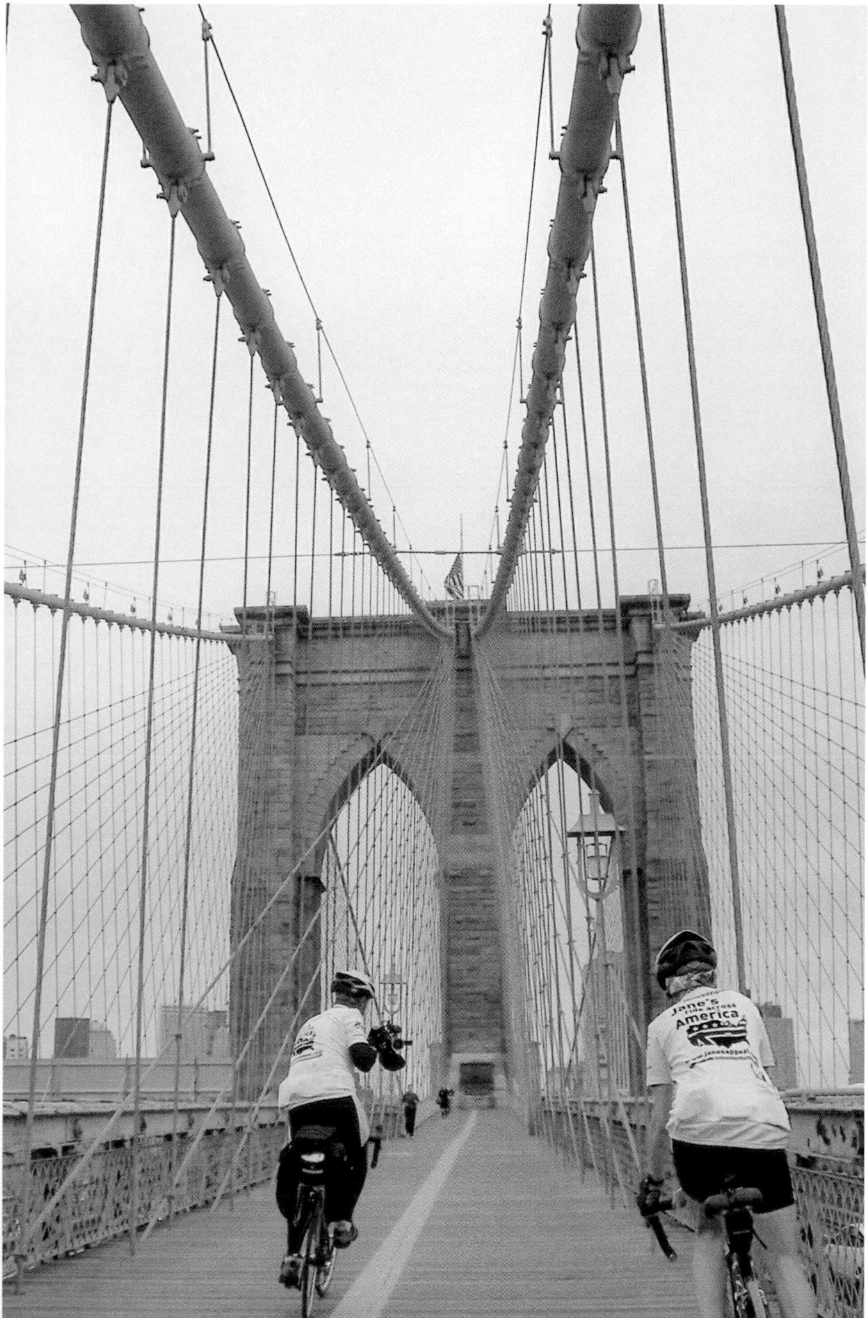

The moment Jane had looked forward to from the outset – Brooklyn Bridge.

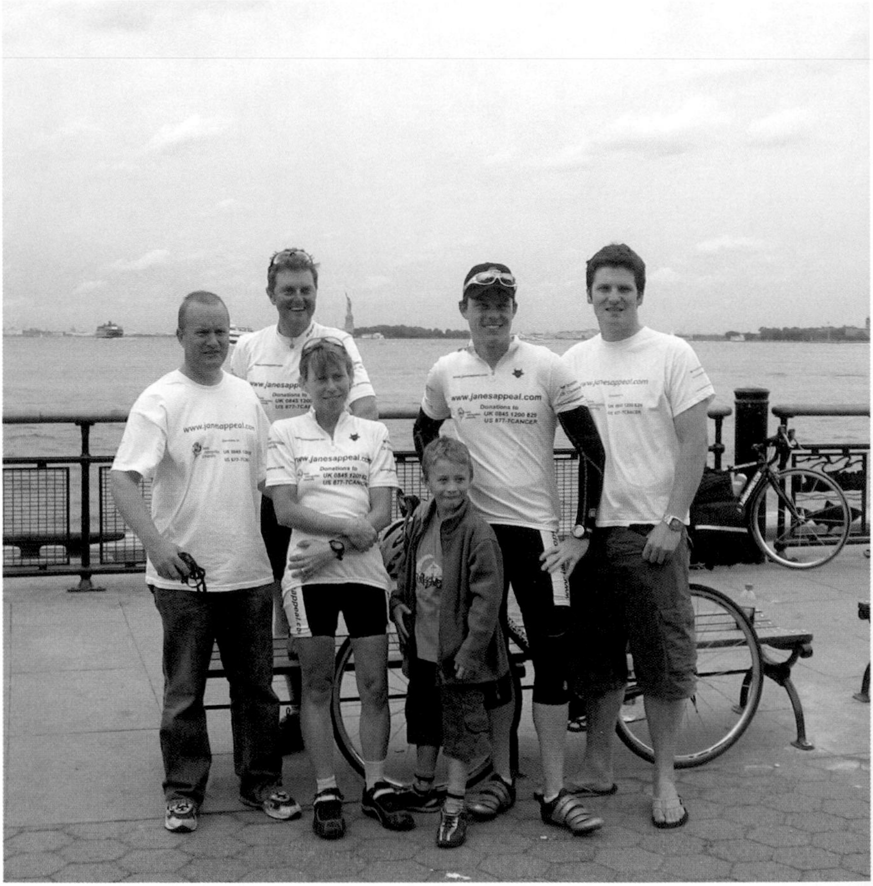

Mike, Martyn, Jane, Steven, Ryan and Michael: proves that cyclists don't need Weight Watchers.

the company of a boy of a similar age for the first time in a month.

Dolores itself was a town geared up for tourists, it was full of cycling shops, cafés and small independent stores. Later that morning, we were lucky enough to find a dentist and for $40 he confirmed that the tooth was chipped but it was okay to leave it until we returned to England.

Jane was sceptical. She thought the dentist had just made an easy $40 and she was in pain, but she had little alternative than to accept it.

When we returned to the RV, Jane looked as though she needed this rest day to stretch out for a month. Steven had gone out fishing, Rebecca and Jodie were helping Ryan cook the tea so I stretched out a map across the table. A two-page spread showed the whole of America.

'What do you think?' I asked.

Jane looked at it and bowed her head, her expression showing little emotion. 'Martyn's map is better than this, we should borrow his.'

I put my hands on hers to stop her getting up.

'Apart from that, what are your thoughts?' I said.

There was no escaping the fact that despite three weeks of cycling, we'd not really covered too much ground. Here we were, at the start of Colorado but looking at the map of the USA it seemed that we'd covered little more than a quarter of the journey. The rest of America spread out in front of us. Jane looked forlorn. I could envisage her looking down from the plane when she flew over from New York to San Francisco and realising the vastness of the Mid-West plains as well as the extent of the Rockies and the Appalachians.

'There's nothing we can do until we get to Pueblo,' she said. 'I'm too tired to do this.' She climbed slowly to her feet, moved to the door and opened it, checking for Steven. Suddenly, he and Joey's animated voices filled the air as if they'd burst into the room. The door slowly closed behind Jane. My head slunk into my hands.

There was a subdued atmosphere at tea, Ryan had received news of a death in the family and was clearly lost in his own thoughts. It hadn't stopped him serving up the best meal of the trip. The table was spread with portions of chicken, bowls of rice, salad and bread. Steven, however, saw the meal as an inconvenience, an unnecessary interruption to his fishing. Jane, I noticed, ate but not with the ravenous appetite of someone who was burning so many calories a day.

'Are you looking forward to going home, Jodie?' I asked. Rebecca and Jodie were flying back to the UK in a week's time.

'Can't wait to see my family, but I'll miss being here.'

'Yeah, right,' Rebecca said. 'Desert heat and RVs, my grumpy dad – who are you kidding?'

'What day do you fly?' Ryan asked.

'Next Wednesday.'

'How are you getting to Denver?'

'Don't know.'

Rebecca looked at me and everyone followed.

'I'd like to go to the airport with her,' Jane said. 'I want to say goodbye.'

'How will you manage that?' I said. 'It's seven days away which means that you won't get any rest.'

'Well, if we don't get another rest day until then, so be it.'

'Jane, you can't go on like this, you're not well enough,' I said.

She looked directly at me. 'We have no choice. We'll follow the route to Pueblo as planned, have a rest day there so I can go to Denver to see Becca off safely.'

'That's not a rest day!' I said, putting my fork down on the table harder than I'd intended. 'This is complete madness. Six, seven days over the Rockies, huge climbs, one day off and you're making a road trip to Denver. You'll not make it.'

There was a silence around the table. Finally, Jane said quietly: 'You've had your say, Mike. It's not constructive so shut up. I agree with you, but that's what I want to do.'

I wouldn't give up. 'We've got to increase the number of rest days.'

Jane just looked at me. 'After Becca goes we'll sort it out, but not until then.'

Day 22 – Thursday, 20 July
Dolores, Colo. – Telluride, Colo.
58.6 miles – 6 hrs 48 mins
Total covered – 1295.0 miles
Highest altitude – 10 222ft

JANE

I rolled my tongue around my teeth. Although there wasn't anything to suggest the dentist had been wrong in his diagnosis, my doubts remained.

I was nervous about today's stage from Dolores to Telluride. Most of it, apart from a couple of short bursts, was a long steady 3000-foot climb from shortly after the start up to Lizard Head Pass, which at 10 222 feet would be a challenge. The climb was, according to the maps, thirty miles. Once over the top we would plummet twelve miles to Telluride.

Having been forced into the decision to increase the number of rest days and therefore shorten this stage of the journey I felt a little more relaxed. Ten consecutive days in the saddle was too much and I was just too fatigued. I reached inside my toilet bag and grabbed the nasal spray to try to ease the symptoms of a dry nose, which was caused by the high altitude. Although we were still only at 7000 feet I'd been increasingly nauseous and it was hard to sustain any appetite.

'Are you good to go, Jane?' said Ryan.

'Yes, two ticks,' I said. It felt good to be getting on the bike and moving further across the country. Ryan was wearing a black cycling top out of a mark of respect. I looked at him itching to get his legs moving, pushing the tension on one pedal.

It was just gone half past six and the weather was cool but fine. With the forests and mountains around us, the sky appeared darker than we had been used to. We set off out of the campsite on to an empty road, turning right to follow the Dolores River towards Stoner. It was absolutely stunning – a majestic backdrop of high mountains blanketed with dark green trees, while all the time the rapidly flowing river kept us company at our side. At various points, we came across little dams where the water level would drop by twelve to eighteen inches. Then the water would be calm again.

Beavers had created these magnificent structures. The size of large rats, they were incredibly shy but also seemed nosy. They were curious as to what we were doing. We'd see one for a fraction of a second and then he'd disappear. Most of the time we didn't notice them until we saw the tail vanish into the water.

'How are you doing, Jane?' Ryan said.

'I'm fine, this is very pleasant and a change from stifling heat.'

Content that I was okay, Ryan moved effortlessly away. Just after an hour we passed through Stoner and the gentle climb started. It wasn't too long before the roads started to get fiercer, not the gradients I'd been used to in Europe but a gentle unremitting uphill climb. We stopped at Rico a further twenty miles on from Stoner, where Mike and Cindy were waiting.

Mike had a concentrated, concerned look on his face, an irritability brought on by worry over me.

'Are you all right?' he asked, frowning.

'Yes, I'm fine,' I said.

He looked at me, wary. 'Are you sure?'

'Yes, for Pete's sake, Mike.'

We didn't stop long, just enough to have a quick drink, comfort break and a look at the route profile.

It was a twelve-mile climb from Rico to Lizard Head Pass. The day was quite chilly and the further we climbed so the blue sky started to disappear and the weather became overcast. The prominent rock formation which looked like a lizard's head actually reached 13 113 feet and was suitable only for experienced mountaineers to climb thanks to its crumbling volcanic rock. It dominated the horizon and there was a little snow left in the sheltered areas. The closer we got to the pass so the gradient got steeper.

As we rose, my breathing began to suffer. I started to try to take large gulps of air but still it made little difference. I began to feel light-headed and it was a relief to see the two RVs at the top of the pass. Ryan was 200 yards ahead, while Martyn kept me company as I struggled with the final approach. Behind us, the mountains were beginning to become shrouded in rain clouds and I was grateful to be wearing both long leggings and a cycling vest. The lush grass made a change from the arid landscapes of previous weeks. The area was geared up for outdoor tourists, especially those on horseback.

Mike had organised coffees and pastries.

'Hi, Jane,' Jodie said, putting her book face down on the table. Steven didn't look up from his Nintendo DS, while Rebecca sat with her headphones on.

'Mike is the water on?' I asked, while the RV was moving the water pump was switched off.

'Becks, flick the water on,' he said from the bedroom. But Jodie was first to move.

'Are you all right, Jane?' she asked.

'I'll be glad when we drop altitude. I'm really beginning to get seriously affected. I feel quite nauseous.'

'Anything I can do?'

'No.'

I went into the bathroom and splashed some water over my face to freshen myself up. If there was one room which felt claustrophobic it was the toilet. There was a real lack of privacy and I felt a moment's sympathy for Ryan and Cindy. This couldn't be easy for two adults.

It was good to get warmed up as, despite the effort to get to the top, I'd felt shivery for the last couple of miles of the climb.

Within thirty minutes we were starting the descent to Telluride. We could see the thunderstorms ahead of us and we knew that we'd need to have our wits about us. We put our covers and waterproofs on and said goodbye to Mike.

A fast descent on a greasy road with a loose surface was fraught with danger but my adventurous side came to the fore. We dropped like a stone the six miles to Howard Fork. The descent was absolutely stonking and soon my speed was up to 40 mph. It was really wild as we shared the road with motorbikes that were hurling around the corners with us. Occasionally, a big logging lorry would draw alongside and your life would flash in front of your eyes.

I had my bum in the air, my shoulders and head down, keeping my eye on the line of the road so that I didn't miss the corners, feathering the brakes when necessary. I gave a slight touch on the brake to slow myself down because I couldn't stop. I looked down at the speedometer as it touched 44 mph; it was a pure adrenalin rush. The previous two hours' cycling was worth the twelve minutes it took to cover the six miles, but as I saw the road rise steeply again I realised how sore and tired I was.

'I've had enough,' I screamed into the rain, the droplets splashing my face. 'Fuck, fuck, fuck,' I shouted, as I tore into the climb. My legs were stinging and I just wanted to climb into bed. Fortunately, the sharp rise was not long and we were soon descending quickly into Telluride. I gritted my teeth and tore into the descent, passing gated communities before dropping to a road on the San Miguel River.

Thanks to our quick descent, we arrived before the RVs who'd set off at the same time. However, it wasn't long before they arrived. Telluride was placed at the bottom of a horseshoe of mountains, with one road in and out. The rain was coming down like an English drizzle. Rather than climb into the RVs we cycled the couple of miles into town. The town was gorgeous; the main street was lined with brick-built shops which was very unusual.

'How was that?' Mike asked.

'Fantastic. I'm shattered now. I need to eat.'

He handed me a recovery drink.

Martyn appeared. 'Wasn't that just brilliant?' he beamed. 'Have you seen Lia, Mike?'

Rob had left the ride in Blanding to return to the UK for a family holiday. Sky News had sent a new reporter, Lia, accompanied by her boyfriend Dan, to assist Martyn but Rob would be returning in a couple of weeks.

'No, sorry, Martyn, although I know she will be here somewhere as she was ahead of us on the road.'

'It's a good bet that this town will have a reasonable choice for food.'

The RV park was back up towards Lizard Head Pass as

Telluride was way too upmarket to allow mobile homes in the vicinity. It was a beautiful campsite in a country park maintained by the county, set in the heart of a beautiful forested area, just off the road. There were lots of mosquitoes around but a nice little stream ran by the side of the RV, which quickly turned into a more torrential stream when we had another downpour.

We had a barbecue that night but with the inclement weather it wasn't hugely successful. In any event, we were above 9000 feet. I had no appetite and what I did eat came back within minutes. There was no doubt that the cancer was making the altitude symptoms more acute.

I grabbed my toilet bag and headed off for a shower to try to clean up. I let the water run down my body, warming it like a comfort blanket, and pressed the button every fifteen seconds to allow a continuous flow. It was a joy to be clean. The nausea was a distant memory. I got dressed as quickly as possible. Speed was of the essence as the insects were huge. Once finished I wandered off to soak in the tranquillity of the surroundings. I vigilantly watched the undergrowth and didn't go too far as it was difficult to see where your feet were going and I didn't fancy a close encounter with a snake.

It was a long night in the RV and I never settled. Getting up, I was sick for a fourth time that night and as dawn was breaking I wandered outside so as not to disturb the others. As I strolled by the stream three does walked past without a care. It was a truly beautiful sight.

Day 23 – Friday, 21 July
Telluride, Colo. to Montrose, Colo.
63.3 miles – 4 hrs 57 mins
Total covered – 1358.3 miles

MIKE

'Don't forget the cowboy hat,' Jane whispered as she departed for the day's ride. She'd seen two pink cowboy hats in Telluride which she thought would make perfect goodbye presents for Rebecca and Jodie.

'Okay,' I said, turning over in bed and pulling the duvet up over me. It had been really cool in the RV in the night and for the first time I'd needed it. Jane, meanwhile, had sweated through two pairs of pyjamas.

'I'll be really disappointed if you don't,' she said.

'Yes, yes, yes,' I mumbled.

'Mike. Just make sure you don't forget.' Her emphasis was on the word 'forget' as she bent down to give me a kiss. I swung my hands around her waist, my hands slowly rising upon the cycling top.

We'd not been able to find an RV park in Telluride so we'd stopped in a campground just off the top of Lizard Head Pass and over ten miles back up the road Jane had cycled along. At just below 10 000 feet, the altitude had caused us all to lose our appetite. Jane had already suffered a couple of nose bleeds and her altitude sickness symptoms were generally more acute. Of all of us, it seemed unfair that she should be the one suffering.

I stood at the kiosk desk at the entrance watching two humming birds feeding just above me. They hovered just by a bird feeder, their brown, yellow and green colours blending perfectly with the vegetation surrounding them. It was a magical sight. I stood transfixed momentarily, my mind emptied from the chores I was there to complete.

'Graceful, aren't they?' the park attendant said, noticing I was entranced.

'Totally beautiful. I'll tell you what, to see them in the wild, it kind of makes this trip worthwhile.'

She smiled. 'Do you get them in Australia?'

'We're British,' I said.

The altitude was making it difficult to adjust but our surroundings were so beautiful. Snow-capped peaks, steep wooded slopes, wild flowers every shade of yellow that seemed to flourish in the bountiful rainfall, deer walking through the park. I wouldn't have missed this for the world.

I delayed our departure for as long as possible. Although the air was rarefied and made me feel a little queasy, it was a joy to be out of the intense heat. That said, knowing that we wouldn't have to sleep at this height again was some solace. I seriously doubted Jane's ability to continue functioning at this altitude. She was shedding weight at an alarming rate, already unable to take on sufficient calories, and was losing too much fluid because of the night sweats. Last night she'd barely touched her food and drank so little.

The drive to Telluride was exhilarating. I'd forgotten what it was like to use low gears to control a descent. We'd been informed that celebrities such as George Clooney and Oprah Winfrey had homes in the Colorado town. That Sotheby's have an estate agent's in the town should tell you all you need to know. With average property prices topping a million pounds, it was as stark a contrast as could be imagined to the living conditions we'd seen since Sacramento.

Surrounded on three sides by snow-capped peaks, Telluride is a winter playground for the rich and privileged. Stunningly beautiful, the landscape surrounding it only emphasised its grandeur. In the winter it must have been a wonderland but summer seemed just as spectacular. All around were posters for forthcoming attractions – film, blue grass jazz and wine festivals. When Bob Dylan comes to play in a town of 2000 people, you know it's something special.

Telluride had a history, too. When in June 1889 Butch Cassidy committed his first recorded major crime by robbing a bank here, he could never have predicted its future prosperity. Indeed, it wasn't until ninety years later that it started proving the cliché that money attracts money.

However, Telluride seemed to want to keep us out. With narrow roads and hardly any parking spots large enough to park the RV, it was clear our lumbering and somewhat inelegant presence didn't quite fit in with the rest of the town.

Convinced I'd find pink cowboy hats later, we headed off towards Montrose. I loved the idea of arriving in a place which shared the name of one of my favourite rock bands.

After driving fifteen miles I noticed the bikes propped outside Sandy's Sunshine Kitchen in Ridgway. The cyclists had already completed the one sizeable climb of the day – the Dallas Divide at 8970 feet – and were now on the long fast descent into Montrose. I pulled in, parking next to a battered red convertible on a dusty strip. We were back on the high plains. Two hardy shrubs were the only vegetation to be seen and the small capped peaks of early morning had vanished after leaving Telluride.

'Yo, Steven,' we heard a voice come from the passenger side of a four-by-four Dodge that was driving past.

Steven, recognising Joey, his fishing buddy from Dolores, called back: 'Yo, yo, yo!'

In the café, Jane was sitting with Ryan, Martyn, Cindy, Lia and Dan and was surrounded by empty plates and mugs.

I sat down near to her. 'How have you been?' I said.

'A little sore.' She looked across at Steven. 'You should try some of the chocolate, its lovely.'

'I'm all right.'

'It's really nice, you should try it.'

'Honestly,' he said, sternly, 'I'm fine.'

'You had a good morning?' I turned to Ryan.

'A bit hairy,' he said. 'Only a couple of times as people tried to drive us off the road.'

Every few miles in Colorado I'd notice road signs featuring a cyclist and the words: 'Share the road'. All the literature I'd read about this area had enthused about how the cyclists were welcome. I'm not quite sure who they were trying to convince as clearly it wasn't a view shared by the truck or four-by-four drivers.

'Did you get what I needed in Telluride?' Jane asked.

'It was impossible, we couldn't get parked.' Jane raised her eyebrows in frustration. 'It *was*, honest,' I pleaded.

'I knew you wouldn't. It wasn't something you were bothered about so it didn't get done. Honestly, Mike.' She turned her head away in disgust.

'We'll get some in Montrose.'

'We'd better, you're running out of days.'

'This is a neat little town.' Ridgway was in the fertile plain with the Uncompahgre River. 'Did you see the True Grit café?' I asked.

'Yeah, but this looked a lot more enticing.'

'They filmed it here.'

'What.'

'*True Grit*.'

'What are you talking about, Mike?'

'*True Grit*, the John Wayne film. Did he get an Oscar for it?'

Jane shook her head.

'Come on, guys, let's roll,' Ryan said, scraping his chair across the floor, his cleated shoes sounding like an uncoordinated tap dancer. His urgency was not mirrored by Jane and Martyn, who methodically reapplied some sun protection, repositioned their bandanas, took final slurps of drink and slowly stood.

'Bye, love,' I said, giving Jane a peck on the cheek, which was cold and clammy, before going to join Rebecca, Jodie and Steven. Upon leaving the café the heat hit you like walking into a steel furnace. Within a couple of minutes of leaving the car park we turned on to the 550. Despite driving for three weeks and covering over a thousand miles I was still flummoxed by the intensity of traffic and the junctions. Some days we'd been lucky to encounter another vehicle at all. Now, approaching Montrose, there was more than one lane to choose from as well as traffic lights and turning vehicles. It was like learning to drive all over again.

The state of the road was shocking, debris and litter seemed to cover every inch of the shoulder and I feared the amount of punctures the cyclists would get.

Entering Montrose on the 550, the strip mall spread out for over a mile on the right-hand side. Many of the major US franchises were next to each other and it seemed sacrilege to see the town swamped by the familiar lurid signs. None of the buildings seemed to have been built with any thought as to their consequences or architectural design; they were just quickly and cheaply erected warehouses with vast floor spaces. Most of the character in Montrose had been flushed out, but that didn't curb our excitement at seeing a Wal-Mart and Borders. Of all the produce we needed, it was the drinks that needed replenishing the most. Our appetites may have been suffering but quenching thirst seemed to be our main priority. So two shopping trolleys were suitably loaded with water, Coke, iced coffee, tea, coffee and milk.

As we were leaving the three cyclists were riding past, dwarfed by eighteen-wheeler trucks whose tyres they barely reached up to. Grid systems in American towns made navigating easy and we counted down from South Twelve Street to Main Street. Main Street was a four-lane road with vehicles able to park on each side, well maintained, attractive, with small trees despite being in a dustbowl environment. Single- and double-storeyed stone buildings stood at either side but it still didn't bustle with pedestrians as the locals preferred to park outside the shop they were wishing to use. It did make you wonder how badly the strip mall had ripped the heart out of the town.

The Stars and Stripes drooped on flag poles, which were mounted on an immaculate small lawn next to an immaculate block consisting of an immaculate shop. From the military pollution of Fallon to the slag heaps of Ely, the miniature wreck yards at Baker to the strip mall of Montrose, everywhere seemed tarnished somehow. Yet the journey had shown us untouched beauty in abundance. The only spoiling factor was human pollution.

Day 24 – Saturday, 22 July
Montrose, Colo. to Gunnison, Colo.
62.2 miles – 6 hrs 56 mins
Total covered – 1420.5 miles

JANE

Mike moved slowly on to his side, his arms reaching out of the bed. He blinked, his eyes unaccustomed to the early morning light. He knocked a pile of coins over. 'Shit,' he muttered.

'What are your plans?' I whispered. Everyone else was still asleep and I didn't want to wake them.

'I think we're going to look at Black Canyon,' he whispered back. 'It's meant to be an awesome gorge. I should be able to get the RV up there.'

'Drive carefully,' I said, planting a kiss on his lips as he rose to his feet.

'Don't worry, we'll just head straight to the finish at Gunnison, so we'll see you there. Have a good ride.'

He stepped into the main part of the RV.

'What are you doing?' I said. 'There's no need to see us off.'

'I'm not. I need to get on with some work.'

As I passed through the RV, I felt an overwhelming urge to climb the ladder to the bed above the cab to look in on Steven. He was fast asleep. I blew him a kiss. 'See you, little man,' I mouthed and left.

The morning started with a tricky fifteen-mile climb from Montrose to Cerro Summit. It was a gradual ascent of 2800 feet but it felt pleasant to be back on quieter roads. The road surface was smoother than it had been yesterday.

The vivid yellow blossoms of wildflowers and blue columbines – the Colorado State flower – decorated the roadside. It was incredibly pretty.

It took us only ninety minutes to reach the top where I took luxurious swigs from my water bottle and stretched my aching back muscles, which had compacted from hunching over the handlebars.

I heard the sound of a vehicle slowing down beside us and turned to see a white state patrol car, indicating to pull in.

'What the chuff now?' I said, under my breath.

'It's nothing we could have done,' Ryan said, watching the car crawl towards us. 'We've been courteous. There've been no problems.'

The car pulled up and parked right alongside us. A bespectacled female officer leant out of the driver's window.

'Are you having any problems?' she asked. She had a warm grin which lit up her face and her fair hair was tied up neatly.

'Absolutely not.' I shook my head, wondering where this conversation would lead.

'We've had a phone call from a concerned lady who'd driven past some cyclists and one was lying on the floor who seemed to be in some difficulty. He was wearing white so I'm guessing it may be one of your party.'

'Oh, that'd be Martyn,' I said. Ryan, who'd discovered that his great aunt had died while we were in Dolores, was wearing black as a mark of respect. I looked across to where Martyn was checking his panniers. 'He's filming the ride so sometimes he lies down to take some shots.'

'Oh, I see,' said the police officer, nodding and reaching down to her right to get her radio. 'If you don't mind, just give me a minute, ladies and gentlemen, I need to call in and cancel the ambulance.'

I looked at Ryan, who smiled. Her passenger seat was a sea of paperwork and as I waited for the call to finish I fully expected to be given yet another warning. We weren't making many friends with the law enforcers. But as she hung up the radio, she turned back to us. 'You folks take care now,' she smiled. 'I hope it goes well.' And with that, she drove off.

'Well, that was different,' I said to Ryan. 'Let's go before we get stopped by another.'

We dropped off Cerro Summit into the very small community of Cimarron before climbing again. The head wind made the 8500-foot climb even more difficult and it was a huge relief when we finally arrived at Sapinero on the banks of the Blue Mesa Reservoir, Colorado's largest body of water. We carried on cycling – there was barely a cloud in the sky and the water was a beautiful azure colour. The roads were clear and we had a perfect view of the Dillon Pinnacles, a stunning set of rock formations formed by volcanic activity. This was as close to perfect as it could get.

'This is more like it,' I said to Ryan.

Day 25 – Sunday, 23 July
Gunnison, Colo. to Monarch Pass, Colo.
56.3 miles – 5 hrs 26 mins
Total covered – 1476.8 miles
Highest altitude – 11 312 ft

JANE

In the morning we were heading for Monarch Pass. It was to be the highest pass of the entire journey and we would reach 11 312 feet.

I felt very sick. At breakfast, all I could manage was a couple of pieces of toast and even that was hard to swallow. My throat and mouth were very dry, my stomach was knotted with nervous tension. Before departing from the UK we knew that I might get altitude sickness and the experience at Telluride had made us doubly cautious. Mike was concerned that the climb might put undue pressure on my heart whose function had been damaged by the use of the drug Herceptin.

I tried to ensure that no one knew how worried I was about it but my stomach turned like a washing machine on its final spin.

We'd agreed to do the climb with both RVs supporting, which reassured me a little. I knew Mike would be keeping a keen eye on me but at the same time I didn't want his nerves getting on mine. It had been an easy thirty-mile cycle across the valley floor from our overnight stop in Gunnison to Sargents, where we'd agreed to meet up before the climb. The six of us sat inside a restaurant at the Tomichi Creek Trading Post preparing for the journey. As the others tucked into food, I could hardly face a dry piece of toast, my nausea was coming over me in waves. I revisited the toilet thinking I was about to be sick but after minutes of dry retching it was clear there was nothing to throw up.

'Come on, let's get on with this,' I said on my return from the toilet for the third time. I caught Mike's worried glance but now wasn't the time to discuss what we were about to do.

We set off at ten thirty and for the first few miles simply plodded our way up the pass. It wasn't too bad; it seemed to be no more than a slight incline which just went on and on and on. We headed into one valley after another. It was difficult to judge how far we were going and it was only thanks to the markers at the side of the road that we could measure our altitude.

Martyn was filming at every vantage point and then scurrying back on the bike to try to race ahead but the climb was so severe it was testing his strength. I looked over at him as he caught up with me from his latest stop and his face was blotchy from the exertion. His mouth was constantly agape, sucking in every ounce of oxygen, and his eyes were focused on the road ahead.

Ryan was constantly on and off his bike looking for the perfect photo and scrambling up the hillside to gain some height. I just stayed on my bike.

Traffic was becoming increasingly heavy with lorries, RVs, pickups and cars. As the altitude increased, so the temperature cooled and the weather began to close in. The unbroken blue sky turned predominately cream and in the distance we could see dark clouds gathering.

Mike and Cindy leapfrogged us every two miles, waiting at conveniently large lay-bys and shouting encouragement. We stopped after five miles with a view to halting again after eight, a couple of miles below the summit to ensure that my heart was fine and not under too much stress.

Each time I had a drink and soaked up the view. By now the sun was almost directly overhead but I planted myself in the two feet of shade by the RV, and pulled in my cheeks as Martyn filmed me. I was still feeling sick but I was conscious that the next few hours were why everyone was here. Could I make it over this monster of a mountain? It was 5000 feet higher than Mont Ventoux. I'd done that. I could do this, too.

Mike was being very encouraging, telling me how well I was cycling, that the gradient wouldn't get any steeper. He hovered around me ensuring that I didn't have to walk, bend or move for equipment, constantly predicting what I needed. Normally I would have been irritated by this but I was desperate to save energy and unnecessary movement.

The three of us got back on the bikes and started pedalling. Until we reached just underneath the snowline I kept my head bobbed down, focusing on the milometer, but every half an hour, we stopped to appreciate the view. At various points, I took my water bottle out and tried to take a swig. But it was impossible to swallow. I was too breathless as the air got thinner. The sun was out and although it wasn't too hot we were soaking wet.

Two miles from the summit I saw Mike's RV.

'Go, Jane,' Mike shouted. 'You're looking really good.' He ran alongside. 'You can just see the summit. You go.'

Steven was screaming, video camera in hand, 'Go, Mum, go, Mum.'

I hadn't the breath to respond, I merely moved the palm of my right hand upwards in acknowledgement.

My legs were burning and I gasped for breath as if each one would be my last. Ryan was fifty yards ahead. I raised my head and saw between the high branches of the tree line a grassy knoll with radio masts. I'd agreed to stop there but couldn't face losing my momentum so as the wheels inched round I continued past the others without even the energy to acknowledge them.

'Keep going, Jane,' I heard someone say. I gasped, my eyes now transfixed on the GPS on my handlebar, a visual indicator of what my body was telling me, that the air was thinning and my breathing was suffering.

I carried on, onwards, upwards to where I could see Mike and the RV waiting for us. It seemed to take for ever. I could see a green sign indicating that the summit was some 100 yards past the RV and a cable car station saying 'Scenic Ride'. Next to it was a car park with motorbikes, cars and the two familiar Cruise America RVs.

'Jane! Stop! You're there!' I heard Mike yell but I carried on, determined to reach the second sign which was fifty yards on. 'Jane! Stop!'

'No, no, you're wrong!' I shouted. 'I'm going to the pass, I'm going to the pass!' I felt my face crack open with a huge smirk when I saw Steven running towards me. This was the highest altitude I'd been in my life and I'd got here under my own steam. Realising his mistake, Mike was suddenly running himself, belting alongside me as I pedalled towards the second sign.

For once, Martyn and Ryan were behind me, playing catch up after I'd passed them at the knoll. 'I'm going to get there before you lot,' I thought, and with every muscle pumping I sprinted the last few yards to the top. I'd done it.

'Fantastic, Jane!' Martyn said as he pulled in alongside me. 'What a ride! I was struggling to keep up, I thought I'd lost you in that last mile or so. I don't think I've worked any harder on the bike.'

I was too breathless to speak. I sat at the bottom of the sign and looked at my watch. We were an hour ahead of schedule.

'How good is that?' I thought, stretching and straightening the back muscles that had been curled over the bike saddle.

'Well done, Mum,' Steven said. 'Can we go on the chair lift, please.'

I straightened up and laughed. 'Yes,' I said. 'Just give me a minute!'

My hands on my hips, I let my head fall back and I looked up at the sky. There was hardly any blue remaining and the temperature was cooler than anything we'd experienced so far.

'I need my fleece,' I said, wheeling the bike to the RV and grabbing my jacket from the wardrobe. I came out into the cool breeze and sat on the step of the RV recovering. My thighs felt like lead weights but I felt alive.

'Are you all right?' Mike was gently rubbing my shoulders. 'You should eat. The café in there is very – and I mean very – basic but you need an energy burst as soon as possible.'

I nodded, still too tired to talk, but I eased myself up on to my feet and started to walk towards the café.

Once inside, I felt disorientated and incapable of making the simplest decisions. Steven buzzed around like only a 9-year-old boy can do so I slumped into a chair.

'Just get me anything. A coffee? But I don't fancy any food.'

This morning's nausea had still not subsided and the high altitude was exacerbating the problem.

Mike returned with some beautiful home-made vanilla and chocolate fudge and black coffee. I devoured the fudge, the sugar hitting my bloodstream almost instantly. It was just what I needed.

As a group we'd become fragmented, with everyone off doing their own thing.

'Can we go on the ride, Mum?' Steven repeated.

'Yes. Mike, will you get people organised?' I asked.

As we'd finished so early we decided to take the afternoon off. The Monarch Cable Car ran from the mountain pass where the road cut through to about 800 feet higher to the summit at just over 12 000 feet.

'Ha ha! You'll have to go as well,' said Steven to his dad. Mike really hates heights, particularly those over which he's suspended in the air by a cable.

'Come on,' I said. 'You'll enjoy it.'

We bought our tickets. Steven sat by Mike and I sat by Cindy and we proceeded up the mountainside, the cable car swaying from side to side. In the car below us were Ryan, Martyn, Rebecca and Jodie.

But almost as soon as we'd left the cable car hut for the first pole, it was apparent that the weather was closing in very quickly.

'Look at that,' said Mike. He was sitting opposite me and was pointing to the sky up behind my head. I looked. Day was turning into night.

Tap, tap, tap – hailstones began to attack our metal cage and Mike's face turned white. I could only imagine how he'd react if the ride came to a sudden halt.

'Nearly there,' he said, possibly expecting comforting reassurance from me. Normally I'd have teased him mercilessly but Steven is predisposed to take on his dad's worries. The stones were coming with increasing ferocity, the car started to sway heavily and in the distance you could see lightning flashes.

'I'm glad I'm not in Becca's car,' Steven said, looking over his shoulder to the car behind.

A few minutes later, we approached the top cable car station and I could see the colour returning to Mike's cheeks.

'We have a problem here, folks,' said the man, helping us off at the other end. 'There's a big storm and you need to move from the platform and on to the second floor where you'll be safe.'

With that, he slammed the door shut and the whole ride came to a shuddering halt.

'What about the people behind?' I said.

'You were the last ones,' he said, peering over his big-rimmed glasses at me. His hand clutched a walkie-talkie.

'There's four people from our party in the car behind,' I said, rattling the words out.

'Hey, Steven, Becca's car has stopped,' said Mike. 'She'll be really scared now.'

Steven's eyes widened. 'Yes, she will, should we ask them to leave her there?'

The man wandered off to the front of the building and peered out as lightning lit up the sky.

'Please,' I said. 'There are four people in the car behind.' He pressed a button and the engines juddered into life and within a minute Rebecca, Jodie, Ryan and Martyn's car had arrived.

'You okay?' I said, as they stepped out.

Rebecca pulled a face.

The sky blackened and with no lighting it was only possible to see the outlines of people until another bolt lit the room. The cracks were really loud. Steven snuggled up close into my shoulder on the verge of tears.

'Don't worry, young man,' said the cable car operator. 'We get one of these up here every so often. It'll soon be over.'

'I'm scared, Mum,' said Steven.

'We're safe here,' I said, and at that very second a bolt hit the building itself. The cable car operator, who had moved to the room's edge and had been standing with his back to the window, instinctively jumped forward a yard, his body crouching, head dropping down and shoulders hunching up as if he was protecting himself from invisible blows.

'Woah, this is as big as we've ever had,' he said, trying to regain his composure. 'The café say all the light bulbs have been blown.'

'He's not exactly reassuring us, is he?' Rebecca said.

'We're doomed,' Mike said, mimicking Frazer from *Dad's Army*. I glared at him.

'Mum, I'm really scared,' Steven said, snuggling in closer. Another bolt hit the building, rattling every window and shaking the floor, and the cable car operator jumped again in a more exaggerated fashion.

Steven whimpered and a silence fell over the room. It was the storm's last hurrah. Within twenty minutes blue sky started to appear again.

'Jane, have you seen the road?' Ryan said.

I looked out of the window. The hailstones had completely covered the surface of the road. Patches of mist hung over the trees throughout the lower levels as if tens of forest fires had begun. 'Highways will have the snow ploughs out soon enough,' the cable car operator said. 'It can be awfully treacherous in these conditions. If you look there,' he pointed down the road, 'they're still clearing up a car wreck from yesterday.'

His walkie-talkie crackled into life and he held it to his ear. He turned to us. 'I'm sorry but the storm's frayed the cable. It's gonna be out of action for some time. You can either walk down, which I wouldn't recommend, or come down in a four-by-four.'

Steven's face lit up. 'A four-by-four!' he said.

Day 26 – Monday, 24 July
Monarch Pass, Colo. to Westcliffe, Colo.
61.0 miles – 4 hrs 34 mins
Total covered – 1537.8 miles

MIKE

The rock tumbled slowly down the rock face like a meteor, with smaller debris following in its wake. Its trajectory brought it to a standstill a few yards in front of the RV; simultaneously my foot slammed on the brake.

'Fuck!' I swung the RV to the right but the near-side tyre hit the rock and the RV started shuddering.

'Dad! Dad!' Steven shouted from the back, as I gripped the steering wheel as tight as possible, causing my whole upper body to shake. To the right, the rock face looked intimidating and to the left was a wall with a fifty-foot drop to the Arkansas River. We weaved towards the verge, leaving the tarmac, and the whole RV rattled like a derailed train. Steven screamed. The rock face loomed as I turned the wheel trying to ensure that the rig didn't topple over.

We ground to a standstill with the sound of metal tearing against the concrete. My arms were rigid against the wheel.

'What's happened, Mike?' Jodie said, jolting me back to reality.

'It's all right, Steven, we're okay,' Rebecca comforted her brother. I undid my belt, waited until there was a gap in the traffic and left the vehicle.

'You can't leave that fucking rig there, you asshole,' a red-faced man shouted out of the open window of his pickup. 'Some fucker's gonna get killed.'

'I'm just checking the damage!' my voice croaked.

'Move the fucking RV, you motherfucker.'

I was aware that my body was shaking as I walked in front of the RV and saw that the passenger wheel was shredded, only the flimsiest remnant of rubber remained. In the background was the constant drone of 'Move the fucking rig, motherfucker'. The man pulled into a lay-by across the road and exited his vehicle. I looked under the RV and there was a pool of liquid. I tried to reach far enough to touch it, sure it was water from the air conditioning but I wasn't 100 per cent convinced.

The main RV door opened. 'What's happening?' Rebecca said, with Steven beside her on the step.

'Get back inside!' I screamed, but within seconds reconsidered. 'No, no, forget that. Let's get across the road to where we'll be safer.'

After shepherding them to safety, I looked for a convenient

place to move the vehicle. The pickup driver was now directing traffic around it, but this didn't hinder his ability to continue hurling advice in my direction.

Within a couple of minutes, a Highways officer pulled up. 'Good day,' he said to me, before adding 'Hiya' to the kids. Strangely, the pickup driver had stopped shouting.

'What's the problem?' asked the officer, walking over to where I was standing. His brown uniform blended in with the rock face behind so that his body looked as though it had been carved out of the rock face itself.

'A blowout as a result of the falling rock,' I said.

'Wooahh,' he said and bent down to inspect the tyre.

The pickup driver called over, 'You need to get him to move that goddamn rig or there'll be an accident.'

'Not sure whether we can, there's liquid underneath,' the officer said. He radioed in while walking across the road.

'How are you folks?' he asked the children. Tears were streaming down Steven's cheeks.

'We'll have you sorted out soon enough, don't worry.' He turned to me. 'Have you arranged a breakdown truck? You'll need to say you've got a small RV.'

'I'm just gonna phone,' I said. Not unusually, the Verizon mobile had no signal. I extended the aerial of the SAT phone but with the huge rock face in front of us, I had to walk 200 yards up the road until one bar lit up. The Cruise America emergency line was a call centre and I joined the interminable queue. After ten minutes the phone crackled into life.

'Hello?'

'Hello? We've had a blowout on a busy road and we're blocking it,' I said.

'I can't hear you too well. Ring back.' The phone beeped and went dead.

'Fuck,' I muttered and wandered back. A county sheriff's car with two officers pulled up alongside the Highways guy's.

'What's occurring?' the passenger asked his colleague from Highways.

'A blowout. They pulled over and got out.'

'We're responding to a stabbing but it'll have to wait. You ordered a truck?'

'No, the British guy is just ringing the breakdown company.'

'You say you need a big rig,' one of the county sheriffs said, while his colleague went to help with traffic direction. 'You've got a big rig so you'll need a suitably equipped breakdown truck.'

'I can't get through.'

'We need to get this rig moved.'

They all moved back across the road, examined the liquid and the sheriffs decided to allow me to drive across to the small verge where the kids were standing. Within minutes they'd phoned their centre and arranged for a breakdown truck to attend.

'It's gonna take some time, they're sixty miles away,' the sheriff said.

For forty minutes I unsuccessfully waited for Cruise America's emergency call centre to answer their phones.

Jodie, Rebecca and Steven were now safely back in the RV, although without the air conditioning the temperature was becoming uncomfortable. While one sheriff directed the traffic, the other stood with me chatting about our journey as well as his time in Europe while in the forces and the state of America. It was with some relief the SAT phone started to beep.

I phoned Cindy. Her phone was off. I left a message. I also left messages with the cyclists hoping that the other RV would return to collect Rebecca, Jodie and Steven.

When my phone rang, I presumed Cindy had listened to her voice mails and was getting in touch. So I was a little startled when I heard a man's voice.

'Hello, Mike, it's John Shanley. How are things?' John is the chief executive of Sparks, one of the benefiting charities and Michael's boss.

John was sitting in his London office at the end of the working day, trying to catch up with us on our journey. I quickly appraised him of the situation.

'Leave it with me,' said John. 'I'll call Cruise America and try to contact Jane and Cindy.'

'Progress?' the sheriff asked, as I put the phone down.

I nodded. 'I hope so. It was someone sensible in London with a land line so we should get some progress.'

'You know if you were French we wouldn't help you, would we, Tony?' he shouted across to his colleague, who was busy pointing and gesticulating to drivers.

'What?' he shouted.

'I said if they were French we wouldn't help.'

'God no, we would certainly not.'

'Why?' I felt compelled to ask

'Can't stand the French, no friends of America, not like your President Tony Blair. Now that's what we call a fine man, a real friend to America.'

'It's a beautiful place, France,' I added.

'I went to Paris once, never met as rude a people anywhere. No, the French are not welcome here.'

A police motorcycle approached, its side panniers gave it the width of a small car. It glided towards us and halted. The sheriff turned to me. 'This is a state patrolman, he'll be in charge now. You need a state patrolman to agree for a breakdown truck to attend because they won't come to calls from the public for their own safety and to ensure they get paid.'

The motorcyclist lifted his leg over the bike like a modern-day John Wayne; a gun in its holster hung just over his hip. His pristine blue shirt, gleaming insignia and spotless bike suggested more a military presence than one of law enforcement.

'Where's the truck?' he said, after checking out the RV.

'It'll be an hour,' Tony said.

'An hour? Where's it coming from?'

'There's not a breakdown outfit locally that'll cater for a big rig.'

'Big rig? I'll show you a big rig. I've a sixty-footer at home. This is – what . . .' He moved away to peruse. 'Thirty feet,' he shouted across. 'This is a small rig. It just needs a normal truck. Any problems, you tell control I told you.'

The sheriff rolled his eyes. 'It's big,' he whispered.

The patrolman came over, formally introduced himself and went to check the road.

'Where's Highways? This road needs cleaning, get them here now,' the state patrolman barked at the sheriff. He turned to me. 'You were lucky. A lot of people out here could have ended up in the river or the rock face, well done. This often happens after rains like yesterday, especially after how hot it's been.'

The accident form cost us $20 and once he'd checked my insurance, driving licence and passport he showed Steven around his bike.

Steven repeated a request he'd made to the two sheriffs for an interview. They'd told him they were unable to do media interviews but the patrolman had no such restrictions.

The satellite phone beeped again. I answered it.

'Mike, it's John. I can't get through to Cruise America; there's no answer, it's just a long call centre queue.'

'Some emergency system. They've been less than useless since day one.'

'I have spoken to Cindy, though, and the cyclists are on their way to you.'

Within a minute, the second RV appeared, followed a minute later by Lia, who pulled up adjacent to the stricken RV and on the northbound carriageway. The patrolman, Randy, shouted across, 'Move that goddamn car.' Lia looked perplexed so the patrolman marched purposefully towards her. 'You! Lady! Get that goddamn vehicle off my road.' She looked shocked and a moment later he barked 'Now, woman' with such ferocity that I felt surprised it didn't cause another rockfall. 'Now or I'll book you.'

His hand moved towards his holster and Lia, looking very confused, moved on. Within a couple of minutes she'd gone up the road, turned round and returned, trying to squeeze the car on to the outer edge of the lay-by where there was just slightly not enough room.

'You!' said the patrolman again, pointing at Lia. 'You move that goddamn vehicle or I'm going to arrest you now, woman.'

Lia looked like a rabbit caught in the headlights. She inched away down the road before disappearing completely.

As Jane approached, I could see the alarm register on her face. 'I was worried,' she said. 'All you said in your voice mail was you'd had an accident.' With the relief came the tears.

Steven looked up. 'It's all right, Mummy,' he said, as she hugged us both.

The patrolman thrust his card into my hand, informing me if the breakdown truck didn't arrive in an hour I was to phone him. In the event, there was no need, as within ten minutes the mechanic arrived.

'Who called this in as a small rig?' were his first words. 'I don't have the tools for a rig this size.'

Across from us in the river, a dog barked and leapt about in the torrents.

'How far have you got left to cycle?' I asked Jane.

'About ten miles,' she said. I could imagine how frustrating this detour was for her. She should have finished two hours ago and now she was hanging around in cold, damp cycling gear knowing that whatever time the RV was fixed she would have to remount.

'You could call it a day.'

'We'll see what time we get away. We'd already done some unnecessary miles because we took a wrong turning so it has just been a completely frustrating day.' Making unnecessary detours on a 4000-mile trip was always going to be inevitable over the nine weeks but they still led to friction.

It took four hours from the near-miss to finally getting back on the road and by that time my nerves were shredded. I'd not eaten anything or hydrated sufficiently and was shaking as I got back into the driver's seat and took the wheel. My confidence had evaporated and with excessive caution I inched down the road to the frustration of other motorists.

We reached the RV park, which was a little way outside the town of Westcliffe, at 4 p.m. The park was in an isolated area a couple of miles from the town. The mountains some miles over the plain were a looming presence as the clouds hung low in the sky and the lightning flashed.

We were relieved to know this was our last major day of

mountains. We always felt that once the Rockies had been crossed that the hardest part of the ride was over.

Yet in the back of my mind was the fact that although Colorado might almost be finished, the worst of the journey still lay ahead.

CHAPTER 5

Day 27 – Tuesday, 25 July
Westcliffe, Colo. to Pueblo, Colo.
55.1 miles – 4 hrs 18 mins
Total covered – 1592.9 miles

MIKE

'What are they laughing at?' Rebecca said, referring to a group of motley individuals standing at the entrance to the street.

'Us, I think,' Jodie replied.

Since leaving the Interstate 25 the area had become grim, tacky and dirty. We were surrounded by prefab houses and trailer parks with drab industrial land spread out to our right.

'Are you sure we are on the right road?' Rebecca asked.

'Well, I suggest not getting out and asking,' said Jane. She was sitting in the passenger seat. It was odd suddenly having to share the driving space with another adult after several hundred miles with only the kids for company.

'Why?' asked Rebecca.

'Check out the locals. The wheels would be off before we parked.' Around us, were gangs of bored-looking youths, their eyes following the RV like a scavenger would a shipwreck.

'Why are they laughing and pointing though?' asked Rebecca.

'I've a bad feeling about this,' said Jane.

As if on cue, the Tom Tom burst into life. 'You have reached your destination,' it said, as the chequered flag appeared on the screen.

I looked at Jane. 'We could look for another park,' I said quietly. 'But I think we're stuck in this shit hole.'

'I think they're laughing because they know the park,' Jodie said, pointing to the entrance up ahead. It was built like Stalag 15. A high wire fence surrounded a car park the size of six football pitches. Apart from a toilet block and what seemed to be a prison accommodation hut in the centre with several RVs around it, it was empty. We drove forward. At the entrance were stairs leading up to an office. Behind that, was the park's only attraction, a small outdoor swimming pool, although I couldn't imagine anyone wanting to use it.

'I'm not surprised they were laughing,' Jane said.

'It's horrible,' Steven said.

'It'll be all right once you're accustomed to it,' I said. There was a collective groan. 'Come on, it'll be okay.'

'Yeah, right,' Steven said.

'If you're so enamoured, you can check us in, Mike,' Jane said.

'Anyone want to come in?'

'You're joking, right?' Steven said.

It was hard to imagine that only this morning I'd seen a wild bear foraging for food at the side of the road as we descended San Isabel National Forest from Westcliffe to Pueblo. I'd let out an exaggerated girly yelp followed by 'Look out!'

Jodie, Rebecca and Steven, fearing another close encounter with falling rocks, had shrieked and taken a brace position. As soon as the bear had heard the RV engine it had scurried into the forest.

For the last ten miles of the journey, the plains had spread out before us like a fawn-coloured ocean. It was as if we'd descended to sea level but we were still a mile high. The landscape looked as though someone had shaken a sheet and ripples of land spread over miles. Initially there were little ridges and then it became totally flat. We'd known we'd have to get down to the town early to buy a new tyre and then change the spare before travelling to Denver in preparation for Jodie and Rebecca to fly home. For Rebecca, Pueblo was a return to civilisation and a Starbucks, last seen four weeks and a thousand miles previously.

'Hi!' a late middle-aged lady looked up to greet me as I entered the park kiosk. There was a counter at chest height over which were spread dozens of leaflets of local tourist attractions. A few feet behind the counter was an open door to a similar sized office, complete with the familiar accessories of a desk top, phone and calendar.

'Do you have a reservation for Tomlinson?' I asked.

'Are you English?'

'Yes, how do you know? Most people think we're Australian.'

'Howard! There are some people from England.'

A portly man with tattooed forearms came into view.

'How are you?' he said, stretching out his hand. 'Which part of the country are you from?'

'Leeds.'

'Bloody hell, marching on together, eh? Bremner, Hunter and Charlton before your time, I guess.'

His pronounced Essex accent was becoming stronger by the second.

'Not at all. Where do you come from?'

''Ave a guess.'

'Essex?'

'Sarfend to be precise,' he said.

I explained Jane's trip across the USA and said that Steven was filming occasionally for television, 'Would you do an interview for him?' I said.

Howard looked a little perplexed. 'Right, TV you say, what channel?'

'ITV.'

'What you get up norf, Yorkshire is it?'

'Yes, but this may be for the ITN news nationally.'

'Oh, don't know 'bout that, don't want the folks at home to know where I am. No, don't think so, mate.' It was hard to ascertain whether this was humour or a genuine concern.

'He's only nine,' I said. 'The chances are it won't get shown and it's only a camcorder he's using.'

He stood pondering, as if weighing up the options. 'Look, ask him to come down later this afternoon and we'll see.'

Day 28 – Wednesday, 26 July
Pueblo
Rest day

MIKE

The sound of the RV door reverberated throughout the room and I stretched my arm across the bed in the darkness to where Jane's body should be. I recoiled as I hit the damp patch, spreading out like a liquid Turin shroud.

Outside, the sound of Jane retching broke the early morning silence. The noises were so deep that they conjured up images of my grandfather coughing up masses of coal-dust phlegm and spitting them on the open fire. It was a sound that would strike fear into an army.

I pulled back the flimsy curtains but could see nothing. There was rustling in the living area. Jodie and Rebecca must also have heard it.

'Are you all right?' I asked, as Jane returned and sat down at the bed's edge.

'Not really.'

'Are you getting in?'

'It's too wet.' Her hand rustled the pillow. 'Yuk.'

'Here, you have this side.' I turned her pillow over and rolled over as far as possible until I was perched like a diver at the edge of a high board.

'I'll be glad to get out of here,' she said.

'I know.'

'I want to go and get a shower but it just doesn't feel safe.' Although the block was only seventy yards away neither Jane or the girls had the confidence to walk across the almost deserted car park.

Jane sat down tentatively on the bed before inching her legs up, as though they were shackled to the floor.

The drive from Pueblo to Denver had looked simple enough, straight up Interstate 25, but the road surface was the worst I'd ever seen for a major road route. It was littered with roadworks, potholes large enough to have been spotted from space. Jane's back had taken more hammering on the fifty miles of interstate than it had in the last ten days of cycling.

After we dropped the girls off at Denver Airport there was a palpable melancholy in the RV. Jane shed a quiet tear. She moved her hand to wipe her eyes.

'Are you okay?' I said.

'I'd be better if I was on the plane as well,' she said dryly.

'She won't even give us a second thought; she'll not even think to give us a call when she gets home.'

'She will,' Jane said, without conviction. I turned across and gave her a quizzical look.

'Perhaps.'

A low cloud of grey fog hung over the city, which seemed to be emphasised by the clear blue sky around it and the stunning backdrop of the Rockies' eastern edge.

'I'm amazed that a country with so much space is so polluted,' Jane said.

'Maybe it's the space that is the problem, maybe there's too much of it.'

My mind was taken back to Leeds and my morning commutes on days when a similar, if smaller, cloud hung over the town.

We managed to get back to the campsite in Pueblo by mid-afternoon. I called over to see Cindy as I'd asked her to get us some supplies for both RVs.

'Bread and milk.' She handed me a carrier bag.

'Thanks,' I said.

'How's Jane? Did Becca and Jodie get away okay?'

'Yes, they did. Jane's been very unwell. Very nauseous this morning and we haven't managed to get any food down her.

Anyway, she's lying down with a blinding headache. I think it's as a result of dehydration.'

'I'll come and say hello,' Cindy said.

Jane was zonked on the bed.

'Hiya, Jane,' said Cindy. 'Would you like some grapes? Will that help? Mike asked me to stock up and I've got lots of fruit in my RV.'

'That would be kind,' said Jane and Cindy departed. 'Are we stocked up as well then, Mike?'

'Well, not exactly, but let's not go there, eh?'

Jane looked dreadful, as white as a sheet, her eyes struggling to open at all. Her blouse hung loose as if she'd borrowed the clothes from a much bigger woman. She reached for a water bottle and took a minuscule sip.

It was an hour later when a rap at the door announced Martyn's arrival.

'Hello!' he said with a chirpy, childlike grin. Under his arm was a large road atlas of the USA.

'Hiya, Martyn,' Steven said.

After our conversation in Dolores about increasing the number of rest days in the trip, nothing had actually changed. But with Jane's health continuing to decline sharply, we knew we had to take it more seriously. Martyn laid down the atlas on the table in the RV.

'To accommodate more rest days we either need to delay the finish or shorten the journey,' I said.

'I'm not finishing later than the first of September,' said Jane. 'If we fall behind schedule I'm giving up.'

Martyn's smile switched to an expression of studious concern and there was a business-like approach to his laying out the map.

'One of the problems is that it's impossible to get a feel of the route because the area to be covered is too large. You look at one page, follow a route you think is fine then five pages later you realise you're three hundred miles south of where you need to be.'

We all studied quietly as the heavens cracked like the whip

across a horse's backside. I rose to turn on the lights and within seconds drops of rain the size of marbles were pounding the RV.

Jane looked across. 'We need to head north-east in Kansas.'

'I agree,' said Martyn. 'We can definitely save miles. The TransAmerica map takes us across the Appalachians to Richmond. We need to find a gap to the north.'

'I think we need an extra five rest days,' I added unhelpfully.

'If we aim for a rest day every six days as opposed to ten it should sort it and reduce the average miles per day by ten,' Jane said.

'You won't have maps, though,' I said. 'You could follow the original route, finishing a week late.'

Jane looked at me sternly. 'I'm not finishing late.'

'No one will mind if you're a week late.'

'I don't give a fuck about anyone else. I just don't want to miss Suzanne's due date.'

The biblical rain provided a momentary welcome distraction as outside it was as dark as if there was a total eclipse. I opened the door and the park had turned into a lake.

As the maps were ordered into states, it was almost impossible to plot out an accurate route. We needed a huge map of America with all the routes.

Jane studied the maps again.

'So if we follow the TransAmerica route out of Colorado as opposed to exiting Kansas by the south-east, we go northwards to the city.'

'What about the next rest day?' I said.

'Kansas City would be sensible if we could get there by Saturday week,' Jane said.

'What's the point of that? It's ten days' cycling. We're meant to be making things easier, it must be six hundred miles by that route.'

'Okay, get back in your box. We'll fit one in next Monday,' Jane said. The rain was now drowning out the generator and the thunderstorm showed no signs of abating. 'I feel like shit, we need to get some miles in the bag because if I keep deteriorating like this we won't get anywhere near New York.'

'Even so, it's ambitious to try to get to Kansas City by a week Saturday.' I looked at Martyn.

'It's very difficult to work out all the mileages; it's a vast land and we can only estimate.'

I took hold of the atlas and turned to the rear where the whole continent was stretched over two pages. I folded an A4 piece of paper in half and with a pencil drew a straight line from Pueblo to New York. 'If we use that as a basis we won't go too far wrong.'

'I love the scientific approach, Mike,' Martyn said. Jane was looking at me as if I'd lost the plot.

'I'm not saying follow it but if we don't deviate too much we won't go far wrong.'

It was ambitious to think that Martyn and Jane could fathom a new route in an hour when they'd looked at maps throughout the winter. Still, everyone was agreed the original planned route was out of the window and we'd be going to New York as near as possible on a crow's path. Hopefully this would save 300 to 400 miles on the entire trip.

Day 29 – Thursday, 27 July
Pueblo, Colo. to Ordway, Colo.
54.9 miles – 4 hrs 39 mins
Total covered – 1647.8 miles

JANE

Having spent most of the previous day being sick and suffering from a throbbing headache, I was unable to get a real grip on my pain. When I woke up next morning, my back was aching and my mouth felt dry.

'Just fifty-five miles today,' I said, and Ryan and Martyn both agreed without question. I was not prepared to push myself.

The journey would take us out of Pueblo and into the flatlands of eastern Colorado. Pueblo, with a population of 100 000, was easily the biggest conurbation we'd been to since Sacramento.

As we set off, the journey involved riding alongside a busy four-lane highway so there were always two lanes of heavy traffic at our side. Each time we came to a junction we had to stop, look over our left shoulder, and see what oncoming traffic was going to race right in front of us. It was frightening. The oncoming vehicles could just sweep us off the bikes if we weren't careful. Fourteen miles outside of Pueblo the road divided and we left Highway 50 and went down the much quieter 96 and we soon stopped at Boone.

There wasn't a lot there but Martyn managed to come out of the general store smiling like the Cheshire Cat.

'Ryan, Jane, have you seen this?' He clutched a small leaflet.

'What is it?'

'The store owner's quite a character. A Gulf War vet. Anyway, he gave me this leaflet which gives photos of severe weather conditions which we need to look out for.' Martyn held out the leaflet which had pictures of four severe weather formations: Mammatus, Tornado, Wall Cloud and Shelf Cloud.

I took the leaflet from him and scanned it. 'How comforting to know that they have to warn us – and after the storms we've seen in the last seven days.'

I read on. 'If I see anything looking like that,' I said, pointing to one of the pictures, 'I'm off the bike and in the storm ditch.'

As we made our way up the 96 we first passed the Crowley County Correctional Facility before reaching the small town of Crowley where Mike was waiting for us with Steven. As we stopped for a coffee there was a group of people sitting talking in a play area.

'Have you seen the guy in the flesh-coloured T-shirt,' Martyn said.

'He's humongous,' Steven said.

It was impossible to disagree. The man looked wider than he was tall. Martyn surreptitiously put his camera to his eye and from some distance homed in on the group, who were an eclectic bunch of either extremely fat or skinny men with ladies who looked like a collection of bedraggled ageing hippies with scraggly ponytails and tie-dyed T-shirts.

'We need to make a move,' I said. I put my sunglasses on and strapped on my helmet.

'They're coming over,' Steven said. We watched as a few of the group crossed the road, while Martyn moved to the store doorway, camera still shooting.

'Hi there, are you having a good day?' a portly silver-haired gentleman said with a broad smile. His red T-shirt had a logo in a vertical oval containing the words College Heights Baptist Church and three crosses. We quickly exchanged pleasantries and some words about our trip before the conversation moved on.

'We're from Texas, visiting the folks here in Colorado to tell them about how great the Lord is.'

'It seems a long way to come,' I said.

'Well, it's important work and we need to spread the news. Do you walk with the Lord?' he said.

I treated it as a rhetorical question, wheeled the bike forward a little and looked down and smirked at Steven, who was pointing his camcorder directly at me.

The journey to Ordway was quickly completed with only the occasional message of 'Reelect Miles Clark for Sheriff' breaking up the telegraph poles. The roads were good and clean and we were able to use the shoulder to cycle on.

There was a slow stream of traffic but none of it bothered us and the drivers were courteous. As we came into Ordway the skyline was dominated by a rusting grain tower, while trees edged both sides of the road except where a functional light business unit stood.

A green road sign said 'Ordway City limit elev. 4312ft' and to the right a cheaply built slab bungalow stood on a large plot, with a pickup and saloon parked under a car port. The land was dry and dusty, there was a sense that it wouldn't be easy to eke out a living here. Next to it was a rundown property.

We approached the crossroads on the far side of town where the 71 and 96 met and I saw Mike, Steven, Cindy, Lia and Dan. A white six-by-six in front of a scrapyard preached 'STAND UP STAND UP FOR JESUS'. A selection of trucks and trailers were parked up nearby. It was not an attractive sight.

'Hi,' Mike said, as I dismounted on the forecourt of the gas station by his RV. Cindy was just walking back from the kiosk.

'Where's Cindy's RV?' I said.

'Cindy got here first. They said she was getting in the way so was told to move on, so she's parked up round the back.'

As if on cue, Cindy rounded the corner. 'Wow, guys, that was cheap, fifteen dollars for the night or thirty dollars for the month.'

'Climb in, Jane, we'll get parked up so we don't piss off the drivers.'

The RV park was completely empty and litter was strewn everywhere. Mike drove down the rows looking for a suitable plot but each one had its own problem and the site was in a complete state of disrepair.

'This is completely scummy, Jane,' he said, getting out of the cab. He inspected the pitches, checking the electricity, water and sewage, before reluctantly parking in the least inappropriate place.

As we stopped, I opened the door and noticed a sea of red ants crawling like a moving carpet. I stood transfixed and within seconds they were crawling up my legs.

'Urgh, get off, you little buggers.' I shook my legs. 'Steven, shut the door quickly. Mike!'

'Look at this, Jane. I don't think this pitch has been used this millennium. Even at thirty dollars for the month it looks like it's way overpriced.'

'Weren't there any other options?'

'No.'

I went to film the daily blog for Martyn and he quickly departed with Lia and Dan for their motel in Rocky Ford. My heart sank as I walked around the back of the gas station and saw the two RVs parked in what looked like an extension of the scrapyard. Around the side of the park was fixed caravan accommodation. They looked shabby and dirty. Several dogs were roaming around.

'It's only for one night,' I told myself, but we were in effect marooned in the middle of a dodgy area unable to open the RV door because of the insects.

'Hi, Ryan!' I called. He was just attaching the bikes to the back of the RV. 'Make sure they're secure.'

I looked across and noticed a tall, silvery haired man standing just behind some bushes. His hair was just long enough to protrude from his cowboy hat, which was crammed down on his forehead to shade his face. I whispered to Ryan, 'Have you seen that guy?'

'Where?' Ryan followed my eyeline and spotted him. The man didn't move. 'That's freaky.'

The man was dressed in black and looked typecast for the role of killer in a modern-day western.

'I really don't like this place. I think we should just move and write the thirty dollars off,' I said. Slowly, the man moved away, shielded by the bushes, but he continued studying us intensely.

'Nothing normally scares me but I'm really not comfortable here. You won't find me begging to stay,' Ryan said. 'He's spooking me.'

Mike arrived from behind the RV.

'Hi.'

'We should move accommodation, Mike,' I said. His eyes followed mine.

'I see you've found a serial killer,' he said. 'I'll unhook us now and ring Lia and get directions to the motel. Even the car park would be better than this.'

We drove to Rocky Ford where the Sky crew were staying. As we pulled into town, Mike slowed down to ask for directions.

'Are you a terrorist?' The man stared at Mike through the open window of the RV, his eyes scouring for any evidence that he was some kind of insurgent. It seemed an odd response to the question of: 'Can you direct me to the High Chaparral?' which was a surreal enough question in itself.

'No,' Mike said, pointedly.

'Are you sure?' he said with some intensity.

'No, I'm an English visitor,' Mike responded.

He seemed satisfied with that but carried on peering through the window. 'It's a good job you're not French, they're all terrorists.'

Mike raised his foot off the brake and we slowly moved forward and away.

'Wanker,' Mike muttered under his breath.

The High Chapparal was a beautiful motel – in stark contrast to the RV park. We'd been on the road for four weeks so this was the first night we were going to have such luxurious accommodation. We pulled up and the owner allowed us to book two rooms, one for ourselves and one for Ryan. Cindy was happy to stay in the RV.

I opened the hotel room door and immediately felt my shoulders relax. It was a little haven. Just to feel the cool of the air conditioning was paradise. The Savoy wouldn't have felt any better. I had a quick snoop around. I could hardly contain my smile when I noticed the well-sized bath and even a television, all the things we hadn't had for a month. I thought I'd died and gone to heaven.

Steven was especially overjoyed with the television. He ran over, switched it on and just sat there for the whole of the afternoon gorging himself on trashy television.

Without getting bathed or changed, we headed across the road to a burger bar. I felt yucky from the ride and contaminated from the RV park but we needed some sustenance quickly.

California had its In and Out burgers, this area of Colorado had Sonic burgers. I looked at the menu and thought I could eat anything – the cycling had rekindled my appetite and as I'd barely eaten for forty-eight hours there was a large hole to fill.

We sat outside and ordered our food through the intercom. When it arrived, it looked awful. Unappetising slabs of brown meat with congealed cheese, limp lettuce and burnt bun. It didn't matter – I ate the whole thing and practically licked the plate.

Day 30 – Friday, 28 July
Ordway, Colo. to Eads, Colo.
60.8 miles – 5 hrs 14 mins
Total covered – 1708.6 miles

MIKE

Leaving the High Chaparral next morning, Steven and I felt suitably refreshed after our first night in a motel.

'You should stop and get a melon as you leave town,' the owner said, giving me $40 change from a $100 traveller's cheque. At $30 a room, the motel had been cheaper than many RV parks and substantially more civilised. What a joy it was not to have to dump the sewage in the morning and to merely climb aboard and turn the key. 'It's the melon capital of the world,' he added.

I looked at him, bemused. 'What is?' I said, waiting for the punch line.

'Rocky Ford is famous for its melons – cantaloupes especially.'

'Really?' I said. I like a nice melon but at nine in the morning I didn't feel the need to go and hunt one down.

'Oh yes, you'll find various people selling them at the roadside. You can't visit Rocky Ford without trying one, there's nothing like it. We even have a watermelon day at the Arkansas Valley Fayre.'

'I thought this was Colorado,' I said.

'Oh, it is,' he said.

We left but I'd enjoyed the few hours in the town. Dominated by the railway, which ran straight through the centre, we'd watched as goods trains, which could be half a mile long, came through, the driver sounding the horn every few yards, presumably to clear the track as it was easy to cross at any point.

Our route took us back along Highway 50 which we would be saying goodbye to for hopefully the last time.

'There's the "Stand up for Jesus" sign,' said Steven, as we passed back through Ordway. Although it wasn't really much of a town, the townsfolk had clearly not had their faith diminished.

In no time at all we were making quick progress down the 96 and into Sugar City. You would expect the word 'City' to indicate a thriving metropolis, but we'd come to realise that in the USA it could mean little more than two houses with several hundred yards between them.

The Sugar City grain tower dominated the skyline for miles. At only 200 feet high, it was at least 180 feet higher than its nearest challenger. It was a quaint town. A thirty-foot historic

Union Pacific train car was permanently stationed in a small lush park, visible by its immaculate vivid yellow paintwork and red lettering and roof. The sun was shining and there were only the merest wisps of cloud; the conditions were perfect for the cyclists. Although once midday arrived the humidity and wind would rise so it was essential to start and finish early.

Sugar City was named after the town's sugar beet factory. Situated on the Missouri Pacific Railroad, the factory had closed in 1967 and the one-time population of 1500 was now down to less than 300. Lake Meredith to the south and Lake Henry to the north meant it was well irrigated.

I'd naively assumed that we'd have a wider choice of accommodation once we'd finished travelling through the deserts of Utah and Nevada. As it turned out, there was as much chance of finding a local RV park in the Colorado plains as locating an honest man in Parliament.

Our scheduled stop was in Eads, some twenty-five miles from a suitable campsite so I moved ahead of the riders to suss out the town. We passed the cyclists and Jane looked to be cycling comfortably, although the flat stages of the ride would cause their own problems. For one, it would mean Jane would remain in the same position throughout the day, which would result in some parts of her body getting no respite. She preferred some slight hills to allow her back to rest in a new position which would relieve some of the stiffness. But the flipside was that the average miles per hour were increasing and the amount of hours in the saddle was reducing.

Again, dominated by a grain tower, Ead's architecture seemed to be modelled on a five-year-old's Lego set. It would have been hard to design an uglier set of buildings. Many were white-washed concrete slabs with windows blacked out. There were rundown shops whose signs had missing letters and overhead was a mishmash of radio masts, telegraph poles and pylons.

I drove through, not really wishing to spend more than twenty minutes there but settled on parking in the forecourt of the Econolodge – a typical double-storey motel with car parking directly outside its rooms.

'Is this where we're stopping, Dad?' Steven asked, scrabbling to his feet.

'I don't know.'

'It looks okay.'

'We'll see,' I said. It seemed too easy and comfortable. The point of having the RVs in the first place had been to control costs. Corporate sponsorship which Ryan had arranged was paying for the trip, but the more money we saved, the more that would go to good causes and I felt uneasy about another night in a hotel. The fundraising had been abysmal – we'd raised less than £10,000 in the month so far.

'Let's have a peep in the rooms,' I said.

We strolled across the almost deserted car park. Only one silver Buick pickup was parked outside reception.

'What do you think?' I said to Steven as we peered inside the window of a room. The brown polyester bed quilts reminded me of home in my teens. I contemplated the pros and cons, convenience over cost. But I was feeling particularly indecisive so decided to brew up in the RV.

'Dad! Dad! Phone!' Steven handed me the mobile.

'Hi, Dad!' My heart leapt on hearing Suzanne's voice.

'How are you?' I asked.

'Good, good. Everyone's well. Has Rebecca rung or emailed?'

'No.'

'She got home and went up to Settle. She seems well, tired but okay. Jodie's parents dropped her off.'

'Fantastic,' I said. It was typical of Suzanne. She knew we'd worry about Rebecca and I marvelled at her maturity. Rebecca's own thoughts meanwhile would have already moved on to the next thing – summer with her grandma in Settle. 'Thanks for letting us know,' I said.

'We saw Steven's report on the news. How's Mum?' she asked.

'Tired, losing weight, in a lot of pain but in reasonable spirits.' I chose my words like a politician.

'She looked dreadful, Dad. Both grandmas can see. People are worried and everyone's asking.'

'Don't worry, she'll be fine.'

I could hear the concern in her voice. 'Dad, are you sure?'

'No. But I won't let her push herself too far.'

Suzanne laughed. 'Yeah right, like she'll take any notice of you.'

'She hangs on my every word,' I smiled and Suzanne guffawed loudly as I handed her over to Steven.

Jane arrived sooner than expected, only twenty minutes later.

'Is the accommodation sorted?' she asked, taking a huge gulp from the small can of recovery drink.

'It's a shit hole here,' I lied, in the hope that Jane would take the statement at face value.

'We're going to the KOA at Lamar just down the road.'

Jane's face dropped.

'How far?' she asked.

'About twenty-five minutes' drive,' I said, knowing full well that it would take about double that.

'Are you sure it's not suitable here?' she said.

'We've looked, haven't we, Steven?'

'Yes,' he said, without moving his eyes from his laptop. I felt that if we stayed a second consecutive night in a motel, we'd get used to the convenience and costs would spiral.

We set off to Lamar. Twenty-five minutes turned into forty-five and justifying not using the Econolodge was frustrating Jane. Her constant tutting and acerbic comments started to disconcert me.

'How far now, Mike?'

'Two minutes,' I said, knowing it was nearer ten.

'Five miles that sign said.' Jane made no attempt to hide her frustration.

'The camp's a couple of miles this side of town.'

'You mean we're not even in town, so we are marooned on an RV park.'

'It's a KOA.'

'Whoopy do,' Jane said and Steven laughed from the back. 'Mike, this is ridiculous, I'll have to get up an hour earlier tomorrow.'

'Yes, but you wouldn't have settled in that motel,' I said, praying that Steven did not tell her how comfortable it really looked.

Day 31 – Saturday, 29 July
Eads, Colo. to Tribune, Kansas (Kan.)
57.2 miles – 4 hrs 33 mins
Total covered – 1765.8 miles

MIKE

The following morning at 6 a.m., Cindy took Jane and Ryan back to Eads while we set off to Tribune, the next stop.

The drive was monotonously flat. Telegraph poles on poor, dry parched earth marked both sides of the road. We travelled the whole fifty-seven-mile route meeting only two other vehicles, both pickups, on the way.

Towns were sparse, their white grain towers visible for miles. The landscape was uninteresting and mundane with little to feed the eyes.

This area of eastern Colorado into western Kansas suffered an agricultural collapse in the 1930s. Decades of extensive farming, without crop rotation, had caused the fertile soil of the Great Plains to be exposed and laid the foundations for disaster. Agricultural prices in the early 1930s were unstable, giving oxygen to overproduction, and severe droughts dried out the soil.

For these remote small towns, the disaster was continuing. Communities were closing by stealth. It wasn't uncommon for every business to be shut apart from the US postal building.

For a visitor, all the signs screamed 'Don't stop!' But we had little choice. The cyclists would have had to cycle another twenty-two miles to reach Leonti, the next town, and it wasn't feasible.

The aptly named Trail's End Motel in Tribune was our destination. My heart sank as I noticed its sign, wedged on top of a pile of logs, with a picture of a cowboy on horseback, lone-ranger style.

The motel's facilities were highlighted beneath but the wording had faded. It didn't look particularly welcoming but I knew after last night's fiasco that there was no way Jane would want to move on. We stood at the entrance to the motel as the cyclists approached, expansively taking up all the road, uninhibited by other vehicles.

As Jane cycled towards the motel, the strong wind, which had picked up mid-morning, buffeted the wheels. The tops of the trees were arching over and there was the rhythmic clanging of metal chains at the Ampride garage opposite, which only added to the rather desolate nature of the place.

The only sign of life was the remnants of a child's toy car, sitting folornly underneath a gas station sign which looked like a half complete hangman puzzle. It was Saturday afternoon and we were in a living morgue.

'Is this it?' Ryan said, even his continuing optimism showing signs of faltering.

'It's not aesthetically pleasing, I'll grant you,' I said. Jane dismounted from her bike, her bronze arms glistening, she looked a picture of health. She tore off the GPS unit and propped the bike against some logs.

'Have you booked us in?' she said.

'Not yet.'

Both RVs were parked face on to the wind.

'Where's Lia, Mike?' Martyn asked.

'I've not seen her, I'm afraid.'

'Mike,' said Jane, her voice serious. 'Get the rooms sorted, so we know where we all are.'

Two minutes later, armed with two keys and the surprising knowledge there were only three rooms available, I handed a set to Martyn and went to open the second room with Jane.

I unlocked the door and stepped inside. Space and a TV were the only redeeming features. I peered round in the darkness. A team of industrial cleaners would be needed if we were going to stay there. It was grimy, dirty and I would have not trusted the mattress or the bedding. The toilet cum shower was disgusting; the tile grouting was brown so it looked at first sight as though shit had been smeared down the walls.

Cindy appeared in the doorway.

'I'm not staying in this room, it's disgusting,' she shouted.

'It's only one night,' Jane said to me without any conviction.

'I'm happy with it,' Ryan said, turning to Steven. 'Do you want to watch cartoons this afternoon?'

'Yes!' Steven jumped on the nearest bed which rocked and slightly dislodged his baseball cap. '*SpongeBob*!'

I quelled the desire to tell him not to stop bouncing.

Jane turned the light on but it made no significant difference. It was midday outside but in this cell of a room it could have been midnight.

We felt like we'd been mugged as we wandered back to the RV to get something to eat. Martyn was still waiting for Lia to arrive; he was getting chilly in his wet kit.

'Lia's not going to like the accommodation,' he said, joining us in the RV for dinner. 'I imagine she's quite particular.'

'You don't need to be particular, just have a desire for basic hygiene,' said Jane.

'Still, it's good to rough it occasionally,' Martyn said.

Jane and I exchanged quizzical looks before Martyn smiled.

It was a couple of hours before Lia and Dan arrived and we managed to go through some route maps and have a detailed interview with Martyn and Jane in anticipation of a documentary for Radio 5 Live on the ride so far.

'Fancy exploring the town?' Jane shouted from the bedroom. Steven glanced at me and pulled a look of disgust.

'Do you think we should?' I whispered to him.

'Do we have to?'

'Yes.' Jane appeared at the doorway putting on her light purple jacket, her sunglasses already in place. Her recent shower had fizzed new life into her hair. Steven, without further prompting, put on his cowboy hat and grabbed his camcorder.

Although it was still hot and humid outside, the wind took the edge off it. We turned right and headed back towards Eads.

There was no pavement, just a wide gutter and all the buildings on the left were corrugated metal. Parked outside each one were station wagons or pickups, usually black or dark blue, with blacked-out windows as if the town was a celebrity hideaway. I doubted that there was one property of greater value than the vehicle outside it.

Fifty yards further down the road, a sign advertised a drive-thru burger bar. Incredibly, as we hadn't seen any vehicles for some time, there was a queue – an almost antique Merc and a battered pickup.

'Shall we have a burger for tea?' I said.

'I don't think that would be a good idea,' said Jane flatly.

'Why, Mum?' said Steven, but Jane didn't explain. We continued walking, turning ninety degrees every couple of hundred yards until we were just south of the RV park and on the main street. Traffic lights in the middle of wires in the road swung to and fro as music was pumped from outdoor speakers and American flags whip cracked in the wind.

An electric display on the First National Bank said the temperature was 32 degrees, that it was 3 p.m. on a July Saturday afternoon. At home in Rothwell I imagined the park heaving with people queueing for the tennis courts, men carrying armfuls of beer from Morrisons and the distant shouts of 'Howzat!'

We passed a small supermarket with a pickup parked outside. There was one customer, an enormous older lady who was propped against the counter. I studied the local community adverts in the shop windows; mud volleyball was on Tuesday nights, apparently.

We walked on to the town's museum – inevitably, it was shut. A police car drew alongside, its occupants watching us until we turned back towards the motel then it drew away.

Tea was mince and rice, undercooked. It was no wonder Jane was disappearing right before us. Her size zero was turning into negative numbers.

At supper time Steven and I headed across the road to the garage in search of treats. It was clearly a Mecca for local kids because like so many of the bigger gas stations we'd come across, it doubled up as a coffee shop, burger bar, mini-supermarket and youth club.

Inside, there was a collection of boy racers watching their future selves as four mute, huge truckers complete with oil-stained baseball caps made quarter-pound burgers look like bite-sized snacks. It was the most happening scene for a hundred-mile radius. A constant stream of post-pubescent lads arrived to practise their handbrake turns and gravel spins.

Steven watched with a mixture of awe and trepidation. We settled on coffees and ring doughnuts and returned to Jane who was writing in her journal.

Sellotaped on the magazine holder was Cindy's handwritten itinerary for the next three days: 'Sunday July 30th Tribune to Dighton staying in Scott City, Pine Tree RV Park, 702 North Main Street 620-872-3076 water, sewage, elect, no toilets, nor showers, nor laundry.'

You could guarantee there'd be no pine trees either.

It continued: 'Monday and Tuesday July 31st and August 1st Dighton to La Crosse staying in WaKeeney KOA, Wednesday August 2nd La Crosse to Ellsworth staying in Salina KOA.'

'Have you fucking seen this?' I said, tapping my knuckles on the list.

'What?' said Jane, without looking up from her journal.

'This agenda! Tomorrow we're staying thirty miles from where you finish and Monday and Tuesday we're further away. Wednesday, we're staying where we finish Thursday. We're doing more miles than a Middle East peace envoy.'

'I know.'

'We're going over the agreed mileage on the RVs. It's fucking madness.'

'I know.'

'We must be adding an extra two hours to each day. Bollocks. I'm going to ask Cindy to cancel the reservations.'

'You do that,' Jane said, in a slightly mocking tone.

'Are you taking the piss?' I asked.

'I've been telling you about this for days. Anyway, we're cancelling the rest day.'

'What?'

'If we're not in Kansas City next Saturday I'm stopping the ride. This new schedule gets us there on Saturday.'

Jane's feet were stretched across the double seat, the wind gently rocking the RV like a boat on the sea. 'You need a rest,' I said. 'If this wind continues you won't be able to set off anyway.'

'We'll see. But we're all agreed we need to get across Kansas quickly. Martyn and Ryan are happy.'

'I'll go and see Cindy.'

The motel looked like a sleazy brothel as purple fluorescent lights flickered randomly from the sign. I knocked and knocked at Cindy's door but there was no reply. I opened it. Cindy was sitting on the bed, facing an illuminated laptop which was the only source of light.

'Hi,' she said, not moving her head from the screen.

'The guys have decided to cancel the rest day.'

'They didn't check with me.'

'Well anyway, it's a done deal but I think we should scrap the schedule.'

'What?'

'The stops are miles from the finishes and I think it's adding unnecessary strain to Jane.'

'Well, you said you'd prefer KOAs.'

'I do, but not if it means we're crossing time zones. Anyway, don't bother booking anything in future, we'll take our chances where we finish, it can't be any worse than the shit holes we've been staying in.'

She carried on looking at the screen, motionless.

'Well, I don't think that's a good idea. I don't like being disorganised. I like to know where I'm staying everyday and some days in advance.'

I took a deep breath. 'Well, the bookings have been taking you hours each day so you'll have a lot more free time. Anyway that's what's been decided. Have a good night. I'll see you in the morning.' I felt quite small as I left.

When I got back to the RV, Steven was already asleep and Jane was working at the laptop.

'How's Cindy?' she said.

'Extremely pissed off I think.'

'She's not comfortable without a formal plan or structure, is she?'

'It's gonna be an interesting few weeks as I'm buggered if I'm booking anything in advance again,' I said.

That night I was woken by Jane who had dragged herself up and was peering out of the window.

'What's going on?' I said, stretching across to look at my mobile. It was 1.45 in the morning.

'I think the proprietor of the motel is selling a car,' she whispered.

'Don't be so bloody stupid, woman, it's nearly two o'clock on a Sunday morning.'

There were only two cars in the car park and both looked like they'd been scrapped.

'I'm telling you, they're selling a car,' she said.

'Bizarre,' I said, laying back on the pillow. 'Totally bizarre.'

Day 32 – Sunday, 30 July
Tribune, Kan. to Dighton, Kan.
69.7 miles – 4 hrs 54 mins
Total covered – 1835.5 miles

JANE

The wind was battering us from all directions as we lay awake in the RV. However much I tried to persuade myself that I wasn't at sea, it felt like the RV was swaying up and down in a rough ocean. I was really worried that we would be cycling in these conditions the following day.

We couldn't have the air conditioning on – it wasn't safe to do so for a long period – and the night was humid.

'Are you okay?' Mike murmured. I was soaking wet. I'd already been up twice to change my pyjamas but had got up out of bed to change them again.

'I can't sleep,' I said. 'I feel like we're on the sea. And look at this . . .' I lifted the damp material of my top to show him. 'I can't sleep in this.'

I got up and took off my pyjamas, rummaging around for a dry set. I towelled the sweat off my body but it was no use. As soon as I'd wiped it off, new droplets appeared on the surface.

'Shall I sleep elsewhere?' whispered Mike, propping himself on his elbow.

'You don't have to . . .'

'You're not going to get any rest at all if you stay as you are. You get back into bed and have my space, it's dry.'

I didn't argue. He shuffled out of the bed and tiptoed into the main space of the RV so as not to wake Steven.

I crawled back into bed, the dry mattress a welcome relief. Within minutes, I lay in the darkness listening to Mike and Steven competing for the loudest snore. I rolled over and shut my eyes.

Next morning, I woke at five thirty. I'd managed to get a few hours sleep but was anxious about the day ahead. We tried to set off early as we knew the wind would increase as the day progressed but even by six fifteen it was picking up.

The road out of Tribune was littered with potholes. Every two or three seconds we'd bang over one, then another, then another, the jolts shooting straight through my body. I lifted myself up from the saddle, keen to avoid further pain up my back, but using my legs for any length of time expended far too much energy. I knew I'd have to pace myself.

'Oooh look at this, fantastic,' I said, as we turned on to smooth tarmac that felt like velvet under the wheels.

'Don't get too excited,' said Martyn. 'That's where we're heading.' He nodded his head towards a dustier secondary road that had potholes as far as the eye could see.

I took a deep breath and put my head down. We had seventy miles to cycle and there was nothing we could do about it. It was a long day, passing through some very small towns. We eventually got to a little township called Scott City and saw Mike and Cindy's RVs and parked up the bikes alongside.

I banged on Mike's door but got no reply. We presumed he'd gone shopping so I knocked on Cindy's door. She answered it after a few seconds.

'Hi, do you know where Mike is?'

She shrugged. Earlier in the day, she and Mike had had an argument. Mike had asked her to move her RV after she'd parked in a dangerous part of the road and Cindy had taken umbrage.

'He might have gone to church or something, but I'm not sure. The RV was here when I arrived.'

Puzzled, I went back to Mike's RV, leaving Martyn and Ryan with Cindy. I peered through the window. Mike was sitting at the table reading some papers.

'Mike!' I said, banging on the door. He opened it, looking a little surprised.

'Hi!'

'What are you doing? Why didn't you answer the door?'

He moved to one side to let me in. 'I thought it was Cindy,' he said. 'I didn't want to talk to her 'cos she's been so odd with me all day.'

Irked, I sat on the sofa next to Steven and we exchanged a look. He smiled and pulled a face as Mike poured me a coffee and put a pastry on the table. My irritation lifted slightly.

Mike sat down opposite and tore some pastry for himself. 'I really don't see why you're going to cycle any further today,' he said, chewing.

'It's only eleven, Mike. We'd be better off getting more mileage out of the day now. The weather might be worse tomorrow.'

'Well, you definitely shouldn't be cycling if it gets any worse than this.'

He was right but I couldn't help but feel annoyed. The last forty-six miles had been hard work. We were travelling in an easterly direction and a strong southerly side wind was blowing uninterrupted across the plain. Without warning a gust could practically knock you off the bike. And as the hours had ticked by so the velocity of those gusts had steadily increased.

'I can't drive the RV in this wind,' he continued, his face tight, his eyebrows drawn down, his lips narrowed. I was in his bad books. I felt my throat tighten.

'Well, it's not very nice cycling either but you know we've got to do it.'

I got up and reached for my cycling helmet. Waving goodbye to Steven, I looked over at Mike. He was doing his 'I don't approve of this' look.

As I got on the bike, pulling on my gloves and tightening the strap on my helmet, I couldn't believe how immature both Mike and Cindy were being.

Without any lunch, I was beginning to get weary but we still had seventeen miles to go before we reached our destination. And the most stupid thing was that we were actually camping in Scott City so as soon as we'd finished the ride, we'd be getting in Cindy's RV and travelling back over the ground we'd just covered.

A couple of miles from our end point at Dighton, a police car drove alongside us, waving at us to pull over. We braked and pulled up behind the car, ready for a telling off.

The police officer got out of the car, his hat flying off and down the road. He ran to rescue it and my anxiety lifted a little as he retrieved it, brushed it off and walked towards us.

'So what are you all doing here now,' he asked. His manner was friendly, completely unthreatening. 'I've had several people ringing me, concerned for you folks.'

We explained. He listened, nodding, his hat still in his hands. The sun was beating off his bald head. Satisfied with our explanation, he smiled.

'Well, I thought I might come out and just check that you were all right.'

Cindy, who had parked the RV vehicle behind us, came up to him.

'So how long have you lived round here?' she said. Her voice was different, lighter, sweeter.

'I've been here all my life, lady, all my life,' said the police officer.

'Is it always windy like this?' she smiled.

'Oh no, this is one of the windier days,' he smiled back. 'I can tell when it's windy 'cos my hat don't stay on.'

Martyn, Ryan and I sat listening to this for a few minutes more before the police officer turned to us again.

'Well, as long as you are careful,' he said, making a move to leave. 'We have fatalities on the road and we don't want you to become one. You'll find that the drivers will give you a wide berth because they don't want to clip you under their wheels.'

'Thank you, officer,' said Cindy.

He gave a quick nod in her direction. 'Just make sure you give yourselves enough room on the road so that you're not swept off.'

Mike had been right. It was just too windy to continue but we still had this distance to travel and we couldn't be dictated to.

When we came across an area of woodland, I expected the wind to drop but the turbulence was immense and it was even harder to cycle. The wind was rolling around on the road and it was virtually impossible to fight against it.

Gripping the handlebars firmly, I managed to steady the bike and stay in control. Occasionally, a monster truck would thunder by, almost sweeping me under the tyres. I just had to keep myself wide on the road so that I didn't suddenly skip across it and into the path of a vehicle.

We arrived at a sign which said 'Welcome to Dighton' at twelve thirty. I couldn't have been more delighted. Cindy rushed past in the RV and parked up just ahead. We hadn't seen any sign of her since we'd left her chatting to the police officer.

Leaving Martyn in the town because he was staying in the local motel, we climbed into Cindy's RV and she drove us back to the campsite. The RV park was clean but basic with no water or electricity. Dogs seemed to be howling all around.

Mike and Steven had gone to Mass but checking my watch I realised that they should have been back by now. I showered and changed. It was always a relief to get out of the cycling clothes and into something vaguely more human. By 1.30 p.m. there was still no sign of them. I made myself a sandwich because I couldn't wait any longer but as I sat and ate it, my anger and anxiety grew. Tears started to form in my eyes. Where were they? How dare they simply disappear?

I decided to go out and look for them and as I turned the corner out of the RV park I saw them both jauntily tootling up the road, laughing and joking.

'Where have you been?' I said, furious.

'Mass,' said Mike. 'And then we went to get some dinner at Pizza Hut.' As an explanation on it's own it sounded reasonable enough but I knew and he knew that his selfish behaviour was childish.

'It cost ten dollars and I had three Cokes. All the people from church were in Pizza Hut, Mum, it was weird,' Steven said.

'Have you had a good time?' I said, trying not to cry.

'Brilliant, wasn't it, Dad?'

The tears started. 'You could have called me, Mike. You leave the RV and I don't know what time you are coming back. I need to eat. This is just you being a pillock because of what happened with you and Cindy this morning.'

He walked towards me and put his arms around my shoulders.

'Maybe you are partly right,' he said. 'But if you'd checked the phone, you'd realise there's no signal. The SAT phone's in the RV. What were me and Steven to do? Sit in the RV for two hours waiting and wondering whether you were all right? You made the decision to cycle on, which is fair enough. But I didn't know how long it would take you to do the last twenty-four miles and then get back. So I'm sorry if I've upset you but I've done nothing wrong. I'm sorry, my love. I wanted to get to Mass and then we were hungry. Don't read anything more into it than that.'

Day 33 – Monday, 31 July
Dighton, Kans. to La Crosse, Kans.
67.0 miles – 5 hrs 41 mins
Total covered – 1902.5 miles

JANE

That night, all three of us listened intently to the sound of the wind outside. Once in a while there'd be a hush, as if the wind had vanished completely, then one of us would go outside only to be disappointed. As we awoke, the RV was still being buffeted.

'What are you going to do?' Mike asked.

'We'll set off,' I said.

'This is madness.'

'If we have to wait until the wind subsides we might be here for days and if I don't get to Kansas City by Saturday I'm going home.'

I knew the winds were worse today than they had been yesterday. Even as I'd popped outside to check on Ryan in the other RV, strong gusts of air had whipped round my legs. Mike shrugged. I hadn't told him how bad the journey had been from Scott City to Dighton. I didn't need the lecture. I knew if I could travel above 17 mph the wind would keep me stable. If I slowed below that speed, it could be more dangerous.

My legs felt fragile, keeping the bike stable yesterday had put more strain on them than usual.

The journey from Dighton to Ness City – our first stop-off point – was thirty-two miles. It took us just over two hours and we were there just after eight.

We had a quick coffee and another frank exchange with Mike about the conditions. I decided to continue cycling but as we travelled out of town the wind speed was increasing and it was becoming more difficult.

A few miles further on at another small town, Alexander, Mike parked up, facing the wind, and before I could even get off my bike he'd got out of the RV.

'I can't believe you're continuing to cycle in this,' he shouted above the howls of the wind. 'You're putting us all at risk.'

Martyn and Ryan pulled in beside me.

'What do you mean?' I said.

'Because you decide to cycle you're making us drive the RVs and quite frankly it's not safe in there with Steven. We're being tossed about the road, the RV is getting caught like a sail. One minute we're driving safely then we're being slewed to the other side of the road.'

I looked around at Cindy.

'Cindy, what do you think?'

She tipped her head to one side. 'Well, it's certainly windy but it's manageable,' she said.

'Ryan?'

'I think we're doing okay. I wouldn't like the roads to busier but I'm happy to continue. But it's your choice, Jane.'

'There's nothing here, Mike, we need to continue.'

'No, you don't. You *want* to continue because you've got this stupid schedule in your head. We could park up here and move on when the wind subsides.'

'That might be days. If we're here for two days with no sign of it abating, we'll have to set off and we'll have just lost the time.'

Mike looked away, irate. 'Before we came out, you said at any point if I said we should stop, then we would.'

'If I stop here, then I'm going home.'

'That's fine with me.'

'Look,' I said. 'The conditions are tricky, it's far from ideal, but I think it's safe to continue.'

By now both our voices were raised and my last remark was accompanied by some finger pointing, which I knew would infuriate Mike further. Martyn, Ryan and Steven had crossed the road and were out of earshot.

'So it's okay with you but sod me and Steven,' he said, kicking a stone away which flew twenty feet in front of him.

'Emotional blackmail,' I spat. 'That's cheap!'

'Steven's in the fucking RV,' he hissed. 'He goes where you go. The bloody thing's not safe to drive in these winds. You can keep it on the road but all the time you're just hoping that a gust doesn't come along at the same time as an oncoming vehicle.'

'So it's down to me? Well, thanks.' I grabbed my bike. 'Fuck. Fuck. There's no more than fifteen miles left today.'

'Whatever.'

'Don't whatever me. You could at least be supportive.' I knew if I stopped here, we'd be going home.

'And you could at least listen,' Mike retorted, though the power of his voice was lost in a gust.

'We're going,' I said to Martyn and Ryan. Both knew better than to get embroiled in a discussion with Mike and me and we cycled the next fifteen miles in silence. Fortunately we turned left five miles before La Crosse and benefited from a tailwind so covering those miles in no time at all.

Upon arriving in La Crosse I could see that the RVs stood out like a beacon on a black night.

'It looks okay, Jane,' Ryan said.

'They're parked on the town's playing field. They are the only vehicles anywhere in the vicinity. Ryan, we'll be the local attraction for the night. Every idiot in a pickup will drive past; we'll be the animals in the zoo.'

I didn't want to start on Mike immediately but had to say something.

'Is this it?'

'Yep.'

I shook my head. 'Is this another one of your silly games because you didn't get your own way, or is your economy drive plummeting new depths? What is it here? Five dollars a night?'

'Neither. I've moved on from this afternoon. This is the only RV park for miles and miles, but feel free to peruse the map and search for an alternative if you like.'

He busied himself in the RV tidying, wiping down the tables. 'There's a sandwich for you and coffee. Anyway, look on the bright side – we're conveniently located for the town's tourist attraction.'

'He's right, Mum,' Steven said.

Of course. On the map, La Crosse was hailed as the Barbed Wire Capital of the World. For two weeks Martyn had been convinced that there must be more to it than a museum, but I'd disagreed.

Ryan, Steven, Mike and I had to check it out, simply out of curiosity. Clearly in this part of Kansas the excitement threshold was extremely low. Cindy must have been tipped off because she made her own plans for the afternoon.

But hard as we tried, it was impossible to be fascinated by rows and rows of 'the devil's rope', even harder to believe that there are more than 2000 types or even that anyone cares.

The highlight was undoubtedly the 'Hall of Fame'. There, a

collection of grainy head-and-shoulders shots of late middle-aged gentlemen and the odd lady were hanging from the walls in a dimly lit room. All had made their own unique contribution to the barbed wire industry.

By this stage tears were streaming down my face and I was bent over double, weeping with laughter as we approached the exit.

Mike, who'd just about managed to regain his own composure, asked the attendant: 'Do you get many visitors?'

'Quite a few, but you're the first from Australia.'

'We're British, actually,' Mike said.

'Oh, really? We've been busy this afternoon. You're the second group round. You got here just in time, we're closing soon. Are you going to look round the Fence Post Museum next door?'

'No, I think we'll save that so we've got something to look forward to if we come to La Crosse again. Can I ask you something?' Mike said.

'Fire away.'

'We've found quite a lot of antipathy to French people while we've been in America because of the war.'

'Oh, for sure.'

'Is it odd to have a French-named town and how did it come about.'

'Oh, La Crosse isn't a French word,' she said.

We left but stopped on the way out to admire the largest ball of barbed wire in the world.

Day 34 – Tuesday, 1 August
La Crosse, Kan. to Ellsworth, Kan.
66.0 miles – 5 hrs 10 mins
Total covered – 1968.5 miles

MIKE

'You said Kansas would be flat,' Steven said.

'That's what I'd imagined.'

'Well, you imagined wrong.'

We dropped down a little hill into Ellsworth, Kansas, just after lunch. Steven and I had already scouted the town and decided to book three rooms at the Best Western Garden Prairie Inn just on the edge of town. With an indoor swimming pool, spa, air conditioning and a TV there was little more a boy could want – apart from a laundry, which it also had. For the first time on the road, it meant everyone had a room to stay in. The newfound generosity was not borne out of a financial windfall but a need to regroup.

Once again, from the start of the ride, the riders and RVs had been buffeted by incredible side winds, with the strength reaching up to 50 mph. When we turned a corner, the first for several hundred miles, Steven and I cheered and suddenly the riders benefited from the tailwind, which blew them into town. If only we'd cycled from Florida to Seattle.

For three days, Jane and I had argued over whether to rest or continue. Jane's stubbornness won. She'd left me in no doubt that if the wind prevailed we'd be flying home. And after the journey from Pueblo to here that would have been a blessed relief.

There was a sense of euphoria as Steven and I parked just off North Douglas Avenue, hoping that a night of comfort might lift everyone's spirits. It wasn't long before the cyclists, having spotted the RVs, met us. All the cyclists looked as refreshed as at any stage over the last three weeks. What simple joy a tailwind could bring.

'Enjoy that?' I said.

'The last twenty miles were awesome,' Ryan said. 'We averaged twenty-five miles an hour and I got up to thirty-five on the flat.'

'What's the town like?' Jane asked.

'Cool,' Steven said. 'We've got a surprise for you.'

'Will we get a coffee?'

'Probably. We've not looked around on foot. It's a pretty town, well kept, and there's some shops.'

'Is Lia here, Mike?' Martyn asked.

'Not seen her.'

'I think I'll stick with you guys for a while then, she'll turn up eventually.'

Ryan manoeuvred his bike over to Cindy's RV.

'If we stick the bikes in the RVs, we can walk into town and get some food,' he said.

'What's over there?' Jane asked, pointing across the road. A railway track ran parallel to the road we were parked on and on the other side were a series of property fronts, iron figures and descriptions of the town's history. There was the front of the Nick Lentz Saloon which Steven posed before, his shoulders hunched, hands down on an invisible holster. It was part of an open air museum displaying Ellsworth's Wild West pedigree. It seemed every town wanted a piece of Wild West heritage, the Pony Express at Cold Springs, the hanging of people from balconies in Austin, Butch Cassidy at Hanksville, and now Ellsworth wanted to share its blue chip credentials. That Cold Springs was a thousand miles away made me realise just how vast an area the Wild West covered. It also surprised me that most events happened a little over a century ago.

Fort Ellsworth was established in 1864. It was a key point to drive Cheyenne off the route to Denver. It was renamed Fort Harker in 1866 then relocated a year later. Fort Harker was a major supply post for destroying Plains Indians. Ellsworth grew thanks to the nearby fort, providing soldiers with local services, brothels and saloons. Within a couple of years the railroad had arrived, bringing its frontier men and reducing the demands of the local service industries.

In 1868, Wild Bill Hickok ran for sheriff and by the early 1870s wild Texas Longhorn were traded through the streets of Ellsworth. It was a complete cowboy town but it was short lived. By 1875 the cattle pens were closed.

The town was noted for its violence. On 15 August 1873, the inebriated Billy Thompson accidentally but fatally shot the sheriff during a gun fight. He remained on the run for fourteen years before being extradited from Texas and found not guilty. In October 1911 five members of the William Shewrens family were murdered by axe. For a town of 3000 people it bags its fair share of violent stories. I began to understand the American belief that it is every person's right to carry arms.

Without any big franchises, Ellsworth was a reasonably well-contained town, with a couple of convenience stores and cowboy stores, florists, card and gift, pharmacy and liquor stores. We made our way to Ellsworth Antique Mall, which contained a fresh sandwich shop, ice-cream counter and coffee shop but surprisingly few antiques.

'How was today?'

As soon as it left my lips I realised it was a totally inane question. Jane treated it with the contempt it deserved but Martyn was way too polite.

'Okay, we were struggling until aptly named Great Bend.' He moved his sunglasses up, revealing a completely two-toned face.

'Don't take this the wrong way, Martyn,' I said. 'But your face looks . . . I don't know how to say it.'

'Ridiculous,' Jane added.

'What? What?' said Martyn, looking alarmed.

'Have you looked in the mirror recently?' Ryan asked. 'The bottom half is red, your nose is especially glowing and your eyes and forehead are completely white.'

'Yeah, it is, honestly,' Steven added. It didn't help that poor Martyn's face was set against a background of a black and white chequered floor and lurid plastic counters.

'You're joking?' he said, feeling his forehead.

'No. I suggest you give your bandana a rest for the next few days,' Ryan said.

We took photographic proof.

'God, Natalie will be impressed,' laughed Martyn.

'I think we should get to Kansas City by Saturday now,' Ryan said. It had taken little time for both fellow cyclists to realise that Jane's threat of pulling out of the ride if the timescale slipped wasn't just bravado. I wouldn't say it cast a shadow over the ride but mileage, weather conditions and routes were becoming more and more important.

'Have you checked tomorrow's forecast, Mike?' asked Jane.

'Tomorrow's due to be windier than today and a huge storm is forecast for tomorrow afternoon.'

'Funny, Mike,' Ryan said.

'Seriously. I think an early start is called for tomorrow, the winds are going to get up to 60 mph.' Everyone looked a little concerned. 'But not until 4 p.m., so if you get your foot down, put some effort in, you'll be okay.'

Ryan looked particularly worried until he had realised that I was only semi-serious.

'According to the *Rough Guide*, the section between here and Abilene is the windiest interstate in America, with winds heavy enough to blow over a truck. But don't worry, you'll have a lower centre of gravity on the bikes.'

'Oh, it's not us that needs to worry, those RVs will be like sails,' Jane said.

'You're joking, we'll be making a mad dash in the morning to the campsite well before the storm, won't we, Steven?'

He nodded vigorously. 'Yes, we will. You can support yourselves tomorrow.'

Behind the joviality there was a semi-serious nature to this particular discussion. Jane had already vetoed any suggestion that she shouldn't continue riding through Kansas in the winds but I was still very concerned.

However, the attempt to forge some team cohesiveness at the Best Western Garden Prairie Inn by providing rooms for everyone failed miserably. After an initial scramble to bag the washing machines, everyone sought sanctuary in their own room.

Day 35 – Wednesday, 2 August
Ellsworth, Kan. to Salina, Kan.
44.0 miles – 3 hrs 47 mins
Total covered – 2012.5 miles

MIKE

The ride to Salina was uneventful and hard, the corrugated hills giving the riders little respite. It was a race to arrive before the storm broke.

The westerly approaches to Salina were particularly unattractive, mainly industrial and populated by insalubrious looking bars, porn and pawn shops. We arrived at the campsite mid-afternoon. Jane looked washed out so Steven and I decided to go for an afternoon swim. The park's pool was like an oversized kid's paddling pool. Although there was only one other couple in there, they were of such a size that the water lapped over the edges. They were as loud as they were wide, bellowing like an army of pneumatic drills recreating Beethoven's Fifth. Steven rolled his eyes. 'Shall we go back to the RV, Dad?'

'No, let's have a swim.'

The wind continued to gather momentum and trees which once bent slightly now arched over, half their original sizes as the clouds gathered. It was like Judgement Day. Steven and I beat a hasty retreat just before the heavens opened. We entered the RV quietly but Jane was not asleep.

'Did you have a good time?' she asked.

'No,' Steven said. 'We were going to play with the ball but couldn't.'

'Well, never mind.'

'I've thought about taking Steven to Abilene tomorrow morning,' I said. 'We've got the choice of the Dwight D. Eisenhower museum or the Greyhound museum because it's a little known fact that Abilene is the Greyhound Capital of the World.'

She smiled. 'Well, have fun; it does sound like one of those days when cycling is a good option.'

I peered out of the window.

'I see the weather forecast didn't exaggerate the storm,' Jane said as the RV rocked as if being shaken by a rugby pack. The Interstate 70 that towered over the park little more than fifty yards away was no longer visible. 'Another day, another storm,' she added.

Day 36 – Thursday, 3 August
Salina, Kan. – Alta Vista, Kan.
71.8 miles – 6 hrs 38 mins
Total covered – 2084.3 miles

JANE

'Mike was unerringly accurate with his prediction of a four p.m. storm yesterday,' Martyn said.

It was frustrating for all of us, as we should have set off twenty minutes earlier to cycle seventy miles into the middle of nowhere along Highway 4 from Salina. It had rained so heavily in the night that there was a very low-lying mist along the roads and we needed to wait until it was safe enough to set off.

'Yea, but for Pete's sake don't tell him,' I said.

'Absolutely,' he said. 'You look tired, Jane, are you all right?'

'I had a bad night. My back's very sore. I'm still sweating through two sets of pyjamas a night and having to sleep on both sides of the bed. Mike's having to launder the sheets every time he gets to a washing machine.'

'Well,' said Martyn, as he sat astride his motionless bike, 'there's no rush, Jane.' He was right, but delaying the start always put pressure on the rest of the day.

After cycling through Gypsum we reached a road junction where a red and white diagonal sign indicated that the road ahead was closed and that only local traffic was allowed. My heart sank. Even Ryan, who was perennially cheerful, had a despondent look on his face. I sighed and studied the map. A detour would mean an additional fifteen miles and after eight days of continual cycling I doubted whether my body would be able to withstand such a tortuous day.

I'd scrapped the planned rest day in La Crosse with the hope of reducing the daily mileage. I was finding the seventy- and eighty-mile stretches simply too much. The temperatures had dropped to the mid-eighties but the humidity level had spiralled, often making it feel like it was over 100 degrees.

'What do you want to do, Jane?' Ryan asked, looking at the diversion sign.

'I don't know.'

'Chances are, it's the bridge over the creek that's out,' Martyn said, pointing to the map. 'There's a smaller detour, if we cut through part of the roadworks.'

'Let's go for it,' I said, anxious to ensure that the extra mileage was kept to a minimum. Once you've been delayed you are forever losing time and it can mess with your head. The chances of finishing at a reasonable time and being able to rest were disappearing.

As we cycled down the detour we assumed that the route would be paved. But two miles into it we came upon a gravel and rock road. The bikes juddered over thousands of broken stones, at times it was as if I was riding a pneumatic road drill rather than a bike. With each jolt over a particularly large stone, it felt as though my bones would crumble.

'Are you okay, Jane?' Ryan had slowed down and was cycling alongside me. 'You're shaking.'

'I'm scared, Ryan,' I said. 'This is such a slow speed that if we meet any dogs, I've no chance.'

Martyn moved up close on my other side.

'I really don't want to meet a ranch dog on a road which isn't used to having traffic and people coming through,' I said.

'I didn't realise your phobia was as acute as this,' Martyn said. 'If we get the pepper sprays out, just in case, will that help?'

I nodded, keeping my eyes on the road ahead. 'Anything,' I said. 'I just want to get back on some tarmac.'

We carried on cycling, past bushes adorned with a plethora of red, white and blue ribbons. It was becoming a more common sight. As we'd travelled eastwards, it had become noticeably more nationalistic. Stars and stripes hung from flag poles and roofs, yellow ribbons and messages of support were pinned to gateposts and trees.

It was a late finish at Alta Vista, a pretty little town snuck back from the road. That night, once we'd checked our gauges, we realised that we'd climbed 3000 feet that day and gained no altitude.

When Mike told me that we were staying at another state RV park, I let out an audible sigh. We'd gone more than two days without doing any laundry and I could feel myself getting irritable.

That feeling, however, soon lifted when Steven, Mike and I took a stroll along Council Grove Lake that afternoon. The sun glinted on the surface of the clear water, while children still enjoying the late summer afternoon screeched and laughed. This wasn't like any Kansas I'd read about in the tourist guides and, for an hour, it was as though we were on a summer holiday. Just the three of us.

The park itself was surprisingly clean, tidy and quiet too, a perfect holiday waterside destination for a landlocked state.

It had been late when we'd arrived in the town of Council Grove for dinner and we were relieved to find the local family diner open. It was an old town, by American standards at least. People had settled here in the mid-nineteenth century.

The food was typically mid-America – a salad starter with choice of dressing, meat and chips for main followed by dessert. As usual, all our soft drinks were continually refilled and, by the end of the meal, we unable to cram any more in.

'That was fantastic,' Ryan said, leaning back in his chair and puffing out his cheeks.

'No wonder they're full,' Cindy added.

'How much was it, Dad?' said Steven, watching Mike study the bill.

'Twenty-nine dollars,' he said.

I couldn't believe it. 'Mike, are you sure? That doesn't sound right. Twenty-nine dollars for six people, three courses and drinks?'

'No way,' Ryan said.

Mike showed us the till receipt. 'There you are and before you ask, yes I checked to make sure it was right.'

Fit to bust and feeling rather pleased with ourselves, we drove back from the diner in Council Grove to the State Park.

When we got back, Mike and I walked down to the lake's edge, hand in hand, as if discovering each other again. It was a momentary oasis of calm and with the sun setting low over the trees, casting their shadows, for once we were just able to share the time.

'Jane, Jane,' Ryan shouted. I turned to see him standing on the step of his RV, with his mobile glued to his ear. 'Jane, there's Paddy on the phone.'

Paddy? I must have looked puzzled because Ryan added, 'From the Cross Country for Cancer team.'

Of course. Paddy was part of the other cycling team we'd met while riding through the Rockies. Since we'd taken the northern route eight days earlier and they'd taken the TransAmerica cycle route, I'd missed seeing them regularly.

'Hi, Jane,' Paddy said. 'How are you doing?'

'Okay. Kansas has been a struggle, high winds and the terrain has been much harder than we'd envisaged.' I sat down on one of the folding canvas chairs. 'Where are you?'

'We've just got out of Missouri, which is why we're ringing.'

'This sounds ominous,' I said.

'It is, I'm afraid. As I've just told Ryan, we've had numerous dog attacks. Daily. Many have been vicious,' My heart started to race. 'On one occasion there were a couple of Great Danes running around in the street, they blocked the road, barking and snapping. The owners just stood there with their children and laughed for ten minutes before they called them off.'

'No!' I said. 'I'd be going home.'

'The drivers just ignore the fact that cyclists are on the road. It's common to be pushed off or cut up deliberately. It's very dangerous. The worst occasion was when Ezra raised his palm to acknowledge a red pickup but the driver clearly thought he'd given him the finger and slammed on the brakes and reversed back.'

'What did he do?' I asked.

'Ezra ran off the road and put himself behind a tree. The driver popped out of the pickup with a shotgun and screamed profanities at Ezra for a few minutes before leaving.'

'No!'

'It's full of Confederate flags and rednecks. We decided that we didn't want to risk our lives by continuing so we got a lift for the last sixty miles of Missouri.'

My heart went out to them. I knew only too well how hard I'd find it if I had to make the same choice. To be cycling across the country and to miss out a sixty-mile section, not out of illness or injury, would be heartbreaking.

'I gather you guys are sticking to the northern part of the state,' said Paddy.

'Yes, we are heading almost straight between Kansas and St Louis.'

'That may be all right,' he said. 'I'm sure it's further south where the problems lie.'

Day 37 – Friday, 4 August
Alta Vista, Kan. to Topeka, Kan.
63.5 miles – 6 hrs 7 mins
Total covered – 2147.8 miles

Day 38 – Saturday, 5 August
Topeka, Kan. to Kansas City, Kan.
51.2 miles – 4 hrs 38 mins
Total covered – 2199.0 miles

JANE

The fear of dog attacks put me on edge. The ride from Topeka to Kansas City was the tenth straight day of cycling and my body craved a rest. For the last two days we had climbed over 7000 feet without raising any altitude. My back, legs and shoulders throbbed and each time I hit a bump my body shuddered. Sleep was difficult and the nausea was becoming more acute.

We headed out of Topeka and entered the pretty university town of Lawrence which had an abundance of trees and quaint timber-built houses. It was if the town was part of a forest.

We cycled into Eudora. Mike was there waiting for us at the very outskirts of the town. Cindy was lost, unable to find Eudora. I couldn't believe it. We couldn't have made it any easier for her to find – she just needed to come off the freeway and go into the town.

'How did she manage to miss the whole town?' I said to Mike.

Ryan was shaking his head. 'This woman has been on the road with us for so long now and all she has to do is be able to cook and to navigate. What the hell is she playing at? We've found it and we're on bikes!'

'Where is she?' I said.

'She's at De Soto. It's about five miles further on,' said Mike. 'But she's fuming. She's really annoyed that she can't find us and I don't think we should mention it when we get to her. But I don't think she'll find us if we stay put here. She's got a mental block on coming back.'

I heard myself sighing more loudly than I'd intended.

'This is just the pits,' I said. 'I can't believe that this woman is so incompetent.'

Mike came over to me. 'Look, don't get angry. It's just not worth it. Let's put the bikes on the back of the van and go and get a coffee.'

As we walked into the town I was silent, overwhelmed with frustration that not only could Cindy not finish the simplest of tasks but also that she was angry with us when she was clearly in the wrong. We'd given her specific instructions, told her clearly where we'd be heading and she was the only one who couldn't find the damn place.

There were no cafés in sight, only a gas station that sold beef burgers and soft drinks. We bought refreshments and sat at the side of the station, munching them. Just as we were finishing, the other RV pulled up. It was Cindy. We watched as the vehicle slowly pulled into the parking area and stopped. She didn't move from the driving seat.

'Heck, you lot, I don't know where you've been but I couldn't find this place at all,' she called from the window. 'I've been sat down in De Soto waiting for you but you never showed up.'

I counted to ten. 'That's because we didn't arrange to meet in De Soto,' I said. 'There was no way we were going to cycle any further just because you couldn't find us.'

'Well, shucks,' she said. 'What am I supposed to do now?'

I tried to remain calm. 'You do your job now, Cindy. You meet us at the next stop and then go into Kansas City. Do you think you can manage that? We'll finish at the Lenexa barn museum, which should be easy enough to find. Is that okay?'

We got out the maps and pointed at where she would be meeting us.

'Do you guys not need anything to eat?' she said.

'We've already had something. Now are you sure you are going to be able to find this place?'

'Aw shucks yeah, of course I'll be able to make it – you can't miss it.'

I turned to Ryan. 'I bet we don't see her for a little while when we get to the next stop,' I said.

It was an awful stretch of road through to Kansas City. Tiny town roads full of holes and huge bangs in them. Every time we reached the crest we could see more bangs ahead of us and another and another. My heart dropped.

The temperature was soaring. I tried to manage with just the water fastened to my cycling top. Eventually, I called out to Ryan to stop and rest.

As we got to Kansas City, the streets got narrower and narrower and the sun got higher and higher. I was sweating profusely. Each time we thought there would be a little downhill, there was a climb up.

There were various dogs strolling around. None of them had chased us but I could feel my heart pounding in my chest every time one showed any interest in us.

Martyn went ahead. As long as the dogs were in someone's yard, I didn't mind, but if I thought they could get near me I got really twitchy. I had the pepper spray but I was nervous that I would not be able to balance to accelerate away from them or to stand there and spray them.

We got closer to the city and found the main road which would be easier to ride down. We headed down 87th Street and made our way round the very outskirts of Kansas. We saw the signs for the Lenexa barn museum, which had early farm equipment from the Wild West.

Pulling up, Mike's RV was there but there was no sign of Cindy. We met up with Mike and Steven, and I was proved wrong because Cindy was there in Mike's RV. She had followed Mike into the RV park and dropped off hers.

Ryan got a bit uptight about the RV already having been dropped off. 'How am I supposed to manage – I can't use the bike during the weekends, it's too busy around here.'

'Why don't you get a taxi?' Cindy said.

'That's not really suitable, is it?' Ryan huffed. 'We're staying at this hotel and we can't take the bikes with us.' He turned round to Cindy and said: 'You're just going to have to take the bikes.'

'I'll be stepping over bikes all weekend.'

'Well, that's your problem – you sort it out.'

So it was agreed that the bikes would stay with Cindy. Mike and I had booked into a hotel for the night, a real luxury hotel that we'd paid for ourselves, because we were having the weekend off. We weren't going to do any cycling, we weren't going to do any media work, we were just going to be a family.

Cindy dumped us on the pavement outside the hotel and practically threw our stuff on to it. I didn't care. All I could think was, 'Have I got enough stuff for the weekend?'

MIKE

RV parks fell into three categories. The first was the beautiful picture postcard park, an aesthetically pleasing State or National Park. The second was a functional one, usually located far outside a small town. The third and least attractive were the ones in the big cities, usually located in a disadvantaged area where real estate is cheap and there's little more than a car park.

In Kansas City everyone apart from Cindy had decided to book themselves into hotels to enjoy a well-deserved break. We'd pinpointed an RV site a few miles out from the city centre and the cunning plan was to drop off Cindy's RV at the site before meeting Jane at the finish in mine. Cindy would then take this to the RV park for the weekend.

However, on arriving at the RV park, it didn't seem appropriate to leave Cindy there alone for the weekend. It was full of long-term visitors, the accommodation was poor and the residents were not the type of people you'd want to meet on a darkened street. And while it was marginally better than the park we'd encountered in Denver, you'd still want to barricade the windows and doors with grilles.

We stopped near the exit and Cindy wound down her window, tears streaming down her face. 'I can't stay here. I was scared just driving round.'

'No one would expect you to stay here,' I said, trying to calm her down. She was completely distraught.

A lanky man with a sour complexion and the first mullet I'd seen in twenty years approached.

'Hey man, are you booking in?' he said.

'We're just deciding, we won't be a minute.'

'Well move the motherfucking rig,' he barked.

'I'm not sure that attitude is going to entice customers,' said Cindy, through a veil of tears.

We beat a hasty retreat on to the interstate, the Tom Tom rattling off instructions at breakneck speed and requiring us to cross multiple lanes one after the other. Unsurprisingly, within minutes Cindy had missed the exit that Steven and I had taken and her RV disappeared into the distance. It didn't take long to find her again but by then her nerves were shredded.

'It should be a little easier now,' I said. Cindy's face was florid and her eyes bloodshot. She'd always struggled with the navigation and this section of Kansas was extremely demanding. Travelling by herself I could fully understand her anxieties. She was also spending the weekend on her own which I presumed would be unsettling her.

We found another, safer RV park for Cindy and left her RV there.

The cyclists arrived at Letexa – apparently the Spinach Capital of the World – at just after twelve thirty.

After soup and rolls at Panera Bread, an upmarket bakery chain that Cindy had recommended, she dropped us off at our hotel in downtown before departing to the out-of-town RV park.

We entered the hotel. What opulence! A two-night break at a four star hotel. The room was huge, twice the size of the RV, with two king-sized beds and an incredible view over northern Kansas City.

We quickly showered, changed and caught a bus down to the Country Club Plaza, built in the 1920s and the world's first shopping centre to accommodate cars. Obviously it had been revamped since, mainly because of a bad flood in the late seventies. The marketing blurb said it had been modelled on Seville and other Mediterranean cities but it actually looked like a film set. Spotlessly clean, it had mosaic pavements which barely had a brick out of place. But the pristine nature of the place only added to the fakeness.

Weekend breaks had been a main feature in Jane's life since her terminal diagnosis six years ago. Told she had only six months to live, it seemed important to all of us to ensure that every month there was something to look forward to.

Initially, Jane and I had visited Chester without the children, a final lost weekend before chemotherapy started and Jane would lose her hair. Jane had also had weekends away with the children, one at a time, for them to garner unique memories. Despite Jane's hectic schedule, throughout the six years those regular three days of sanctuary became crucial to our mental well-being.

Kansas City was our mid-ride treat – our 'weekend break'. The swanky hotel, albeit the cheapest available in downtown Kansas, was empty as it was outside business hours and it cut us off from the road for a couple of days.

With early evening upon us we scouted for food in the Plaza, settling upon a pub-type diner. Jane was stiff and her body slumped in the chair. The room was packed and everywhere shiny wooden surfaces gleamed. It seemed to have been designed as a ye olde English village pub but without the charm and quaintness, a sanitised version. That said, it was clean, pleasant and the food was wholesome.

'What's wrong with my head?' Jane said, looking at Steven.

'Nothing,' said Steven.

'Well, either I've grown a third ear or you seem to be more interested in what's going on behind me.'

'There's nothing, Mum, honest.'

Jane looked at me. 'You're as bad.'

Steven smiled conspiratorially. Jane looked over her shoulder to where a screen was showing Chelsea vs MLS All Stars.

'Football. Bloody football,' she said and Steven laughed. 'That's why you two dived for those seats. Who's playing? The World Cup finished four weeks ago.'

'No one,' Steven said.

'Well, in that case, you can talk to me. I cycle all day, the least you can do is pay attention at night.'

'But . . .' Steven was mumbling.

'Don't tell me you've taken an interest in American soccer,' Jane said.

'It's Chelsea, look.'

Jane turned her head round to the screen again and then looked back at me.

'Chelsea, bloody Chelsea. It's a Saturday night, we're in Kansas in mid-summer and bloody Chelsea are playing football.'

Football had been an integral part of our journey together, despite her hatred of the game – or more accurately her hatred of my love of the game.

My mind slipped back to an early summer night over two decades earlier as I walked back from the pub with two friends after watching England snatch an unlikely win. Spotting a red phone box I said to my friends: 'You go ahead I just need to make a call.'

In the phone box, I carefully avoided the discarded gum, and ignored the unpleasant smell of urine, as I adjusted the cord on the phone and slotted a 10p into the slot.

Despite – or perhaps thanks to – the fact that I was fuelled with the best part of a gallon of Tetley's finest, my legs went weak as I scoured down in my pocket for the old beer mat which had a phone number written in mascara.

I'd deliberated for five days as to whether to call the beautiful petite girl who'd given it to me in a Leeds nightclub. It seemed implausible that she'd ever be bothered to see me again. It's not like we'd got on the first time, she'd been argumentative and very feisty, so I was staggered when she gave me her number.

Only a few years later Jane was having a breast lump removed on the day of England's World Cup semi-final with Germany. A decade later, during the first match that Steven had ever attended at Burnley, it became apparent that Jane's breathlessness was so bad that even climbing the terrace steps to our seats was a test of endurance, the first major sign of how desperately poorly she was.

I looked back at Jane.

'It's no good,' I smiled. 'You know you'll get no sense from either of us until the game has finished. Why don't you read your book.'

She looked resigned. 'I won't forget this.'

After dinner, we headed straight back to the hotel.

Despite asking for a low numbered floor, we had been allocated a room on the twenty-third, giving a great view of the light displays from the nearby skyscrapers. A few hours earlier we'd been mesmerised by an electrical storm.

With the curtains open, I sat on the bed with the laptop resting on my knees, watching the city's lights, one skyscraper in particular displaying a fantastic show of red, white and blue patterns.

I filed the blogs and the newspaper articles needed for Monday, to try to keep tomorrow completely free, before turning my attention to the emails on the Jane's Appeal website.

There were far too many to answer but I checked them all. The most recent was from a literary challenged Glaswegian, whose poisonous note could at best be described as abusive and at worst threatening. The essence of his criticism towards Jane was that being a woman, how was she ever going to cross the USA when she clearly needed balls. He then launched into a more vitriolic tirade.

Unprofessionally, I composed a two-word response.

The next email was from a man whose wife had died years earlier of cancer. My sympathy for him quickly evaporated as he complained that Jane was merely causing him to relive the experience.

A third email came from a lady complaining that Jane made her feel inadequate. The anger which had been swelling in the pit of my stomach broke forth as I sent a dismissive reply.

Jane appeared from the bathroom looking angelic wrapped in a white bath towel. It was hard not to notice her shoulderblades which rose at right angles almost jutting from her skin.

'What are you doing, Mike?'

'Blogs and emails.'

'Any chance you could put them away for the night at least.' She grabbed a small towel and rifled her hair.

'Of course. I love you,' I said, staring at her. It was hard to imagine that this morning she'd cycled sixty miles yet now she attracted vitriol from complete strangers.

I couldn't imagine another terminally ill person who'd suffered abuse like Jane. Her legs still bore the scars of the violent assault three years' previously, when she was punched by a passenger from a passing car, causing her to hit a house wall. None of the four youths in the car was prosecuted because the police couldn't identify which one had thrown the punch.

I moved the laptop to the side of the bed, while Jane let the towel drop and climbed in beside me before extinguishing the light.

Day 39 – Sunday, 6 July
Kansas City
Rest day

MIKE

Panera Bread was busy even at this early hour. They had a stream of customers who were reading the Sunday morning papers over steaming coffees and pastries.

'Can I go to the toilet, Dad?' Steven asked.

'Of course.' He rose gingerly and set off at a snail's pace across the café floor. Jane's eyes followed him, her sunglasses perched on top of her head. It was unusual to see her without a cycling top, gloves and helmet. She looked fatigued, as if even getting a spoon to her mouth was summoning the last of her energy reserves.

'You sweated as much last night,' I said.

'I know.'

'The room was freezing.'

Jane's eyes watered slightly. 'You don't need to say anything else,' she said, breaking off part of a bread roll, white crumbs falling on to the table.

'It's your liver, isn't it?' I said. 'These night sweats have nothing to do with the cycling.'

'I think we both knew subconsciously that the pain is more prominent. Don't be sad, Mike, please.'

My hand covered my mouth, the pit of my stomach seemed to have disappeared.

'We should go home,' I said. 'You need chemo.'

Jane shook her head slightly. 'We'll see the ride out. Otherwise it'll have been a huge waste of time. We've raised no money, we have to finish. If I don't finish we won't be able to set up the 10k.'

'Let's go home, love.'

'Mike leave it, you're not helping.'

Steven returned. 'Hiya, are you okay, Mum?' He stretched out his arm and put it round Jane's neck. She closed her eyes briefly.

'I'm fine, Steven,' she said.

'*Pirates of the Caribbean* then!' Steven said, enthusiastically.

'If you insist,' she said, knowing that we'd been promising to take him.

Day 40 – Monday, 7 August
Kansas, Kan. to Warrensburg, Missouri (Miss.)
67.9 miles – 7 hrs 30 mins
Total covered – 2266.9 miles

JANE

'Cindy's here,' Mike said. We were standing outside the hotel in downtown Kansas, our suitcases at our feet. Six fifteen on a Monday morning and the business district still showed no signs of waking from its weekend slumber. I felt slightly conspicuous clad in Lycra cycling gear without a bike in sight. The ride out to Saturday's finishing point at the Lenexa barn museum was quick and all of us were ready as planned to set off at 7 a.m. Unfortunately no one had given the weather the same instructions because a thunderstorm rolled overhead.

Despite having had a rest day, I felt weary and the thought of climbing on to the bike and heading into Missouri hung heavy. The phone call from Paddy had made me wary and I knew that dog attacks in the forthcoming days would be inevitable. Last night's sweat had been as ferocious as ever but at least Mike hadn't overreacted, even though he had been chipping away at me about going home.

'We'll wait for the electrical storm to pass,' Ryan said and proceeded to chain the bikes to a park bench. The setting was lovely. There was a little lake, grassland and interesting sculptures but even so it was extremely frustrating not to be able to set off when we'd hoped.

'The best laid plans,' I said, as the skies rumbled.

'We're going to be heading through here at rush hour,' Ryan said.

Martyn moved around. 'Another long day,' he said.

'We can't set off just yet,' I said. 'These storms are just too violent.'

'No, it would be madness.'

It was after eight when we finally set off, but we very quickly passed the border into Missouri. The storm had left a lot of standing water and the road surface was greasy. The constant junctions and traffic lights made progress slow. Our conversation was muted as we all needed to concentrate on cycling. The sense that we were constantly losing time weighed heavy on us all.

We were on Interstate 70, which wasn't a massive road but was incredibly busy. Trucks dwarfed us, their enormous wheels drenching us with spray; the drivers giving us little room for manoeuvre. I felt particularly vulnerable and it wasn't long before we looked to try to find an alternative quieter route.

'Jane, if we take a right and get off the 70 we can maybe make quicker progress,' Martyn said. Ryan stood, his legs astride his bike and taking a sip of Gatorade, as Martyn and I pored over a map.

As we stood there, a sixteen-wheeler truck sent an arc of spray, which made us all duck. We had to get off here. Drivers turned right in front of us without any consideration and it seemed inevitable that one of us would get clipped at some point. I wore my high visibility jacket as much to mark my presence as protection against the rain.

We decided upon a route which we thought would be a short-cut but we discovered it was closed and so we were forced to head back to Interstate 70 and Kansas. Even though we were moving further away from town, the traffic volume didn't seem to be reducing.

'We've travelled less than thirty miles,' Ryan said. 'Five hours on the road and less than thirty miles.'

There was no hiding Ryan's frustration but we all felt the same.

'Shit!' I said, as the yapping of a dog came from behind us. My heart rate went through the roof, my feet hit the pedals hard, my calves pushing with every ounce of effort. I shot across a road junction with barely a second glance. Beads of sweat gathered on my forehead.

'Are you okay, Jane?' Ryan asked. Short of breath I continued to pedal furiously, wanting to put some extra distance in until I felt comfortable. 'It's okay,' said Ryan. 'The dog's half a mile back.'

'We'll be able to get on Highway 50 after Lee's Summit,' I said. 'At least then we may be able to get up some decent speed.'

Today was turning into a marathon ride. My phone beeped, I pulled my bike over and grabbed it from my cycling top pocket.

The screen display showed it was Mike's phone. 'Hi ya,' I said.

'Where are you?'

'Still working our way out of Kansas, near Bryant.'

'Where's that?' I could sense disappointment in his tone. 'Oh I see it. I was on the following page. I'd have thought you'd have got further.'

My throat tightened. 'It's been a bad run, a road closure, a dog attack. I don't need any grief.'

'Look, there's no way you're travelling on Highway 50 today. It's horrendous, Jane. There's no way any bikes can get on it. It's a full-on motorway as mad as the M25.'

'How far did you travel down it?'

'Until Highway 7.'

'Well, we're some way from where we can join Highway 50. We'll see when we get there.'

'I'm telling you, it's way too dangerous. It's bad enough in an RV.'

'I'll have to go, Mike.'

I slotted the phone away. All the clouds had been burnt away and the sun was beating down ferociously and the humidity rising. We headed off down the main route again but within minutes the familiar sight of highway trucks blocked the road.

'What's that?' I said, as we approached some roadworks.

'Oh boy, someone's jinxed today,' said Ryan. 'Did Mike say it was going to be easy?'

'Can we get through?' I asked a workman as we pulled up.

'No, you'll need to detour,' he shouted over the noise of generators. My heart sank as for the second time we were forced back on to a major road – this time the 291 which dropped down to Lee's Summit. We pulled in at a gas station for a comfort break and to have a quick coffee before setting off back down the detour we'd already made. Reversing the route was soul destroying. Every yard would mean two extra. Ryan went inside to buy refreshments. Martyn and I were sitting outside on the pavement when the phone rang again. It was Mike.

'Where are you?' he said.

'Going back up the road we've just been down, more bloody roadworks. We're going to head down the 291 until Langsford Road then join the 50 off the 7.'

'You can't go on the 50,' he said. 'It's way too dangerous, you'll get yourselves killed.'

'Where are you?'

'Just up from Pleasant Hill.' I pulled the map out of the folder and spread it across the pavement. Martyn looked down on me.

'We'll have a look. I'll ring you back.'

Ryan came out with coffees. I slumped with my back against the wall. My bandana felt soggy so I rearranged it.

'Mike says the 50 is too dangerous for bikes,' I said. We looked at the maps, our destination was Warrensburg and we'd covered barely a quarter of the journey. At this rate we'd be cycling at midnight. A detour to where Mike was would add another fifteen miles at least, with more difficult cycling.

Martyn crouched down next to me. 'We should be able to manage on the 50,' he said. 'It loses its interstate status at that point. Have Mike or Cindy seen what it's like?'

I phoned Mike back and asked.

'No,' he said. 'There's no way at all that you can go down that route. You can't take that route at all.'

'We're not planning to go on the motorway part of it,' I said. 'We're just going to go on the single carriageway. Has anybody checked that out?'

'Yeah, yeah, yeah, Cindy's driven down that as far as she could go and yeah it's not a motorway but just as busy, she says.'

I closed my eyes. 'Mike, I'm knackered. This is a huge detour you're asking us to do. You need to be certain.'

'Jane. That road's mayhem. There were three lanes or four lanes but cars, pickups and trucks were going off in all directions. Overtaking in every lane, Cindy had been driven off the road once; how she didn't get cleaned up I'll never know.'

I put the phone down and sighed. Martyn and Ryan both looked up to me expectantly.

'Listen, they're telling me that it's horrendous up there and that we have to go across Highway 7 and come down to Pleasant Hill. It's a bit of a long step, but you know, hopefully, it shouldn't be much longer than the mileage we anticipated so . . .'

'Is Mike certain?' Martyn asked.

I nodded. 'I'm probably unhappier than you at this but Mike's absolutely insistent we shouldn't be travelling on the 50.'

They both still looked disgruntled.

'Look,' I said, 'I'm not having any more arguments with my husband. I'm not willing to put my relationship with him at risk any more for this trip.'

I could tell there was an air of resignation about the situation and they quietly accepted the decision. They could both see that they weren't going to move me on this one.

We set off on the route Mike had described. As we came across where Highway 50 finished we could see that the motorway was quieter.

'What have we done?' said Ryan. 'The traffic's not that busy.'

I knew he was right. The road wasn't busy.

'Well, I've got to go with what I've said now,' I said. 'We can't change our minds. I've agreed that I'm not going down Highway 50 and that I'll go down Highway 7.'

To add insult to injury Highway 7 was extremely busy. There was very little space for the bikes. Cars kept overtaking other cars, oblivious to our presence. By the time we reached the two RVs at Pleasant Hill our nerves were frayed.

The temperature had continued to rise and in the shade by the roadside it was 99 degrees. Martyn was so cross he wouldn't sit in the RV with Cindy and laid down in the shade of it.

I went across to the RV where Mike was playing cards in the air-conditioned cool with Steven.

'Are you okay?' he asked breezily.

I kept calm. 'Just how much of Highway 50 did Cindy actually see?' I asked, my tone measured.

He shook his head. 'I'll go and check.'

He loped out of the RV and was back within seconds 'She saw up to the intersection with the 7, she didn't go any further.'

I was incredulous.

'That's a fucking disgrace!' I screamed. 'I've just made Ryan and Martyn cycle miles out of their way on your and Cindy's words and you haven't even checked the roads!'

'That's not fair!' he said. 'We travelled on the 50 all the way from Kansas and let me tell you it was the most dangerous bit of road I've ever travelled on. It would have been ridiculous to try it on a bike.'

'I told you we weren't going on the interstate! You're just not bloody listening.' I slammed my helmet down and I threw my shoes across the van. 'I've had to cycle an extra twenty miles because you couldn't be bothered to drive another five. It's two o'clock, we've been cycling for six hours and we've still got another four to go and I'm absolutely beat. I can't believe that you've been that incompetent.'

Mike just sat there, silent, looking crestfallen. I couldn't bear to look at him. I got up and stormed out of the van, sobbing and sobbing. I was being suckered and defeated by the people who were supposed to be supporting me.

I stood outside, tears streaming from my eyes. I was completely inconsolable. Martyn still lay quietly thirty yards away, he knew better than to try and console me. My tears turned to fury. I picked up my helmet and hurled it at the wall.

'That's it! I'm going home. Let's get off and go straight to the airport.'

Mike stood up. 'Good,' he said. 'You'll get no argument from me. Get your stuff together.'

Almost instantly Steven burst into tears. He'd been playing on his computer game but had been listening intently to our argument.

'You can't go home now!' he said. 'We're not finished! We've got to go to New York.'

Mike and I went across to comfort him but he was completely heartbroken.

'Okay, Steven,' I said softly, my arm around him. His chest was heaving. 'Let's go and get some food at that Mexican fast food joint because you know how much I like tortillas.'

As we sat and ate, we all realised we had come too far and invested too much time and energy to go home now.

'If you give up, you give up for ever' was the mantra that had kept me going on previous challenges. It would keep me going now.

Day 41 – Tuesday, 8 August
Warrensburg, Miss. to California, Miss.
69.9 miles – 5 hrs 57 mins
Total covered – 2336.8 miles

MIKE

'Look, Steven, there's your mum's bike!'

'Where, where, Dad?'

'By that café.'

The café was halfway down a strip mall which seemed to stretch for miles at either side of a fast four-lane highway going north–south of Sedalia. A minute later I'd parked the RV within spitting distance and, as we approached, Jane exited the café door with Martyn and Ryan. They were preparing to leave.

'You should try some cake, home-made and very yummy,' Jane said to Steven. Steven was quiet.

'Are you all right, Steven?'

'I'm fine, Mum.'

'We're not leaving because you've come, but we'd like an early finish.' Jane looked in my eyes.

'It's okay, I understand,' I said.

'Give me a hug, Mike,' she said. My arms outstretched and Jane slotted into them like a well-worn jigsaw piece. Yesterday's fierce argument had left us both emotionally drained and there was a sense that we were walking on eggshells.

'You get off, Jane,' I said.

'Are you sure? I'll stay for a while if you wish.'

'No, let's have an early finish. California's not far.'

'I wish,' Jane said.

The cyclists left so Steven and I went to explore. Inside the café, it was like an extension of the owner's kitchen, easy chairs, newspapers, the hissing of a coffee maker. The only other patrons were two smartly attired elderly ladies enjoying a mid-week natter. Steven and I ate slowly, soaking in the relaxed atmosphere, an oasis from the strip malls and bustle of the high-way. With some reluctance we eventually decided it was time to return to our thirty-foot eyesore.

'Are you from the UK?' One of the ladies spoke to us with a proper English accent.

I looked up. 'Yes, Leeds.'

'Are you with the cyclists, one of them looked familiar.'

'Yes. What brings you to Missouri?'

'My son is based at Knob Noster and he's just about to be posted overseas,' she said. Knob Noster was just up the road on the way back to Warrensburg and originally we'd mooted staying at the State Park. That was before yesterday turned out to be so shit. I must have looked perplexed as she added: 'Have you not seen the signs?'

'What signs?'

'Knob Noster is home to the Stealth Bomber.'

'Oh, where is your son being posted?' I said.

'Iraq, tomorrow.'

'I presume you must be used to it by now. Still, it must be very nerve-racking as a parent,' I said. The lady looked on the wrong side of seventy so I was guessing her son was no pup.

'No, it's his first posting overseas.' She looked down at her empty cup. 'Forty-eight as well.'

'Wow, that's quite an age to be sent into a war zone. No offence but are the US Air Force running out of qualified people?'

'That's exactly it,' she said. 'His boss is going as well and he's fifty-eight. They're in a right mess. Bush is making such a mess of things.'

I didn't know what to say after that. 'Best wishes to you all. I hope it's a safe posting,' I said, drinking up.

'Me too. How are you finding Missouri?'

'Pleasant, a little busier than we've been used to but pretty.'

Her American friend spoke up. 'There are a lot of social problems in the state, poverty, poor housing and drugs.'

'Really?'

'It's nicknamed the Meth State, be careful as you move through it.'

'Thank you, we will.'

We passed through Sedalia and were soon at our overnight stop of California, Missouri. The whole of the state seemed to be blighted with the most uninspirational names possible and the lack of an RV park meant we were staying in the Motel California, an uninspiring name for a bog standard basic resting stop.

The Eagles' refrain of 'you can check out any time you want but you can never leave' played out in my head. It was a typical American motel, the sort you'd see in cult movies where a hooker, drug addict and homicidal maniac would be holed up in the room next door.

We rented one room and arranged for the two RVs to lighten up a cheerless car park. The motel seemed to be half occupied by long-term guests who were clearly on benefits. Jane rattled off a quick interview for ABC in California with an English journalist working for an American broadcaster who was trying to bang the drum. He'd managed to get Floyd Landis, the recent winner of the Tour de France, to give a quote on Jane's exploits which under normal circumstances would have been a great boost but as he was also trying to explain away his failed drugs test, its value was limited. It seemed to sum up the ride's luck. Dogged by uninterested media in the UK and the USA, it was in danger of being a monumental flop. With Jane's health failing and a flagging Mid-West morale it seemed as futile a journey as ever.

Donations were still minuscule and it seemed unlikely that we'd reach £20,000 for the whole trip. We could all have got temporary work for the summer and earned more. Ryan had looked at generating publicity in the USA and now that we were visiting big towns like Kansas City and St Louis there were opportunities. Jane, though, was sensibly saying that she couldn't fit in media work into her schedule.

It was clear to me that we were understaffed by two on the ride; one more was needed to help Cindy and someone else to go ahead to organise publicity in advance of Jane arriving. Knowing this only increased my frustration.

The heat was beating down as we traipsed across a dusty gravelled launderette car park with two full black bin bags of cycling kit, bedding and clothes. We shared the room with a number of Hispanic ladies with small children, the American underclass. We slumped down on a wooden bench and watched in silence while the whirr of washing spinning and the clicking of jeans' buttons broke the silence.

'I'm hungry,' Steven said. 'Can I have a burger please?'

'If you like,' Jane said. 'Let's eat now, Mike, we can have a sandwich later.'

After six weeks in the USA we knew what we had to do – get in the RV and drive forty yards to McDonald's. The car park was stacked with numerous pickups, red and black, all four seater and mostly pristine. Steven laughed. 'I wish I'd brought my video camera.'

The restaurant was empty apart from twenty men, all aged sixty plus, wearing faded denim dungarees and black and red checked shirts like a look-alike Grandpa Walton competition.

'They all look the same, are they clones?' Steven asked.

'I suspect there's a strong chance they're related,' I said.

'They're unlikely to know it though,' Jane added.

'Can I go back and get the camera, please?' Steven begged.

'No. It's too bizarre, Steven. They'll probably lynch us.'

The county fair was on at the showground in town so after tea Steven and I went to explore but it seemed too busy and coupled with lethargy and tiredness we gave up the ghost and all settled for an early night.

'What's that, Mike?' Jane poked her hands into my ribs. 'Mike, Mike.'

'Errrr.'

'Mike.' A door slammed, there was some shouting. Our door rattled and it felt like someone had joined us in the room.

'Come on!' a female voice from outside screamed. 'Come on, you two!' A child's cry rang out. 'Come on, we can't do anything, the doctors will sort her out.'

'Mum! Wake up,' the child's voice shouted, choking with tears.

'I don't know, but we need to get out of here,' said the same female voice.

'I'm scared, I want my mum.'

'We have to go, there's nothing we can do, the paramedics will sort her out.'

Jane was out of bed and looking out of the curtains.

'What's going on?' I asked.

'There's a woman, who was in next door, fleeing with two kids across the car park.'

'Shut the curtains,' I said.

'Shall we check next door, it sounds like someone's overdosed,' Jane said.

'It sounds like there's an ambulance coming, it sounds like it's a whole lot of shit and dangerous. I suggest you shut the bloody curtains, we wake up early and get out of this shit hole.'

Martyn had described a recent night when he was certain the adjoining room was being rented out on an hourly tenancy.

This ride was turning into one long endurance event in more ways than one.

Jane climbed back in to bed. 'This type of behaviour must be a regular feature with the motel because no one's made the slightest bit of difference and no one's interested. It's just too weird.'

As part of our social responsibility, I asked the owner to check the room before we left but he seemed neither surprised nor nonplussed. The room, he said, was 'fine', although that word was used in its loosest sense.

Day 42 – Wednesday, 9 August
California, Miss. to Hermann, Miss.
75.7 miles – 7 hrs 06 mins
Total covered – 2412.5 miles

MIKE

'Where are you, Mike?' It was always welcome to hear a voice from home and Dave Harrison from Yorkshire Television had been a regular caller throughout the trip.

'Cole Junction.'

'All right, smart arse, a state would be good, still in Missouri I'm guessing?'

'Yep, we're just on the outskirts of Jefferson City, hopefully about to cross the Missouri.'

'Good. How's Jane?'

'It's only three days since the rest day but already she's shot. They'll be with us in a minute.' As if on cue Ryan appeared at the top of a brow ready to descend. At the same time, a railway barrier between us came down and the familiar refrain of a horn hooting announced the arrival of the train. 'Ryan's here now. Well, he will be in five minutes after the train's gone through.'

'I'll get off and call you in thirty minutes.'

'We're okay for five minutes, the train's really long. I think it's the hills that are getting to Jane, her right knee's very stiff and sore and they've been climbing about three thousand feet a day without gaining any altitude. She's got a knee support on today and we'll ice it tonight.'

'Shit, Mike.'

'Yep, the last two days have been a bit grim. Are you still coming out?'

'Yea, we're coming to Washington and staying till the end so it will be in just over two weeks.'

'Flipping 'eck, that's soon. It seems so very close, but Jane's being held together with sticking plaster.'

'Will you give us a ring and let us know if things deteriorate as I'll need to rethink.'

'Of course.'

'Okay, Mike, stay cheerful, our love to Jane. How's the money doing?'

'Absolutely shit.'

'Well, we'll have to give it a good push then. Be good, Mike.'

After a brief stop to refuel with iced coffees and a sandwich they were soon off again. The only crossing point for fifty miles of the Missouri was in Jefferson City, the state capital of Missouri, named after the third president of the USA.

Rob had scouted ahead and was confident a bike could cross Highway 50. Jane was anxious to get across onto the 94 on the northern banks of the Missouri because it hugged the river while on the south the road twisted in and out adding as many as twenty miles.

Jefferson City is dominated by the white domed capitol building and its presence drew Steven and I like a magnet. Conscious of our cycling responsibility we grabbed a quick snap before trying to race across the Missouri before the cyclists.

The road was a 'share the road with a bike' road. The legislators had put up a big yellow sign to say as much then the cyclists endured a game of chicken as the trucks and four-by-fours got as close as possible.

The whole conurbation was limited to the south side of the river. To the north, was agricultural land and forestry except for an out-of-town industrial building where we pulled off to regroup.

Jane's cycling top was open in a V and beads of sweat glistened in the sunlight, her shoulders protruded at right angles. Her orange and white bandana was underneath her helmet shielding her from the sun.

'Are you all right, Jane?' I asked tentatively.

'The heat is just making my heart thump like a base drum.'

'Really?'

'My body's having to work so hard, I feel really heat fatigued.' Her head bowed as though talking about it was causing her to have the symptoms. 'My head's thumping and I'm taking it really conservatively up the hills as I've just reached that stage where it is so hot that if I do too much I might just fall off the bike and not get up for a few minutes.'

'Well, there's no rush, Jane, although it looks a little hilly to Hermann.'

'I'm struggling, Mike.'

'I know. We'll get to the finish and get settled.'

Although the heat wasn't as great as in Utah or Nevada it did rise to uncomfortable levels in early afternoon. It was rare to see a day less than a hundred. Because the sun was rising later, start times were later and traffic problems with larger conurbations and cumulative fatigue were ensuring finishing times were an average three hours later than earlier in the ride.

Hermann was reached by crossing an old metal bridge that had clearly been built before the Americans started driving monster-size gas-guzzling vehicles. Meeting oncoming traffic while in the RV was a hair-raising experience. It was a bridge with character, something that the replacement bridge that was being built just down stream was lacking. Once across, the road widened like only American roads can, rather like a two-lane highway with a car park at each side.

We made our way to the RV park, which was the State Park. It was a vast green field. Jane had fretted that this would be the case.

'The only vehicles within the vicinity, parked obtrusively in an empty field – a magnet for all the local nutters.' I could hear the words now but as she hadn't arrived I discounted her feelings and parked the RV anyway.

The park had an open air swimming pool. To hear the screams and whelps of youngsters was a joy. There was a baseball pitch occupied by two bare-chested late teenagers, all-American men, whose red pickup was parked adjacent. Everything was spotlessly clean, as if a picture postcard had been airbrushed. After hooking up, Steven and I set off into town to explore and find a pleasant café for Jane to have lunch.

'Why are there so many German flags?' Steven asked.

'I dunno.'

'Is it because the town's called Hermann?' Steven said.

'We'll ask someone.'

At almost every shop premises the Bundesbehorden was flown, sometimes with the Stars and Stripes, sometimes without. The town was dressed up, there were plant pots, splendid greenery and it was generally very beautifully presented. To satisfy Steven's curiosity we called in at the local newspaper offices.

'Well, this was originally a German settlement in the nineteenth century,' the proprietor said. 'There's a big German ancestry, you can tell from the names – Rhineland, etc. There are a lot of wineries local to here. It's steeped in German history, it's something the town's proud of. Until recently the junior school was primarily German speaking.'

'Were there problems during the war?'

'No, not that I'm aware of.'

While waiting for Jane, Steven and I visited the local hairdresser's to get the obligatory grade 2.

'That'll cause them problems with continuity shots,' I said to Steven, referring to the TV footage being taken.

He laughed. We were three times as long as necessary as we chatted to the staff who said that they'd never seen any tourists from any country visit the town.

As evening drew on, Cindy, Jane and I headed out into the

town to visit the banks of the river. It was a beautiful backdrop, the sun was setting low over the trees with the bridge casting shadows.

'I think we should go home now,' I said. 'Leave the ride on a high.'

'I know. I can't imagine it getting better than this,' Jane said.

'We could sneak off in the middle of the night,' I said.

'We could,' said Jane. 'But I know of one little man who'd be bitterly disappointed.'

I nodded and smiled. 'Ryan'll get over it,' I said.

Day 43 – Thursday, 10 August
Hermann, Miss. to St Charles, Miss.
75.3 miles – 9 hrs 01 mins
Total covered – 2487.8 miles

JANE

It was a wrench to leave Hermann. But as we cycled across the old metal bridge out of the town that morning, all that mattered was that it was another day nearer to the finish line and home. Travelling east on the northern banks of the Missouri, large wineries continued up the hilly road.

'I thought Mike said it would be flat today,' Martyn said, as he drew alongside me.

'You should know by now that he's full of bullshit.'

Martyn nodded. 'Yeah, but he sounds so convincing.'

Ryan was pedalling behind us. 'Hi guys. The weather is looking a little foreboding,' he called. Martyn and I glanced behind to see gigantic storm clouds gathering. It was 10 a.m., unusual at such an early hour.

'It's a shame we can't use the trail,' Martyn said. Earlier we'd passed another route marker for the Katy Trail, an off-road cycle path running for 225 miles along the former Missouri–Kansas–Texas railroad. It is part of the Lewis and Clarke National Historic Trail, which follows the route of the second official transcontinental expedition north of Mexico.

'We'd get too many punctures,' Ryan said. 'We're already running short of equipment.'

Today's route was challenging to say the least. Full of short sharp climbs which sapped the energy from our legs. Although we'd attacked the day in a bid to avoid the storm, it soon became obvious that we weren't going to outrun it. As we rounded a bend I heard a couple of quick toots on the horn. It was Mike in the RV. I waved as he slowed down and pulled in a few hundred yards ahead.

'That storm looks awful,' he said, climbing out of the driver's seat. 'Do you want to shelter? I'm sure it's just about to break.'

'I know, we've been watching it,' I said. I looked up as I took a swig from my water bottle. The sky was now grey and threatening.

'We were hoping to try and catch you before it breaks,' he said.

'There's a small town – Defiance – nearby,' I said. 'We'll try and get there.'

'How's your back?'

I'd been very sore as soon as I woke this morning. My lower back felt like it had a pneumatic drill going through my bones and my vertebrae felt like they were about to collapse in on each other like a concertina.

'Just the same,' I said.

We reached Defiance within the half hour and stopped at a pleasant café/diner, while the rain crashed down outside. It lashed the windows but the clouds seemed to be scudding quickly across the sky. It wouldn't last long.

As the storm passed over, we decided to get back on the road as quickly as possible. For the first time in weeks, we donned our high visibility rain jackets. I was glad we'd taken the precaution – the road to St Charles was busy with high-sided trucks and cars. The pools of standing water at the roadside made us extra cautious – one unsteady slip could have sent us crashing under an overtaking truck. Although we took a short detour off the main road, the extra miles and the weather meant we didn't arrive in St Charles until after 4 p.m. and some four hours later than expected.

The RV park looked similar to the one in Denver in that it was nothing more than a car park. Directly under the airport flight path, jets thundered overhead, their landing gear already down. If that wasn't bad enough, it was also underneath an interstate highway and a railway and large freight trains would be chugging by at regular intervals.

Mike was clearly disgusted. 'We could park at Wal-Mart for nothing,' he said. 'This RV park is the most expensive we've had across America.'

'If you think I'm sleeping in a supermarket car park, you're dafter than you look,' I said, although I could see his point.

That night, perhaps thanks to the physical and mental exertion of concentrating on not getting killed, I fell asleep with surprising ease.

Day 44 – Friday, 11 August
St Charles, Miss. to Greenville, Illinois (Ill.)
70.5 miles – 6 hrs 45 mins
Total covered – 2558.3 miles

JANE

When I awoke with the alarm at half past five however, my back was in agony. I reached for the towel and wiped the sweat from the top half of my body. Once again, Mike had been forced to sleep on the couch in the main room as I'd drenched both halves of the bed. I could hear Ryan outside unchaining the bikes, checking the tyres and lubing the chains.

'Morning, Ryan,' I said, as I crept out of the RV. He looked up, removing the flashlight he'd been holding in his mouth.

'Good morning, Jane,' he said, his voice flat. I was immediately suspicious. I could always rely on Ryan to be cheerful, even at this early hour. Normally he was like a child waking up on Christmas Day.

'I'm going to throttle Cindy,' he said quietly. I waited for him to elucidate but it seemed as though the words were stuck in his throat.

I walked over to him. 'It can't be that bad.'

'You'll see,' he said. 'How simple is it to get the breakfast in? How hard is it? *You* have peanut butter on bread, banana and coffee. *Me* Cheerios, toasted bagel, butter, banana and coffee.'

I knew where this was leading. 'Is something missing?' I asked.

'All of it,' he said. 'I could absolutely throttle her. I'm staying outside as honestly I've had it with her.'

I let out an involuntary laugh.

'It's not funny, Jane.'

'It is,' I said. 'How many hours did you cycle yesterday?'

'Seven hours.'

'See? That's where the problem is. There wasn't enough time to get the groceries for a busy support team. We need to slow down.'

He smirked. 'Well, you do try hard,' he said, before kneeling down again to see to the tyres.

'Touché,' I left him smiling and entered the RV. 'Morning, Cindy,' I said. She was standing at the kitchen unit, rinsing a plate under the tap.

'Morning, Jane,' she smiled. 'How are you today?'

'My back's sore,' I said, easing my way into a chair.

'We're out of groceries,' she said matter-of-factly. 'There are a couple of pieces of bread.'

I let a beat pass before I looked over at her and said as calmly as I could, 'Cindy. We're cycling long distances. We need to make sure that there's sufficient food in every day. It's not really good enough to have just a couple of pieces of bread. Breakfast is so important.'

She said nothing, continuing to clatter around the kitchen like a chastised child. I opened my medicine bag, removing pills from the foil packets and laying them out across the table.

Ryan came in. 'I think we'll shorten today's distance, Ryan,' I said, swallowing the first of the pills. 'We're due to do seventy-four miles today but we'll do it tomorrow and do fifty today.'

A wave of concern spread over Ryan's face. 'Are you not feeling good?' he asked.

'My back's sore and I'm feeling very nauseous.'

'No problem, Jane, but I'm a little concerned.'

'I just need to get some decent rest and the only way we can do it is to finish early. This park isn't exactly conducive to rest.'

As we left St Charles the air was thick with moisture and soon every garment was dripping. We'd be crossing the Mississippi, the route dictated to us by the number of bridges we had to cross. We agreed to meet Mike at West Alton a few miles short of the river just in case the bridge didn't cater for bikes. Sure enough, Mike was waiting for us at a green in the centre of the town.

'There's a little problem,' he said, as I pulled up alongside him. 'Look at the sign.'

The road sign indicated a height restriction which was significantly lower than the RV.

'We've done well to get here without this happening before,' he said.

'Is there an alternative?'

'I'm just checking the maps.'

'These workmen will know,' I said, looking at a couple of people pottering along. I walked over.

'That rig won't get under there,' one of the men said.

'Is there an alternative route?'

'Where are you heading?'

'The Mississippi.'

He looked across the road, straightening his glasses. He was in his late fifties, early sixties.

'You may be able to go down there,' he said, pointing to a road running off at a ninety-degree angle, 'but there's a dual carriageway and I don't know whether you can get on it. I've never been down that road.'

'Oh, sorry,' I said. 'I presumed you lived here.'

'Lived here all my life, just never been down that road,' he said.

Mike tooted the horn of the RV again. He'd found a route. I was grateful – the thought of having to send the RVs back through St Louis and effectively cycle without any support for the day was not one I wished to contemplate for long. Minutes later we were on the cycle path of Clark Bridge crossing the Mississippi. The river's sheer size was awe-inspiring though, judging by its colour, it was easy to see where the 'mud pie' came from.

Psychologically, however, it was a boost. We were in the second half of the ride. We'd covered over two and a half thousand miles but the river seemed to divide west from east in my subconscious. Suddenly, the seventy-four miles we'd previously planned to cycle that day looked possible again.

A few miles after crossing the river, we came across Mike and the RV parked in the small town of Hamel, waving furiously for us to stop. My heart skipped a beat and I sprinted towards him.

I couldn't see Steven so squawked the words out, 'What's up?'

'Nothing urgent, it's just that you're crossing Route 66.'

'Oh,' I said, nonplussed. I vaguely recalled a song or was it a book, no a song. 'Is that it?'

'It's interesting,' said Mike, a little deflated.

'Really?' I said. 'I need the loo anyway.'

'Mind how you go in.'

'What's happened here?' There were glass jars, pans and vegetables strewn about. Cereals had been glued to the floor by a bolognaise sauce which had spilt from a broken jar. The sauce had sprayed its trail up the sides of the cupboards and fridge. The bin which was wedged in the door of the shower had emptied its contents; toiletries lay across the bathroom.

'It looks like there's been a localised tornado,' I said.

'It's his fault,' Steven said.

'Oh, you little so and so,' Mike said.

'What happened?'

'We were just travelling into town and Steven starting shrieking like a three-year-old girl.'

'Didn't.'

'He spotted a spider, started shrieking like a banshee and I slammed on the brakes and here's the result.'

Jane looked at the both of us. 'Well, it looks like you're going to be busy.'

Day 45 – Saturday, 12 August
Greenville, Ill. – Effingham, Ill.
52.7 miles – 4 hrs 52 mins
Total covered – 2611.0 miles

MIKE

Camp Lakewood RV Park in Effingham was idyllic. Situated just out of town, it was set on the banks of Lake Pauline. Quiet, clean and secluded, the pitches were set in among dozens of tall trees. It was a temperate day and Steven, who'd been nagging all day to use the fishing rod we'd recently bought him, finally got his wish. The lake was surrounded by trees, which allowed plenty of shade from the late afternoon sun. Steven was standing on the bank of the lake casting his line contentedly. Driftwood seemed to be the biggest obstacle for him and I had my doubts that his cheap rod and bait would catch anything substantial. But just at that second, I was proved wrong.

'Steven! Steven!' I shouted with increased urgency. 'Your line's caught on a log.' I threw down my writing pad, got up from the canvas collapsible chair and started to rush over the fifteen yards towards him. 'Don't pull it, you'll fall.'

His line was caught on a huge chunk of tree which was pulling away from him.

'Dad!' Steven shrieked.

'Shit!' Just as I was arriving, Steven's body lurched forward, his feet still rooted to the floor. In a split second his hand reached forward and he was half soaked. He stood, rooted waist high in the moss-covered water. I held out my hand to help him back up.

I tried to suppress a smile.

'Don't laugh, Dad,' he said. The edge of Lake Pauline was a green swampy affair and bits of moss hung to Steven as though he'd been gunged. I pursed my lips, trying not to laugh. 'Dad, please, it's not funny.'

'You're mum's gonna go mental.'

'It's your fault,' Steven said.

'How do you figure that?'

'You should've chosen somewhere more suitable for me to fish.'

'Clown!' I said, steering him away from the edge.

'Useless dad,' he retorted.

Frustrated, I packed up all the paraphernalia I had just lumbered down to the lake's edge and we both walked back to the RV. I crammed the chair into the store at the rear but it became jammed on a number of green plastic bottles. Ryan had negotiated a fantastic amount of equipment from Gatorade and they had supported the ride with drink, sachets, towels and bike bottles.

The trouble was there were enough bottles to supply a battalion and every time I opened a cupboard one of the bastards would get in the way. Whenever I was out of Ryan's sight, I jettisoned some, leaving them strategically placed in prominent places, gaps in walls, on a signpost like a child leading a paper trail. But just like sand after you've visited the beach, we never really got rid of them all.

'Come on, you buggers,' I muttered and finally lodged the chair in place.

The campsite was well positioned at the side of the lake, although the ground was bone dry. The trees provided some good shade and the foliage was extremely colourful. It was Saturday afternoon and a popular spot for recreational campers having a barbecue and sinking a few beers.

'Mike! What the fuck are you doing?'

I'd been conscious that Jane's bed was directly above the store where I was trying to cram in the chair and I'd tried to be quiet but appreciated there had been some rattling.

'Fucking tosser.' I heard her foot hit the floor inches above my head. 'What happened?' I then heard her say, as Steven went inside.

'It was Dad's fault.'

'Get out of those clothes now. Careful. Do it outside, Steven,' she said and as she wandered round to the back of the RV to find me, I went round the front.

'Where the hell are you?' she snapped.

As we met by the door, Jane's clothes were drenched in sweat and I could see it was taking some effort to keep her eyes open. I could tell I was on the brink of receiving a dressing down of seismic proportions. Jane was practically in tears.

'It's all right, love,' I said, soothingly.

'Don't "It's all right love" me,' she said, turning on her heels to resume her rest.

The saying an army marches on its stomach could equally be applied to a cyclist pedalling on his or hers. That evening we ate at the picnic table outside the RV, but once again, the food was uninspiring and poor. Jane, who'd been copiously sick yesterday, was barely taking on enough calories to get through the day without exercising. After eating, and in fading light, Steven completed his weekly interview with Jane for television.

It was Saturday night and the smell of barbecued meat drifted through the air; piercing alcohol fuelled songs provided the night-time melody. Jane sat silently writing her diary. She looked across at me and her face beamed a smile that could have melted an ice cap.

'Are you all right, love?' I asked.

'Yes.'

'You're nearly there,' I said.

Her face fell. 'Do you realise how annoying that is?'

'No, but I've got a feeling I will in a minute.'

'You know when you've just run twenty miles in a marathon and you're knackered, your legs have gone and then some clown says you're nearly there . . .'

'No,' I smiled, and Jane chucked her pen playfully at me.

'I love you, Mike. I can't wait to go home.'

Day 46 – Sunday, 13 August
Effingham, Ill. – Terre Haute, Indiana (Ind.)
74.8 miles – 6 hrs 48 mins
Total covered – 2,685.8 miles

MIKE

On Sunday morning, there was little stirring in the campsite apart from the clink of bike chains going through the sprockets as the cyclists set off on the seventy-five miles to Terre Haute. We were closing in on the East Coast. When the Illinois to Indiana state line was crossed today we'd have entered our final time zone.

I'd tried to Google a Catholic church the day before to see if Steven and I could catch a Mass. The experience was confusing and it was impossible to find directions or Mass times. It was clear that fundamental Christianity had a large part to play in middle America. Effingham's rather ostentatious demonstration of its faith was a 190-foot cross on the intersection of Interstates 70 and 57.

I contemplated driving out of town to find a church but thought the chance of meeting a collection of total nutters was too high so we scuttled across to Terre Haute with some haste. We stopped at another strip mall and grabbed a burger. My desire to sit down with a Sunday joint seemed overwhelming.

'Are you the folks cycling across America with the woman who's got cancer?' the cashier said, noticing the T-shirts.

'Yes, how did you know that?'

'I saw it on the *Today* show.'

'That was weeks ago.'

'I wondered whether you'd be coming here,' she said.

I scratched my head, Stan Laurel style, and grabbed the local paper from the rack. I liked to peruse the local papers as it was usually a good barometer of the district. The headline was about racial disadvantage in Indianapolis for black Americans needing regular work. The back pages were enthusing about the visit to Terre Haute of the Indianapolis Colts for a pre-season friendly.

We were soon to discover we'd not actually yet arrived at Terre Haute but at West Terre Haute, separated from its much bigger neighbour by the Wabash River. We headed eastwards and there were some stunningly imposing properties, set back some distance from the road with huge drives and manicured lawns in extensive grounds where clearly the American dream was alive and flourishing.

Our RV park was within a stone's throw from Interstate 70. Terre Haute was deceptively big but uninviting. When Jane arrived we spent two hours poring over maps and trying to work out mileage for the remaining days to New York.

Day 47 – Monday, 14 August
Terre Haute
Rest day

MIKE

After seven weeks together there was a desperate nature to the ride. Martyn was under increasing pressure to deliver TV packages and podcasts for Sky while editing the documentary. Ryan's challenge was catching up with work on his PhD, while Jane, Steven and I needed some family time. Cindy was excited at potentially seeing the Colts. For the first time since leaving Britain, we decided to have a day out as a family. We visited the covered bridges of Terre Haute, the town's main tourist's attraction – the area was naturally the 'Covered Bridge Capital of the World'.

It was a joy to have the real life Jane in the front passenger seat of the RV. For the last two months we'd only had Jane, the disembodied Tom Tom's voice, which had been giving us directions for weeks and verbal admonishments during the day.

Wearing a cotton shirt and blouse, she looked human again. The sweat glistened on her neck, a sign that even now, her liver was working too hard.

As we headed up from Brazil to Mansfield, agricultural land spread out flat to both sides of the road.

'Have you seen the guy on the right, Mike?' said Jane.

An aged man in denim dungarees and checked cloth shirt sat at the roadside cradling a shotgun.

'Weird,' I said as I parked the RV upon entering Mansfield. There wasn't another vehicle or person around. It was completely deserted but stunningly beautiful. Immaculately painted wooden buildings lined the streets and a welcome centre was adorned with flower baskets hanging from the first floor balcony. Everything was immaculately tended. The covered bridge straddled the river as if it had been levitated. Underneath the abundant water turned white as it gushed past over the rocks.

Many of the buildings were built on elevated wooden stilts climbing twenty feet above the ground and a shutdown chair lift ran parallel to the main street. It was clear that this deserted paradise was geared to cater for huge crowds. Across the bridge there was car parking that would have put Silverstone to shame. But every shop, food outlet and facility was shut. Had this been November, it would have been understandable but it was 14 August. There was no indication of when the town would be occupied.

'We won't get any dinner here, Dad,' Steven said.

'I wish we had a picnic,' Jane said.

'We could fix something up in the RV,' I said.

For a moment we just stood there, taking in the view.

'There's something a little freaky about this,' said Jane. 'It's like we're trespassing. A completely empty town in an idyllic setting.'

Steven was close up to Jane. 'I don't like it, Mum.'

'It's very beautiful,' I said.

'It's weird,' Jane said.

'It is, Dad,' Steven agreed.

We left the life-size model village and headed off to Rockville over ten miles away in search of food. Rockville was dominated by a Parke County Court House which took centre place in the town square. Small shops and units were on all four sides, a welcome change from the strip malls of most towns. Dozens of posters with the words 'Gary Cooper for Sheriff' adorned walls and lampposts.

'Look at that,' I said. 'Gary Cooper for Sheriff!'

'And . . .' said Jane.

'Gary Cooper for Sheriff.' I said again.

'So what?' Jane said, but I couldn't be bothered to explain.

As we drove around the streets, we spotted a number of men in orange jumpsuits being loaded into transport – prisoners being returned to the correctional centre, which was just out of town. We'd seen a number of correctional facilities, from the deserts of Utah to the plains of Kansas and it was becoming a regular feature of the trip.

We parked up and looked around. Jane managed to find presents for Jodie and Rebecca, which seemed to ease her conscience and gave my ears a rest. We stopped to eat lunch at a wooden building, which like many others wouldn't invite much passing trade but was well supported by locals who'd tipped us off.

The fare was typically American – starter salad followed by meat and chips. It occurred to me that in a country so vast, the regional varieties in diet were almost non-existent. It was akin to travelling from Glasgow to Tehran and finding everyone ate haggis.

The atmosphere in the restaurant was convivial. Jane, Steven and I sat in silence, transfixed by a conversation orchestrated by a brash charismatic Caribbean American woman that was enveloping the whole room. She was a stout lady with an enormous chest whose primary role seemed to be to ensure that every patron cleared their plates.

'Yo, young man, you need to finish or you'll have to help in the kitchen,' she rounded on Steven, who had been eating non-stop for twenty minutes.

Steven looked up sheepishly.

'You don't get to leave until you finish,' her voice boomed out, 'and your mom needs to eat as well. Look at your dad's plate.'

'He's had a lot more practice,' Steven said and the lady guffawed.

CHAPTER 6

Day 48 – Tuesday, 15 August
Terre Haute, Ind. – Martinsville, Ind.
64.3 miles – 5 hrs 56 mins
Total covered – 2750.1 miles

MIKE

In the corridor of the hotel, I watched as a little girl of around ten held her brother's hand and yanked him across the carpet towards me.

'Hi,' I smiled at them both.

'Hiya,' she responded. She was part of a large family occupying about four rooms on our corridor. We'd noticed that there was constant toing and froing of children swapping from room to room.

'Are you on holiday?' I asked.

'No, we're living here. Our house burnt down. Doug, stop it.' She dragged her brother back.

'Oh, that's tough. Were you all okay?'

'Yes.'

'It must be hard living here.'

'Oh, its okay, we've got cable,' she said, and with that they were off through the rear fire door.

As we'd discovered over the last few weeks, any self-respecting American town always applied a 'Capital of the World' label to it. Abilene – Greyhound Capital of the World; Rocky Ford – Melon; La Crosse – Barbed Wire; Parke County – Covered Bridge. With

Martinsville it was the Goldfish Capital of the World, apparently, because the first successful goldfish farm in the USA was opened here in 1899. Sadly, the goldfish were not the most famous pond life in the city. Martinsville, we discovered, was still notorious throughout the country for the racist murder of a 21-year-old black woman, Carol Jenkins, in September 1968. There was a 34-year-old assumption that it had been racially motivated and there had been a police cover-up. The murderer was finally discovered in 2002 when implicated by his daughter, who had witnessed the killing. He had links to the Klu Klux Klan, although he'd never lived in the town of Martinsville itself.

Whether the town was a victim of a racial slur or it simply had a very unfair reputation based on historical inaccuracies is uncertain. But in the 2002 census there were only eleven black residents in its 11,698 total. Certainly, there was no evidence of racism to the passing visitor.

Day 49 – Wednesday, 16 August
Martinsville, Ind., to Rushville, Ind.
59.7 miles – 6 hrs 30 mins
Total covered – 2809.8 miles

MIKE

'Dad, Mum's here,' Steven said, coming through the fire door having loaded his bag into the RV.

Jane had set off for the day's cycle twenty minutes previously, but the weather had been inclement.

'It must be the mist,' I said. There was an autumnal feel to each day now with more modest, mild and accessible temperatures. Today, the sun was taking its time to burn the mist away. Jane appeared. It was rare to see her in her luminous yellow bike jacket – I'd grown used to the white 'Ride Across America' cycling top over the last seven weeks.

'Are you helping Dad pack, Steven?' she said.

'No,' he laughed.

'We thought we'd rather come back and grab a coffee here

than have a frustrating wait at the roadside,' Jane said. She had set off a little while ago but clearly there was little point trying to navigate these big roads in these conditions.

'Good,' I nodded. 'It makes sense.'

'Are you all right, Mummy?' Steven asked.

'Yes.'

'Are you scared this morning?'

There had been a number of dog attacks on yesterday's ride which had destroyed Jane's confidence. We knew she wasn't keen to climb back on the bike today.

'It should be more suburban today,' she said. 'So hopefully it won't be too bad.'

It was good to have a little extra time with Jane in the morning but all the cyclists were anxious to get off as soon as the mist lifted. By eight thirty, the three of them were back on their bikes.

'I'll see you in Franklin,' Jane called and they were off.

Steven and I quickly loaded the RV and went to grab some breakfast. Within half an hour we'd set off and passed Jane. In no time at all were parked up in Franklin. Twenty minutes later, Cindy arrived.

'Why's she parking there?' I said. We'd parked at the start of the town in the car park of a selection of shops while Cindy had pulled up a hundred yards away, nearer to the oncoming cyclists.

'Dunno,' said Steven.

As we moved into the more densely populated areas where there was more than one road, it had proved something of a problem for Cindy. She'd spurned Steven's offer of help with the Tom Tom – perhaps out of pride – but as a result, her support to the cyclists had become, well, patchy. She'd programmed the satnav herself and stuck to its instructions with almost religious zeal. It didn't matter if the maps – or the rest of us – said there was a shorter or quicker way, Cindy was having none of it. It meant that on several occasions, the cyclists turned up to a meeting point before she did, which didn't go down well.

Fortunately, today we were on a straight road with no turn offs. Minutes after we'd parked up, Jane arrived and pulled into Cindy's van. It was fifteen minutes before she came to say hello to us.

'Good of you to come and say hello to Steven,' I said.

'I didn't see you parked up and Cindy only just told us you were here. Why aren't you parked together?'

'Ask Cindy. We were here first.'

'And you couldn't have driven down?'

'That's not the point.'

'No, you'd rather sulk.'

'I'm sorry but we've done nothing wrong, have we, Steven?'

'No,' he responded dutifully.

'If you're not happy with Cindy, go tell her. You're paying her wages. Sort it.'

With that, Jane stomped out of the RV, her cyclist shoes thudding on the ground before she slammed the door which bounced open again with the force.

'She's happy,' Steven said.

We set off to the next stop, Shelbyville, on a road that was practically straight all the way and we were there in no time. There seemed little point in supporting the riders because Cindy had it covered so Steven and I decided to go bowling. With the American kids back at school, the lanes were empty so we spent an hour or two playing, planning on heading out of town to the final stop at Rushville to find accommodation. But as we were leaving Shelbyville, Jane was just cycling through it so we pulled up. Jane's front wheel wobbled as she arrived and I could immediately see tear tracks down her cheeks.

'What's up?'

'Steven, go inside,' Jane said and Steven knew better than to protest.

'I've been worried sick after this morning,' Jane said. 'And then you don't appear here for the rest stop. It's fucking pathetic, Mike.'

I was a little surprised. 'We've only been bowling. What's the problem? Steven's had hardly any time for fun on this trip.'

'You only had to say . . . to let us know where you were – I was worried about you.'

'I did. I phoned Cindy.'

Jane frowned. 'She never said anything.'

'Well, I apologise, but she knew. Steven heard the phone call if you need corroboration.'

'Fuck,' Jane spat and climbed back on the bike. She was caught between tears and anger and as she moved off her legs buckled and slowly but surely the bike's front wheel slid and she crashed to the ground. I knew better than to rush over to help. There were speckles of blood down her elbow.

'Look what you've done!' she hissed.

'Me?'

'Cindy then,' said Jane, brushing grit from her arm. She was shaking her head. 'I'm sorry, I know it's not you.' And with that she burst into tears. 'Look, there's been a lot of dog attacks. I'm sick of bloody dogs.'

I moved towards her hesitantly. 'Martyn and Ryan will sort them,' I said.

'I know, I know, I'm being stupid but I'm terrified. I'm so scared I don't want to cycle another 1000 miles with dog attacks.'

'Don't worry,' I said, and held her tight, blanketing the sobs. 'You've been through heat waves, mountains and crickets. Don't be beaten by dogs.'

Her shoulders heaved in my arms. 'I've had enough, Mike.' I knew the anger would pass but a wave of guilt spread over me. I wasn't the one cycling, just the one causing the problem.

Jane looked down the road to Martyn and Ryan who were standing with their legs astride their bikes. 'I need to get off, the guys are waiting.' Her legs turned slowly, hesitantly, not wishing to repeat the fall of seconds earlier.

Day 50 – Thursday, 17 August
Rushville, Ind. to Lebanon, Ohio (O.)
76.5 miles – 6 hrs 58 mins
Total covered – 2886.3 miles

MIKE

Today would be a long day, nearly eighty miles, but the saving grace was that it was flat. The scenery was pleasant although a little uninspiring. As we'd moved east so the land quality had improved and in turn there was more wealth in the local communities. There was also more openly nationalistic support of the troops with the frequency of red, white and blue or yellow ribbons or placards and messages. Many properties displayed the Stars and Stripes – it was akin to England once every four years in the middle of a World Cup final. We'd passed a smoking timber-framed building earlier in the morning with a fire crew still attending. It brought home that many of these properties were not built to last.

We drove casually down the road. Steven sat reading in the RV while I watched the fields roll by.

I turned the radio on.

'. . . my dad said he'd cover my student costs, he lied,' a young lady's voice crackled over the radio.

'And how bad are your debts?' the presenter responded.

'They are quite large. I'm so mad with my dad, we aren't talking.'

'And is your daddy walking with the Lord?'

'No, he's not walking with the Lord.'

'Well, we shouldn't be cross about the debt, but engage with your daddy and get him on the path to be with the Lord. I'll pray your daddy finds the Lord again.'

Steven and I looked at each other, clearly thinking the same thing. As we'd travelled across mid-America so the religious fever had increased. Some small towns could have as many as eight or nine varieties of church – often they were huge, with stadium-size car parks which became completely full on a Sunday morning. It had become a highlight of the trip for Steven and me to look out for and read the churches' slogans. 'Exposure to the Son may save a burning' or 'The soul's insurance policy' were just two of our favourites.

'What a freak,' Steven said.

'This is Christian debt-free radio,' said the voice. As far as I could see the aim was to clear the debt to enable people to be able to donate more to the church.

'They're all nutters,' Steven added and then watched me lean over to push in my CD. 'Oh no, not Journey again,' he moaned. But it was the only one we had with us. Our destination was Lebanon – Lebanon, Ohio that is, as no discerning state was without a town called Lebanon. Jane had picked a route around the cities of Dayton and Cincinnati and once again she'd set a deadline of clearing Ohio by Sunday so it meant seven consecutive days each of eighty miles.

We caught up with the cyclists at Germantown; they were easy to spot as a Japanese film crew was directly in front of them; the cameraman was sitting in the open boot of an SUV like a suicide jumper. There were a number of cars, some included irritable drivers, tailing them, and after fifteen minutes we got past them and stepped out and got Steven to film the film-makers.

'We're going to have to say something, sir,' Ryan said to me as he passed.

Jane soon followed. 'Don't tell me I'm going to have to say something to them,' I said.

'It's your job to control the media.'

'How's it going?' I asked.

'Good but someone's going to get killed. I'm not doing a ten-minute interview until after I've showered and changed and eaten.'

'No problem.'

'Ten minutes, that's all they get.'

'I understand.'

'Do you?'

'Take a chill pill.'

'Careful, Dad,' Steven said.

'Get off and I'll sort it. They seem like a nice bunch,' I said.

'They're lovely, really polite but I'm just too tired to do any more media. Washington and New York and that's all.'

'Any dogs?'

'Not too bad. I love you,' and she pushed off.

'You too.'

After the initial *Today* show and the hassles of Cedar City Jane had decided she didn't want to do any media at all. At the bigger cities there'd been opportunities to do breakfast shows but Jane had quite rightly refused to compromise start times for the days' rides. The ride had become a real test of endurance and there was no strength left to do media interviews.

Jane was wrecked by the time she arrived at Lebanon but like a true professional she completed her commitments to Fuji TV, which took nearly an hour. They'd brought gifts for her and were extremely thoughtful, but it still meant that Jane didn't get as much rest that day and so only re-emphasised the need to do no further media until Washington.

There were only fifteen days left but she still had to cycle the length of Britain, over the challenging Appalachians. Her confidence had been severely dented by the dog attacks and she was looking worse than ever. Never had the ride looked less like being successful.

Day 51 – Friday, 18 August
Lebanon, O. to Chillicothe, O.
73.3 miles – 7 hrs 18 mins
Total covered – 2959.6 miles

MIKE

It wasn't often Steven was awake when Jane departed so he stood outside and watched her go off.

'Enjoy your day!' she said. 'Are you excited?'

'Yes,' said Steven, with a vigorous nod of the head.

'Good morning, little man,' Ryan said. 'Enjoy the tennis.'

Within seconds, the three of them were off, soon to be followed by Rob in his SUV. The success of Andy Murray beating Roger Federer at the Cincinnati Masters Tennis Tournament had drawn our attention and as we were passing within twenty miles, I thought it would be a treat for Steven.

When originally planning the trip to America, we'd envisaged that Steven and I would have a road trip across the USA, sometimes leaving the ride for two or three days at a time so we could take in some of the country's highlights close to the route.

But with Jane's health failing and conditions for the cyclists being more extreme than we'd anticipated, this plan had failed to materialise. Only on a couple of occasions had we not been supporting the ride and today was a rare day out.

We arrived early and the stands were sparsely populated. The show court was huge, steeply tiered but with a great view. We watched a men's double but were enjoying a close encounter between Nadal and Ferraro when the weather started to close in.

'I'll try your mum again,' I said to Steven.

'Is she not answering?' he said.

'No,' I said, as the rain started to trickle. 'Should we head off and go and meet your mum?'

'What time is it, Dad?'

'Two o'clock. But your mum will be finished soon and she'll have to wait for us to get back before she can rest properly.' It was still early as far as the tournament was concerned and most of the day's play would stretch on until late in the evening. It hadn't really given Steven the flavour of professional tennis I was hoping.

'Sure,' he said. Steven was as pragmatic as ever.

'Have you had a good day?'

'Brilliant. Can we go to Wimbledon?'

'One year, yes,' I said. 'At least it's not hard to find the RV, Steven.' The huge lump of a van was parked amidst a sea of gleaming cars.

'Dad, it's embarrassing,' said Steven.

As we inched our way down the track towards the exit, I noticed all the parking stewards messing about by a canopy. Many spectators had not arrived yet so the odd car was coming in but we were probably the first people to leave for the day. They all had their backs to us.

'What was that?' Steven said, as we felt a thud. I touched the brake and stopped. The passenger wing mirror of the RV had hit something, causing it to bounce against the RV and shatter. I jumped out of the driver's door and walked round to the front of the RV. My heart stopped as I saw a young girl lying on the grass. For a few seconds, time stood still, as I ran towards her.

'Are you okay?' I asked, rushing to kneel down next to her.

'Yes, I'm sorry,' she said, attempting to get up.

'It's okay, stay still,' I said. I turned to an elderly woman who was standing watching transfixed. 'Can you phone for some help?' I said before turning back to the girl. 'Please, please, you'd better stay still.'

'I'm fine,' she said, rising to her feet unaided. She looked about fifteen, slim, five six with long brown hair. 'My arm hurts a little, but I'm good.'

I was aware of my heart beating furiously. 'Just don't do anything,' I said. The elderly woman had radioed for assistance and within a couple of minutes an official from the tennis centre had arrived.

'Honestly, I'm fine,' said the girl. But the official insisted she be checked out at the medical tent.

'Do you need me to stay?' I asked the official as they headed off.

'No, she's fine. I'll just take her back and give her a drink,' he said. 'You get off and enjoy your day.'

'Here,' I said, 'these are my contact details.' I scribbled my telephone numbers, vehicle registration and web address down on a scrap of paper.

A little shaky, I got back into the van and looked at Steven. We didn't speak a word. Within minutes we were heading down the road. The absence of a passenger side wing mirror made overtaking and pulling out onto major roads even trickier. Rather than follow the cyclists' route, we detoured to an interstate so we could travel straight to the campsite.

'Hi, Jane,' I said, having phoned her. 'We're approaching the RV park. Do you want or need anything from the shops?'

'Oh, Mike, we've had a bad day,' she sighed. It was just turning four o'clock. With a seventy-mile cycle I'd have expected them to have finished a couple of hours ago, but the background noise sounded like they were still on the road.

'You've had a bad day?' I said. 'You should try ours.'

'No, it's been really bad. Where are you? Still at the tennis?'

'At the RV park, just about to pull up.'

'Ryan, Mike's at the RV park.' I could hear Ryan in the background.

'Oh shit, how's he found it?' he said.

Jane came back on the line. 'How did you find it?'

'It's called using a map and a Tom Tom.'

'Cindy couldn't find it. We've had to cycle on to Chillicothe.'

'What do you mean? Why are you cycling on?'

'It's just been an awful day. Just after we left we came to the road where RVs were prohibited. The camber would have turned it over so Cindy had to take a detour and got lost, so she missed the first two support stops.'

'Why?'

'She got lost, very lost.' Jane sounded like she was on the verge of tears. I sighed.

'Then she was a little late arriving at the third one. At the finish we stopped at the agreed point and waited for Cindy to come and pick us up. Cindy was meant to have checked in and come and met us. But she couldn't find the RV park. So after hanging around for nearly an hour, and by this stage we very tired, hungry, cold and wet, we set off again. There's nothing more desperate than having to start cycling again after you've finished for the day. I'm absolutely wrecked.'

'Where are you heading?'

'Chillicothe.'

I looked at the map. 'I see it, that's about fifteen miles further on. Where are you stopping?'

'Cindy's gone on. She's going to book us some accommodation, but I'd bet my life she stops at the first hotel however shitty it is because she's so damn lazy. We can't do this, Mike, it's ridiculous. We've had no support all day, we're finishing late and we're tired, wet and miserable.'

'Well, I'll see you there. We'll head down the interstate. We'll be there soon.'

Our sister RV, with its picture of the all-American adventure family – all teeth and false smiles, on horseback – had never looked more out of place pulled up at the front of the motel.

Chillicothe looked like a town which was down on its heels, the streets were dirty, the buildings run down.

Jane and Ryan had clearly just arrived as he was still organising the bikes. When he saw me he didn't say anything, just shook his head like a football fan whose side had just taken a 5-0 drubbing.

Almost as soon as I reached the RV, I felt my energy drain as if someone had opened a tap in my heel. I knocked on Cindy's door and entered. Jane was sitting on a chair, still clad in her cycling gear. It looked like she'd got a chill. Cindy was busy washing up some cups. 'Tough day?' I asked, but there was no response. Jane stood up.

'See you later, Cindy,' I said.

'Bye.'

'What happened to the wing mirror?' Jane asked as we got inside our RV. The last thing I needed was to recount the story but silence wasn't an option. Jane moved onto the bed and I slowly relived the day.

'Do you want some paracetamol?' she asked.

I nodded. 'Yes, if Cindy could phone in the accident that would be a great help. And see when they can repair the RV.'

'What a shit day,' said Jane, as I lay on the bed next to her. She hugged me, her wet hair resting against my chest.

'Oh, to be home.'

Cindy was incredibly efficient and made all the calls that evening. When she discovered that it was unlikely the mirror would be replaced this side of Christmas, she headed off to the auto discount shop across the road to see if a mirror could be bought. We'd booked one room in the hotel which Cindy was to have while the rest of us would sleep in the two RVs at the motel front.

'The motel manager has asked us to move the rigs around the back,' she said later when she'd returned. Under instructions we parked as requested down a back alley. To me, it looked like one of those streets in a US cop show where naked bodies were recovered from dumpsters.

'We shouldn't leave the RVs unattended here,' Ryan said. 'They'll be wheel-less in ten minutes.'

'We should move on,' Jane agreed. 'There's a group over there on another planet, Mike.' As she spoke, a semi-naked bloke walked past the RV. 'They're looking at the RVs like vultures.'

I rose and looked out of the rear window. 'Yes,' I said, 'none of us would sleep here tonight. I'd need a twelve bore to feel safe.'

To pack up and find new accommodation after nine at night in the darkness was a situation no one wanted. But we moved off without a word being exchanged. I got the feeling that even the smallest of sparks would have led to the tinder box exploding and words being exchanged which couldn't have been taken back.

CHAPTER 7

Day 55 – Tuesday, 22 August
Marietta, O. – New Martinsville, West Virginia (W.Va.)
60.4 miles – 5 hrs 12 mins
Total covered – 3128 miles

JANE

Fog clung to the banks of the Ohio River, but I ate up the miles with ease. The journey took us up the western bank of the river until a crossing at New Martinsville, the only town within a day's cycling distance. Once across the Ohio, the landscape changed. Ryan cycled up alongside me, my wheels parallel with his, as a dog barked in the distance. Recently, it seemed that there was always another bark, always another dog.

'It's okay, Jane,' said Ryan. 'I don't think that one will be bothering us.'

Experience had taught me that one barking animal was usually providing an early warning system for every other beast within audible distance.

'There's always another though,' I said.

'I'm today's bait, Jane,' Ryan said and he cycled off effortlessly down the road, putting distance between us.

Another loud bark and my heart stopped again. I looked around, concentrating on where the four-legged fiend would spring from. This constant vigilance, waiting for the moment when my heart would race, my legs pump and adrenalin surge through my body, was mentally exhausting. I was fed up with feeling like I had to keep fleeing for my life. My familiarity with the roads had not eased my fear. I knew that the next dog attack would be inevitable. My legs pushed down as the road climbed steeply. From ahead, it sounded like a pack of hounds was patrolling in the distance, the sounds swirling and bouncing off the trees. Ryan was a hundred yards ahead, Martyn behind him, just packing up his camera. I felt vulnerable.

There was a sharp bark. I looked over my shoulder and a large dog was tearing up the road, its jaws agape. My legs pushed down on the pedals as hard as I could but the bike began to stutter, the gear was wrong. I began to slow. The dog closed in on me, forty, thirty, twenty yards. A click of the chain and the forward momentum took me to the top of the climb and I fell away as if I was on the top of the big dipper. My heart rate slowed but I'd had enough.

Just as I thought I wanted to get off the bike and sit and weep, from out of nowhere a second dog appeared from the right, twenty feet away. For an instant, we matched pace as it slavered away at my side. The road dropped for another fifty yards before climbing again, if I got the gear change at the bottom wrong then I was convinced part of my leg would disappear. But weeks in the saddle paid off at this point. I changed gear perfectly and in no time I was out of the saddle attacking the short climb.

We cycled on, Ryan and Martyn staying very close at my side. But I was drained.

We all arrived at the stopping point at the delightful town of Martinsville at just after one o'clock. Mike, Michael – who had rejoined us – and Steven had travelled together in one RV, Michael an extra pair of eyes to replace the wing mirror. Cindy's role was to drive ahead to the following night's planned stop as the maps proved inconclusive as to whether Route 50 was suitable for cyclists.

'Is there anywhere to eat?' Ryan asked.

'Everyone is recommending Quincy's,' Mike said.

'Is it on Main Street perchance?' I said.

'Where else?'

Inside Quincy's, the fare was a buffet at one price of $7.95 and you could help yourselves to as much as you liked. A sign, though, warned that there would be a one dollar surcharge if anyone wasted food. It was hard not to be impressed with the incredible selection of pies, casseroles, ham with pineapple glaze and the most incredible amount of vegetables.

'Proper food,' I said. 'After three thousand miles, we find the most tremendous selection of protein. If only the whole of America had been the same.'

We tucked in heartily though it was impossible not to note the selection of puddings. There were at least fifteen different home-cooked pies laid out on wooden tables. Why anyone in New Martinsville would cook at home I didn't know. As we gorged on the food, Michael looked up.

'Have you seen the sign?' he asked.

'Where?' Ryan asked.

'The one on the wall which says that all patrons have been videoed and recorded.'

'Freaky,' I said and our eyes skimmed the ceilings and upper walls. Steven looked under the table.

'I think there's a religious aspect to this restaurant. You should see the walls in the ladies'.'

There were numerous letters from children praising the Lord. It was clear that faith played an enormous part in the owners' lives.

The owner came across to talk to us, interested in why we were in West Virginia.

'Are you Christians?' he asked me.

'Catholic,' I said.

He looked at Steven. 'Are you walking with the Lord?'

'No,' said Steven. 'I'm walking with my dad.'

I sucked in my cheeks, trying not to laugh as the owner walked away leaving Steven muttering, 'Stand up for Jesus, all praise the Lord.'

'Steven!' I said, trying to admonish him but failing miserably.

'They're weird though,' said Steven.

'Watch the cameras,' Michael said. 'They'll be coming after you, you heathen.'

'I'm a kid,' said Steven.

Cindy had told us that there was only one hotel in the town and had booked the cheapest room. At $184 it blew five days' budget but there was little we could do. Who had the hotel room had always been a source of friction. Mike's view was that I should have first refusal and obviously this benefited him, too, unless I thought I'd be better off alone. My back was giving me terrible jip and the night sweats in the RV were uncomfortable at best, but my view was that we were one team and no one should get favourable treatment.

Ryan piped up, 'I'll have the room, I can get on with my PhD' and reached for the lone key.

As usual it was decided that all of us would shower in the room before heading back to the RVs and when we got there, the room was the size of a four-bedroom house. It had two enormous beds and a couch. Someone suggested that Michael or Cindy should share the room, too.

'Where is Cindy?' Ryan said.

'She rang when we were going into Quincy's to say that she'd get some dinner and then she'd be back,' Michael said. Ryan was still in his cycling gear and all his belongings were with Cindy.

'But that was three hours ago.'

'I'll ring her again,' Michael said.

'She's only gone forty miles down the road,' Ryan said, shaking his head.

Michael returned a couple of minutes later.

'She's about an hour away.'

'An hour!' I said, voicing Ryan's frustration. 'A fucking hour! It's only an hour away at best. What the hell has she been doing?'

Ryan kicked the leg of the table, his lips pursed.

'She's the bloody limit,' Ryan said.

'She got lost,' said Michael.

I laughed. 'She's got a Tom Tom and there's only one road.'

'Sorry,' Michael said.

'It's not your fault.'

'I'm going to get a shower anyway,' Ryan said and stomped off into the bathroom.

Day 56 – Wednesday, 23 August
New Martinsville (W.Va) to Grafton (W.Va.)
65.1 miles – 6 hrs 52 mins
Total covered – 3194 miles

JANE

We set off from New Martinsville as early as we could next morning but a heavy moisture hung in the atmosphere. There was no rain but you wouldn't have guessed from how damp my clothes were. After leaving New Martinsville, the road had been shrouded by thick forestation and the trees attracted the mist.

We'd slept in the RV on the banks of the Ohio and I'd sweated profusely overnight. By breakfast it felt like I should be finishing for the day, not starting. The fear of a dog attack was at the forefront of my mind. Ryan and Martyn cycled alongside me as closely as they could but even with their protection at either side, I was very jittery.

We'd been riding in peace for several minutes when we heard a whole load of hounds baying at a house nearby. None of us could tell if they were fenced in or not. I began to slow down.

'Martyn, please can you go on and look ahead and see what there is?' I said, fearful that if we got up too close, we'd be attacked by a group of marauding animals. Martyn was not afraid of the dogs but he could see how upset I was.

'I will,' he said. 'But that just might arouse them and then we might never be able to get past them.' I took his point. 'If you just stay a little bit ahead then and I'll keep cycling behind you. Have you got your pepper spray ready?'

'Yeah, I'm all sorted for that.'

My legs were shaking as I continued to make my way down the track, my eyes darting between the houses trying to catch a glimpse of where the animals lay in wait. We got to a wide clearing in the road where we could see what looked like a static caravan and beside it was a series of pens which looked like they'd had more money spent on them than the house. For the owners, this was clearly their way of earning a living. They would breed and keep these dogs and rent them out during hunting season.

'Don't worry,' Martyn yelled from his position about 20 yards ahead. 'Not one of them is free – you're all right, Jane, you're all right.'

Ryan kept close to me. 'You can do this, Jane,' he said. 'It's not hard. Come on, I'll cycle alongside you just to make you feel safer, but they're not going to get you.'

My heart was thudding violently in my chest and my mouth was bone dry. At every yelp or loud bark, my stomach flipped and my shaking got worse. I could feel tears prick my eyes.

'Come on, Jane,' said Ryan as we continued to pedal. 'We're past them now. Look, they're behind us, they're not coming after us.'

I couldn't respond. Keeping my head down I carried on cycling, my legs like jelly, until we came to a low wall in a clearing about a mile ahead.

'I need to stop,' I said, pulling in and throwing the bike down on the ground. I stomped over to the wall, waiting for the trembling to subside but by now, the tears that had welled up in my eyes were pouring down my cheeks. I sat and cried while Martyn and Ryan stood astride their bikes, watching helplessly.

'I don't want to go on anymore,' I sobbed. 'Those dogs are penned but the next dogs might not be.' I gulped in air with each sob.

'Jane, they're not going to let their dogs out onto the road,' said Ryan. 'They're really valuable to their owners – they're their livelihoods. They're not going to let them loose – you'll be okay.'

'But what about wild dogs then?' I said. 'I just can't face it, I just can't.' I wiped my damp cheek with the back of my hand.

Martyn and Ryan just looked at me.

'Shall I phone Mike and get him to come back?' said Ryan. 'He'll get you in the van and get you home.'

I nodded, my head bowed in my hands. 'Yeah,' I said quietly. 'I think I want to go home now. I've had enough.'

The two men got off their bikes and came to sit nearby on the wall. While they chatted between themselves I sat there sobbing and sobbing, unable to actually make any sense of what my body was doing and telling me. 'What the hell am I doing?' I thought to myself. 'Why am I here? Nobody cares. We're not raising any money. Why the hell am I putting myself through this?'

Sensing my utter despair, Martyn came over and sat next to me.

'How are you feeling?' he asked gently.

'I just don't know why we're bothering,' I said. 'We're not doing anything, we're not going to achieve anything. Nobody's nice to us and it's just the most horrific experience of my life and I just don't want to do it anymore.'

Ryan came over and sat by Martyn.

'You know, we've been cycling now for over eight weeks,' he said. 'Do you really, really, really want to give up now, having done eight weeks solid cycling? You've only got another thirteen days or so and it'll all be over and you can go home, you can be in your house, in your bed, in your bath. It can all be normal again.'

I looked up. I knew he was right. Of course I didn't want to give up but just for one day I would have given anything not to be here. Rothwell and home seemed such a long way away in both time and distance. I honestly didn't know if I could make it through another two weeks.

Martyn and Ryan sat with me, gradually calming me down with soothing words.

The impasse continued but it soon became clear that Mike would not be returning in the short term. I looked at the bike lying at the roadside. How many times had those wheels turned round over 3000 miles? Abandoning, climbing off, giving up, losing – whichever way it was said it meant failure and I wasn't prepared to accept failure. Whatever it takes.

'Come on, let's get off,' I said.

Martyn and Ryan didn't need to be asked twice. We were soon on the road.

We cycled in as close a formation as we had throughout the journey, like two prison officers escorting an inmate, only the handcuffs were missing. We'd travelled no distance at all before cycling down a long straight road. I saw the back of the RVs. Banks of trees stood behind and to the left of them. The clouds were lifting and the sun was casting its early morning shadow.

Mike was standing outside 'Connies', a diner which looked like a converted fire station, painted red and with an American flag hung limp over the red porch. The three support crew were already in shorts and T-shirt.

'How are you?' Mike asked, concerned.

I recounted the previous half hour.

'If you'd only done that in Kansas,' was Mike's educated observation.

'I just want a few minutes on my own,' I said and wandered off for a quiet walk a few yards down the road. I didn't wander too far, I didn't trust my luck not to have a dog attack and I knew I couldn't outrun one without the bike. When I got back, Mike was deep in conversation with Ryan.

He didn't notice my return, but when he spotted me he said, 'Have you a minute?' We walked a few yards away.

'Are you okay?' he said.

I nodded. 'Just tired, so very tired.' But then I cried and broke down in his arms. 'I'm all right, it's just a silly moment.'

'Ryan and Martyn will look after you,' he said.

'It's not that, I'm just desperately weary and the constant dog attacks are destroying my confidence. But I'll be all right.' I stayed in his arms for a few seconds longer before taking a deep breath and drying my eyes again.

The others had gone into the diner. As we joined them, the smell of the homemade cinnamon swirls hit me. On the wall was an article about an appeal for money to help rebuild a property for a local family whose home had been lost in a fire. The article highlighted the plight of families living in rural areas of West Virginia where incomes were modest. It also reported that a significant proportion

(30 per cent) of children in the state were living below the poverty line. In turn, we all got up and read the piece.

I approached the counter.

'Hiya,' Connie said, at least that's who I assumed it to be. 'Where are you guys cycling?'

I briefly explained the purpose of the trip as I held out a few dollars to pay for the food.

'Oh, I don't need any money,' she said, wafting her hand in my direction.

'Are you sure?'

'If I can't give coffees and pastries to people cycling across the country for charity then there would be something wrong with the world,' she said. 'I'd like to think people would do that for me.'

I put the dollars away in a side pocket of the purse I kept for when people made cash donations to the charity. It was the first money to go in there since arriving in America.

As we left, Martyn came up. 'You look a little happier, Jane.'

'A homemade cinnamon swirl, coffee and touch of unexpected act of kindness was all I needed.'

Day 56 – Wednesday, 23 August

MIKE

Jane's voice crackled over the phone line. The further east we'd travelled, the better the phone coverage but it was sod's law that the moment she rang me was the moment I'd driven into a poor reception area.

'What was that?' I said, not quite sure I'd heard her correctly.

'We've lost Martyn,' she said.

'Congratulations.'

'We were coming out of Lumberport, just after we saw you and he went off to get a shot and we haven't seen him since.'

'Have you been looking?'

'Ryan's been back to search.'

'He'll be all right,' I said. 'We'll drive back. In the meantime, I'll phone Rob.'

Part of me was surprised that the cyclists had managed to cross the USA without losing each other before. While there was never more than a couple of miles between them, Martyn would often go ahead to set up shots or would be left behind while packing up after one. One wrong turn or an untimely puncture could cause a problem. Clarksville where we'd pulled up in the RV was a largish town in the bottom of a valley. Route 50 ran through the centre and was the most direct one but it was unsuitable for bikes.

The tension which had been building over the last few days as a result of the continuous dog attacks seemed to have disappeared. After Jane's little breakdown on the road up from New Martinsville, I knew she would now be okay. This was just her way. She would let fear or nerves build and bubble underneath the surface but that would spur her on to dig deeper into her limitless reserves.

She'd treated her cancer in very much the same way. Any sign of fragility or weakness was often kept deep inside, and while she'd often articulate her fears, in the same breath she'd dismiss them.

Despite this, today was turning into one of the ride's most difficult days.

Communication with Martyn was soon restored, he'd taken a different right turn but by now he was some miles further up the road than Jane and Ryan.

The day's ride was Grafton. The sign for the town read: 'Welcome to Grafton, the birthplace of Mother's Day, May 10th 1908'. Cindy's job had been to go ahead and find accommodation. Michael, Steven, Rob and I waited on the eastern side of Grafton, just off the 50 at a DIY shop in a strip mall. Two fire engines were half a mile further up the hill attending an incident and traffic was backing up.

The early afternoon heat had intensified and it was close to 100 degrees. Martyn soon joined us and lay spreadeagled on the ground, exhausted. It was a good hour before Jane and Ryan cycled into view.

'Where's the campsite?' Jane asked. She was seated in the passenger seat of the RV as we followed Cindy. We'd been driving for forty-five minutes and Jane's irritation had been rising with each mile, knowing full well that tomorrow morning we'd have to do the journey in reverse in order to be able to get back on the bikes from where they'd finished.

'Fuck knows,' I muttered. Since Grafton we'd been lost twice.

'Has she got no common sense at all?' said Jane.

'At least it's your last night in the RV,' I said. Tomorrow, Michael and I were going to head off to Winchester to collect a hire car. Then, on Friday, Michael and Cindy would be driving to Newark to return one of the RVs and ease the burden on the last week of the ride. We'd be staying in motels.

'I can't tell you how lovely that feels,' Jane said.

'No regrets. You don't want us to keep it a little longer?' I asked.

'I can honestly say tonight will be the last night I ever spend in an RV,' she said.

'Hopefully the campsite will be beautiful, our last campsite meal in idyllic surroundings,' I said, not entirely convincingly.

Jane gave a snort. 'If we don't get there soon, Mike, I won't be responsible for my actions.'

It was approaching an hour since the cyclists had finished when we finally caught sight of the campsite entrance. For a moment, my hopes were raised when I saw that it was in a pretty location, set next to a lake. But as we drove into the park, two large dogs appeared on the road in front of us.

'What the . . .?' said Jane, furious. 'I don't believe this!'

I decided to remain silent, driving as far as I could away from the animals, who showed no interest in us at all.

The pitches weren't level so I parked the RV on a twenty-degree slope, our legs would be pointing downhill tonight.

Steven scurried out and Jane and I followed and began to empty our RV of all nine weeks' belongings, tins of food bought in Oakland still untouched, chillies, beans and jams. A pile of goods rose like a bonfire on 5 November outside the RV as picnic chairs and bedclothes joined it to go to the rubbish.

'You'd better dump, Mike,' Jane said.

'Do you want to help, Steven?' I said.

'No.'

'It's the last time.'

'Is that meant to tempt me? Do I look like I'm mad?'

I walked round the side of the vehicle, attached the plastic pipe to the RV, locking the clips for the last time. Dumping had not been such a terrible exercise, partly because I'd been vigilant about allowing people to take number twos in the RV. Unless they had a pained expression, they could wait until a toilet stop.

The drain was up slope of the RV connection, subconsciously I knew that gravity would not be defied. I opened the valves and as none of the sewage flowed, I closed them, contemplating unhooking the water and electricity in preparation for moving the RV a few feet.

I smiled, reflecting how I'd managed to drive for nine weeks without setting off once while connected to a drain. Deciding to do the job right, I pulled the plastic sewage pipe from the drain.

It required a little more force than normal because the pipe was lower than the RV, so I tugged and there was a glug followed by effluent spilling out on to the grass. Slowly the brown liquid began to flow and glancing around I kicked the pipe underneath the RV. As I did an arch of fluid hit the white RV.

There was surprisingly little fluid so rather than go through the performance of unhooking the valves, I thought what harm could there be in opening them and emptying the remainder on the ground – scummy yet efficient.

Glancing around again I bent down and opened both valves, one for effluent, one for water. Within seconds fluid started to flow. I watched in increasing alarm as it seemed that there was to be no sign of the flow stopping.

Panic set in and I decided to wash down the van's paintwork. I turned the water pipe on the effluent which was now flowing down the RV's front and making its way to the lake. I washed my hands and chucked my T-shirt on the pile of RV waste.

'What's the water under the RV, Mike?' Jane asked.

'The water hose wasn't coupled up correctly,' I lied.

'It seems a funny colour.'

'There was such a lot of water, the ground's turned into a quagmire. Let's be grateful we're not on a water meter.'

'As long as that's all it is.'

I shrugged and shook my head.

'Dad, Mum, tea's ready,' Steven said. 'Why is it wet?'

'Because it is,' Jane said and I wandered across to the other RV where the wooden picnic table was laid out ready for the six of us to eat. It had been a little while since we'd eaten together. The maxim of 'A ride that eats together, stays together' had long since expired.

There were six buns on a tray and Cindy appeared with a pan.

'What's for tea?' Ryan said.

I looked at the table which was devoid of rice or salad, which had been a mainstay of the trip.

'Well, I don't really have a name for it,' Cindy said, 'but when we were growing up, my mum called it "shit on a shingle".' She slopped out some mince covered with white sauce onto one of the buns and handed it to Jane. Cindy went back into the RV to tidy the kitchen area.

'Perceptive was she?' Jane said as the mince oozed over the side of the bun. Ryan looked across to her and rolled his eyes. The mixture looked similar to the substance I'd just dumped from the toilet of the RV.

'Do I have to have any?' Steven said.

It echoed my own thoughts but I knew we had no other choice. 'Eat it up, it's all you're getting.'

'I'd rather go hungry.'

It was hard to argue. Jane slid her plate away from her. 'That's totally disgusting processed mince on a bun,' she said. 'How are we meant to cycle on that?'

'What's she been doing, Michael? A campsite miles from anywhere? Shit on a shingle?'

As if on cue, two dogs came up behind her and began to sniff the plate.

'And fucking dogs . . .' By now Jane could hardly contain her rage.

'It's okay, Jane,' I said, trying to placate her. 'I was speaking to a police officer today and he says once you're through West Virginia you won't have any problems with dogs.'

'Why?'

'Each state has its own laws. Some say that the owners are liable for their dogs' actions, others aren't. West Virginia and a few other states fall into the latter.'

Steven was prodding his plate with his fork. 'Do I have to eat it, it's horrible?' he said.

'No,' said Jane, getting up from her seat. 'I'll make some sandwiches.'

Day 57 – Thursday, 24 August
Grafton, W.Va. to New Creek, W.Va.
69.3 miles – 7 hrs 45 mins
Total covered – 3263 miles

Day 58 – Friday, 25 August
New Creek, W.Va. to Winchester, Virginia (Va.)
61.2 miles – 6 hrs 19 mins
Total covered – 3324 miles

MIKE

The two days' cycle from Grafton to New Creek, then on to Winchester, Virginia, over the Appalachians, were extremely gruelling. Two days of cumulative 7000-foot sharp climbs sapped an already beleaguered Jane but fortunately the police officer's words were true and the dog attacks had lessened.

As we arrived in Winchester late Friday afternoon there was a real sense that we were nearing the end. We'd seen a sign that had said 'Washington 82 miles', which meant that the capital was within a day's ride. I could sense that it had lifted the spirits of the cyclists.

Rob had asked whether we wished to join him and Martyn for a meal in the town. The day had clouded over and there were signs that there could be another storm. The nights were drawing in, the dark green leaves hung heavy on the trees. Steven walked ahead, his hands clutching his Nintendo DS, the silver stripe on his Geox trainers standing out in the slight gloom.

'Have you heard from the insurers, Mike?' Jane asked, as we walked towards the restaurant.

'No, I spoke to Michael and he said Cindy's heard nothing.' I'd received an emotional email from the father of the girl I'd hit with the RV and was keen that the insurers were in conversation with the girl.

'How did they get on today?'

Cindy and Michael had headed up to Newark to get rid of one of the RVs.

'They didn't get to Newark until half past four. They've got to now battle through the traffic leaving Philadelphia so they're not expecting to be back by ten.'

'New York,' sighed Jane. 'I can't wait to get home, Mike.'

'Nine days and we'll be back in Leeds.'

'I just want to see Suzanne and Becca,' she said. She dabbed her face, sniffing slightly before regaining her composure.

'One week,' I said.

'One week,' she nodded and then stopped, turned to me and put her arms round my neck. 'Thanks for being here.'

'I've done nothing.'

'I meant the last six years.'

'There's nowhere else I'd have rather been.'

'Urgh,' Steven said.

'Shut up,' we said in unison before clinching harder.

Day 59 – Saturday, 26 August
Winchester, Va. to Washington, DC
75.1 miles – 7 hrs 09 mins
Total covered – 3399 miles

Day 60 – Sunday, 27 August
Washington, DC
Rest day

MIKE

'In the Blue Ridge Mountains of Virgin . . . on the trail of the lonesome pine . . .' Steven had heard me and Martyn singing the Laurel and Hardy classic, picked up the chorus and was trilling it happily as he perched on Rob's shoulders.

We were waiting for the cyclists at a hilltop lay-by in the mountains. An elderly, portly twitcher decked out in black jeans and shirt, his white hat matching his beard, was sharing the spot with us. He was sitting on a fold-out canvas chair, his binoculars hanging from his neck, a camera and tripod adjacent. The top of the hill was like most of the Appalachians, dense with trees and ideal for bird watching.

For the last few days, the Blue Ridge Mountains which divided Winchester and Washington had beckoned the cyclists. In truth, having done more serious climbs over the last few weeks, these particular mountains were more like hills – 600 feet over fifteen miles – but even so, they held a more tantalising appeal – the last of the ride's serious climbs. It was no wonder that Jane, Martyn and Ryan wanted to get them out of the way as soon as possible.

There was a sense of euphoria about the day. As Martyn, Ryan and Jane joined us at the lay-by we were all chatting excitedly about how we'd be in Washington by mid-afternoon for the last rest day. After that, there were only four real cycling days left before the glory leg into Manhattan.

As this was likely to be our only time in Washington we decided to treat ourselves and stay in the Marriott. It cost more than most of the hotels we'd stayed in but as Jane was feeling better, our main priority was to keep her well and not overtire her by staying miles out of the city centre.

Jane beamed as she cycled the last few yards to the finishing point at the British Embassy, just out of town. This had been a long day in the saddle for Jane on the back of the six hardest days on the bike since the Rockies. Steven and I stood back while news crews from Sky prepared to interview her, but we were soon joined by a police car. Clearly the Embassy had noted our presence.

'I'm tired,' Jane said, she rifled her hair with her gloved hand. Her faced looked flushed, her eyes dark. 'Can we wrap this up as soon as possible?'

'Are you all right?' I said.

'I need to be away from here. Speed things up. Get everything organised.'

Ryan came up to her. 'Well cycled, Jane,' he said. 'It was a good effort today.'

Steven put his thumbs up and smiled, while Jane busied herself professionally rattling off three interviews and chivvying everyone to call a finish to the day.

My head was thumping. At the back of my mind was the girl I'd bumped into in Cincinnati. I knew she was okay and suffered only a sore arm but why were the insurers not telling us what was going on?

Each time I thought of her, I had a view of her lying on the grass. The fact that she got up within seconds of me hitting her, practically uninjured, was of little consolation.

The stop-off in Washington, the ride to the White House and then to Baltimore had been strategically planned to coincide with the bank holiday in the UK, to gain as much media coverage as possible. Hopefully it would set up the ride's finish into New York perfectly. There was set to be an influx of UK media personnel arriving over the next few days. Although Jane would be pleased to see some people we got on with, she wasn't relishing the inevitable increase in pressure on her.

The fundraising was still extremely poor and only £16,000 had been raised online since we'd set off. We knew this would account for 90 per cent of donations. This was our last chance to make any success of the ride and I now started to chase down media contacts in the UK to see if they would help.

The advantage of being in central Washington was that for once we could eat something other than burgers or chips. So we chose a pub-styled venue which cooked very traditional English-based dishes with vegetables. Even so, Jane's plate remained untouched.

'You've not eaten much,' I said.

'No, but you're not one to talk,' she replied.

'My head's banging, I'm afraid. I'll be fine.'

'It's just stress, about the accident,' she said. 'Forget it.'

'Hiya!' Steven bellowed, his arms waving. I turned and saw Dave Harrison and Phil Iveson from Yorkshire Television coming towards us. We'd not seen them since day four of the trip.

Jane got up and hugged each in turn, 'I can't tell you how good it is to see you both,' she said.

Dave and I shook hands.

'Hiya, mate,' he said. 'You look worse than Jane!'

'He's stressed,' Jane said, pointedly.

'What's he got to be stressed about?' Dave laughed. 'It must be hard driving fifty miles a day sitting on your arse, getting a tan and doing a bit of shopping as well. I bet you're not cooking either.'

'Are you going to tell them?' Jane said.

Dave, sensing a story, came in closer. 'This sounds good,' he said.

I recounted the nightmare of Cincinnati. It was not a cathartic experience, reliving the tale.

'They're very litigious in the USA, you know,' he smirked. 'I wouldn't be surprised if they don't let you out of the country. They're hot on things like that.'

'Dave, you're not helping,' Jane said, her face straight. She then cracked into a smile.

'Do you want to talk about it, Mike?' Dave said, his face beaming.

'No, I fucking don't. I'm absolutely gutted. We came out to do a charity bike ride to save kids' lives.'

'It'd be a good interview. A chance to get your side of things across,' he said. Then he looked over at Phil. 'We'd come over and cover the trial, wouldn't we?' He could barely contain his laughter.

'Fuck off, Dave.'

Dave and Phil ordered food while we all had more drinks. It was still only eight thirty. Before long we were discussing the finish of the race. We would finish on the Friday but the flights were booked for Sunday. I had an idea.

'I really fancy leaving on Friday, as soon as we finish,' I said to Jane.

'I'm happy for that,' she said. 'I don't fancy two days in New York.'

'Good plan,' Dave said. 'Less time for the warrant from Ohio to come through.'

CHAPTER 8

Day 61 – Monday, 28 August
Washington DC – Baltimore, Maryland (Md.)
58 miles – 7 hrs 21 mins
Total covered – 3457 miles

JANE

Mike had planned for us to be in Washington on what was August Bank holiday in the UK. Having dealt with the press for the last four years he knew it would be a slow news day and that we'd be in with a chance of more media coverage. While I could appreciate his point, it also meant that we'd have to reroute.

The more attractive route around the major East Coast cities which had been recommended by the specialist cycling maps was no good for us if we were to make it to Washington in time. I'd pored over the maps for weeks. Originally, I'd planned a wide arc around the towns heading into Pennsylvania, but as my health became increasingly fragile so the arc contracted and now we were following a straight line up the coast.

I awoke early to fulfil a commitment to do some TV interviews before Michael Creighton gave me a lift to the British Embassy where there was to be a reception for us.

A large sign on the wall outside the Embassy said 'Welcome to DC Jane Tomlinson'. A couple of bikes were parked under it.

Eleven of the Embassy staff had volunteered to join us in

cycling from the Embassy to the White House and on to the city outskirts.

'I think they're doing it to make sure that we get through Washington safely, it's security by proxy,' Ryan said.

'What makes you think that?' I said.

'A couple of the staff have said that some parts of the city are no-go areas and they're quite concerned that we won't be safe.'

'Really?'

'Yes. It would be embarrassing for everyone if something happened to you today.'

At the front of a light and airy room the Union Jack and Stars and Stripes stood on brass stands. The wooden floor gleamed and the windows overlooked Massachusetts Avenue, where we'd stood on Saturday afternoon. I was introduced to everyone and handed an envelope containing a handwritten letter from Tony Blair, who had recently visited the Embassy.

Within minutes, fourteen of us were leaving the Embassy – or trying to – as the exit barrier failed to rise.

'Apparently we failed the security test,' said one of the staff, as the barrier rose and fell nearly giving two of the cyclists a headache.

We cycled at a relaxed pace on the short journey to the White House via Dupont Circle. Apart from early on in the trip, we'd been unaccompanied on the road and it was lovely to share it with other cyclists. We pulled up on the road leading to the front of the White House and set off in formation with the Embassy staff behind me and Martyn and Ryan flanking either side with cameras. I could see a wall of media with Mike and Steven in front of the building. It didn't feel right. I thought the three cyclists should be coming down this path together. My mind flicked back to when I was cycling into Leeds at the end of 'Rome to Home' and I thought of my brother Luke.

After a brief interlude of media interviews at the White House we continued our journey. Pneumatic drills, car engines, sirens and a cacophony of city sounds overloaded the senses as we cycled down Pennsylvania Avenue, the resplendent white-domed Capitol towering in front of us. The Embassy staff led us out and it was there that I began to suspect that Ryan had been right all along.

'This is a shit hole,' I said to Ryan as we went through a run-down area.

The Embassy staff led us out to Riverdale where we were able to join a cycle trail similar to one we'd used on entering the city. We passed Laurel Park Racecourse and Maryland House of Corrections. I'd lost count of how many prisons we'd now passed.

Today, the mileage had been cut down because I knew that with a heavy media presence it would be a long day. As we got to the outskirts of Baltimore it was already dinner time. We stopped and perused the maps and Martyn took a call.

'You'd better have a word with Rob,' Martyn said, passing me the phone.

'Hi, Jane,' Rob said.

'How are you, Rob?' I asked.

'Jane, I'm really worried about you cycling through Baltimore. This is one scary place. I don't think you should come through here, it's not safe.' I was silent and within seconds Rob continued, 'I went in to get some petrol and started filling the car and within a minute, the car was surrounded by a gang of burly, mean-looking locals.'

'Are you all right?' I said, imagining the scene with Rob standing by his £40,000 SUV full of camera equipment as the gang circled him like sharks around bait.

'Jane, I'm telling you I only got out of there because I was able to pay by card at the machine. If I'd gone to the kiosk I don't know what would have happened. It's really freaked me out. I've never been as scared as that.'

'I think we'll need to push on, Rob.'

His voice was deadly serious. 'Jane, I think you should consider putting the bikes in the car and letting me drive you across the city. This is really not safe. I'd rather you got across without risking your lives.'

I listened and knew that Rob wouldn't scare easily. 'We'll have a look at the maps, Rob. I've cycled all the way across. I'm not getting in a car. That's not going to happen.'

'I've got to consider Martyn's safety, too, because he's out here working for Sky News. I'm really uncomfortable with him cycling through here,' Rob said.

'Thanks, Rob,' I said and I handed the phone back to Martyn. We studied the maps but there was no easy route round and I wasn't well enough to contemplate making a detour which would involve another twenty miles.

'I think we should plough on,' I said. 'What do you think?'

Ryan straightened up after looking at the map. 'We're going where you go, Jane,' he said. 'It's whatever you think best.'

I folded the map up and put it back in the wallet. 'Let's cycle on,' I said.

Baltimore's streets were indeed gloomy, menacing and intimidating. At every red traffic light I felt we were being watched by dozens of pairs of eyes. We travelled down Hammonds Ferry Road and Washington Boulevard but noticed a short-cut which took us into a brand new redeveloped plaza by Baltimore Harbor. The difference was incredible. This was as beautiful as the suburbs had been grim. Large stores, cafés and souvenir shops surrounded the harbour. The USS *Constellation* loomed large over the quay. And there it was – the sea. The first time we'd seen it since Vallejo. Tears came to my eyes.

'Now then, Yorkshire lass,' said Martyn, looking out across the water.

'Now then, Yorkshire lad,' I beamed.

'We've made it, Jane, we've made it,' said Ryan.

'We could go home now,' I said.

For the Cross Country for Cancer lads we'd met earlier in the trip this was indeed the finishing point. I wondered what their reaction had been when they'd arrived here. Had we not previously arranged to travel further on up to New York for the cameras, I could have happily ended our journey here too. We'd done it after all. We'd cycled from coast to coast.

I looked at Martyn and Ryan who couldn't take their eyes from the water. There was something special about sharing this time alone with them, without the assorted media and the razzmatazz. A moment for time to stand still.

'Come on,' I said and freewheeled slowly to the harbour's edge. I dismounted and dipped my wheels in the Atlantic Ocean, followed by Martyn and then Ryan. Whatever happened now, nothing could take away the achievement.

'Fantastic, Jane,' Martyn said. 'Unbelievable. All the way.'

'Awesome,' said Ryan.

'Hey, shorty,' the barman said to Steven. 'Ready for more Coke?'

The bar was quiet. Mike and Steven were sitting at their table watching football on the TV screen above the bar. A few seasoned drinkers sat at their stools like the regulars in *Cheers*.

'Give the boy a drink, Frank,' said one of them as I walked in unobserved.

'How did you get on in court, Frank?' said a newcomer to the barman.

'Don't get him on that,' a man with an enormous beer gut said, his trousers up around his nipples. I walked up to Mike and Steven.

'Hey, shorty, is that your mom?' said the barman. Steven turned round.

'Hi, Mum!'

'You just cycled across the country, lady?'

I nodded. 'Yes.' A group of people at the bar clapped.

'That's one helluva job, lady. What about that, shorty? Your mom's cycled the States!' He came across and shook my hand. 'I've been in court today and a two-bit thief mother walked away from justice. But this goes to show there's good in the world. Can I get you a beer?'

'No,' I said, smiling. 'But a coffee would be good.'

'Sure,' he said. 'Shorty, more Coke?'

'Are you okay?' Mike asked.

'We made it,' I said. 'Coast to coast, dipped our bikes in the sea at Baltimore.'

'Fantastic,' Mike said, leaning over and giving me a hug.

'Get in,' Steven shouted, 'get in. Drogba!'

'What are you watching?'

'Chelsea versus Blackburn from Saturday,' said Mike.

'How do you two manage it?' I said. 'Chelsea again in Baltimore on a Monday afternoon.'

'It's a gift, Mum,' said Steven.

I stood and laughed.

Day 62 – Tuesday, 29 August
Baltimore, Md. to Newark, Delaware (Del.)
57.8 miles – 6 hrs 21 mins
Total covered – 3515 miles

MIKE

I stood peering through the glass counter of a deli in Bel Air, just north of Baltimore, eyeing up the delicious looking morning pastries. Jane was next to me wearing her yellow fluorescent jacket, helmet in hand, looking impassively at the offerings. 'Do you want something to eat?' I asked Jane. We were parked up at today's first stop. Ryan and Martyn were seated a few yards away, both quietly taking sips of milkshakes. The cakes and pastries under the glass counter looked tempting to all but Jane. She was barely more than the size of a skeleton.

'No, I'm fine,' she said.

'Have you eaten anything today?' I asked.

'I'm not Steven.'

'No, I have some influence on him.'

'If I eat, I'll vomit, so there's little point.'

'Only three days now,' I said, smiling.

'One day at a time, Mike,' she said softly.

For five years I'd watched Jane compete, and she was never more alive than during an event. Even on Ironman day in Florida, two years ago, she'd found unexpected energy after sixteen hours of swimming, cycling and running. That glint in her eye and the mischievous grin had been her trademarks.

But the ferocious heat, the gruelling distance and the hostile terrain of America had seemed to suck the life out of her. That determined glint was now a distant memory. Yesterday's ride through Baltimore had proved particularly difficult because of the constant stop-starting at road junctions and traffic lights.

My mobile bleeped.

'It's Rob,' I said, looking at the display screen. The café was noisy so I got up and walked out into Main Street. Opposite stood a life-size model of a buffalo outside the Rip Walk Tavern.

'Hi, Mike. Sky's newsroom have just rung to say they've heard that ITV are putting on a documentary about the ride next week,' said Rob. His voice seemed strained.

'News to me, Rob.'

'They're talking about taking Martyn off the ride and getting him to edit straight away. There's no way they'd let ITV go out first, not after the resources Sky have put into this ride.'

I laughed. 'Rob, that's ludicrous. They can't be seriously thinking about taking Martyn off the ride three days before the finish. He's cycled four thousand miles. Clearly the guys in London have no concept of what he's achieved.'

'Mike, I'm with you. But the newsroom have it on good authority.'

'No, Rob,' I said. 'If ITV were doing a documentary they would have to clear it with us and I can one hundred per cent guarantee there's not even been a mention. Dave Harrison would have said something and I completely trust him. But I will put a call in.'

'Do you know where Martyn is?' Rob said.

'No, Rob, I don't,' I said, turning my back on where Martyn was sitting with Ryan. 'And I'm not passing a message on. This can be sorted out within an hour. I'll call Dave now, but you guys know that it's not our way of doing things. We were committed to Sky a year before this ride.'

'I know, Mike, but London are anxious.'

'I'll sort it, Rob.'

I put the phone in my pocket and went back inside the café. I suspected that Rob would have already tried Martyn so I put Jane in the picture.

'Martyn's not gonna climb off the bike now,' Jane said.

'Whatever Sky say, I'm not finishing without him.' It's what I expected her to say.

Within minutes the cyclists had headed off to Rising Sun just over the Conowingo Dam on the Susquehanna River. It plays host to a large hydraulic plant which while an impressive sight was not aesthetically pleasing.

The confusion about ITV's documentary was soon resolved when Dave Harrison said they had no such plans to produce a programme. After tea, discussion revolved around tomorrow's ride through Philadelphia. We felt apprehensive about Philadelphia. Whenever we'd mentioned to any locals that we were planning on crossing the city, they'd looked at us with an expression close to alarm. Most of the eighty-mile ride would be through the sprawling city and after Monday's stop-start experience, it would be a longer day than usual.

'My friends say Chester is just too dangerous to go through,' Ryan said, his sunglasses perched on his forehead, his arms resting on the table. The Pennsylvania map was spread out in front of us. 'That it's just like a ghetto. I really don't think we should do it.'

Jane looked pensive. She studied the route, leaning over the Pennsylvania map, and then opened up a New Jersey which was larger scale.

'There's no other way, we need to keep west of the Delaware River and cross the Schuylkill. If we don't cross by exit 36 of Interstate 76 we'll have a huge detour and be in the city centre. I haven't the strength to do any longer than eighty miles in a major city.'

Ryan nodded silently.

'Jane,' I interrupted their planning. 'You've another interview to do for Dave.' Jane's face sank.

'Let's go for it then,' Ryan said. 'I'm sure it won't be that bad.'

Jane rose wearily to her feet and shuffled across the floor, her legs rising barely an inch from the surface, her laces undone, her body too stiff to bend down and tie them.

'Are you going to be all right, love?' My hand interlocked with hers.

She shook her head. 'I don't honestly know, Mike. If we get through tomorrow, yes, maybe. There's nothing we can do, just pray.'

'We're nearly there.'

Day 63 – Wednesday, 30 August
Newark, Del. to Trenton, New Jersey (NJ)
75.1 miles – 9 hrs 54 mins
Total covered – 3590 miles

JANE

'Twenty-four,' said Mike, who was lying on his right side in a foetal position on the mattress opposite. I was in the adjacent double bed, having moved during the night. He slowly pulled back the covers so as not to disturb Steven and walked around towards me.

'It's damp,' I said.

'I figured,' he said and climbed in anyway. He moved to put his arms around me.

'Don't!' I said, rather too quickly. 'My liver is really bad, it's tender to the touch.' We lay still. 'Twenty-four what?' I asked.

'It's how many times you've been up, altered position, wiped your body down or changed your pillow. Although if I unwittingly did get any sleep, I may have short counted.'

'Sorry I've kept you awake,' I said. The night sweat had been particularly ferocious; the pain had been intense all night. On several occasions throughout the trip, I'd used oral morphine to control the pain which had worked to good effect. Last night, however, I'd never felt that I'd had it under control.

'It's not a problem,' said Mike. 'I was just concerned but didn't want to be irritating you.'

I shuffled closer to him. 'What time is it?' I said.

'Four fifteen.' It was another two hours before I needed to be up but I was already aware that getting on the bike today would be a challenge.

'What time did I have the Oramorph?'

'Eleven.'

This was a dilemma. Did I take another dose now to try to facilitate some sleep or did I wait a couple of hours and try to get some relief before I got on the bike? Taking the drugs before cycling wasn't something I was particularly comfortable with but if I was going to get through the day, I had no other choice.

'Why don't you climb in with Steven,' Mike said. 'That way, at least you'll get some fresh sheets and pillows. If you change your pyjamas, it'll make you feel better. Do you want a coffee?'

Before I could even answer he was up and plugging in the kettle. I climbed into bed with Steven but sleep still proved elusive. By the time the intermittent bleeps of the alarm sounded, it was clear I was going to struggle today.

I inched my legs round out of the bed until they touched the floor and it took another three minutes before I could summon the strength to accept the pain of trying to stand. I straightened my back slowly as if I'd aged four decades overnight.

Mike had powered up the laptop. 'Steven, come on, up time,' he said.

'Leave him, Mike,' I said. There wasn't a part of my body which didn't hurt though it was my liver that caused me the most distress. How the hell was I going to cycle, bent over on a saddle for eight to ten hours?

Ryan looked like he'd seen a ghost when I arrived for breakfast. He was already seated at a table for two so I joined him.

'Good morning, Jane,' he smiled. I'd normally have tried to hide the discomfort but even the walk down from the room had caused so much pain that tears were streaming from my eyes.

'Hi,' I whispered. 'Sorry. I'm not too well this morning.' I slotted down next to him. Sitting down was easy, but I winced at the thought of getting back up.

'Can I get you your breakfast?' he said. I had known Ryan long enough to know that when things looked really bad he'd avoid asking difficult questions. I was relieved.

'No, thanks.' I grabbed a muffin and a bowl of cereal but apart from pushing them around the plate, they saw no action. I really needed to line my stomach if I was going to take the oral morphine. A black coffee was soon dispatched though.

Mike soon joined us in the breakfast area with Steven. He'd seen me getting dressed painfully slowly and concern was all over his face. I checked my watch. Six thirty a.m.

'See you out front in twenty minutes, Ryan.'

Mike followed me to the door.

'I'm worried,' he said. 'You're in no fit state to ride and you know support will be minimal today. There's no harm in calling it a day now.'

It was limp effort, even by Mike's standards. We'd decided that as we were travelling through some of the dodgier areas of Philadelphia, Mike would take Steven directly to the finish in the RV with Cindy while Michael would stay reasonable close wherever possible in the SUV.

Even with twenty minutes to go, I didn't think I'd be able to cycle. My liver seemed as though it was filling like a balloon with water. Spasms of pain came in waves, causing me to bend double. I wanted to vomit.

'I'll set off and instruct Martyn to get me into hospital if I collapse,' I said. 'I should go to emergency now but I know if I do they won't release me and I desperately want to go home. They'd have to settle the disease before they allowed me to travel.'

Mike looked at me and shrugged. 'Just ring me, that's all I ask.'

Fortunately the weather was slightly overcast but we had seventy-five miles to cycle and the journey would be punctuated with dozens of traffic light junctions. As I pushed off it was clear that the problems were more acute than I imagined. As the miles slowly ticked over I grew increasingly anxious as the dose of Oramorph seemed to be having no effect. Martyn rode closely by, I'd told him to call the emergency services immediately should I collapse. He looked nervous.

We cycled slowly together over the first few miles.

'Well, we've done it, Martyn,' Ryan said pointedly. 'We've crossed America.'

'Yes,' said Martyn. 'Dipping the wheels in the Atlantic was the finish for me.'

'The rest of the journey is superfluous,' Ryan said.

I could see they were trying to ease the burden if I wanted to climb off. But I wanted to concentrate on ticking off the yards, focusing on a spot in the distance and imagining myself being wound in to it, just like I'd done when I started running. Focus on achievable objects, one at a time.

'How are you feeling, Jane,' Martyn asked. 'Do you need a rest?'

'Yes,' I breathed. I was almost finished, there was nothing left for my body to give. The pain in my liver was so overwhelming that I craved leaving the saddle. It was the nearest to death I'd felt in over five years. I couldn't contemplate continuing. But there was nowhere to stop. This wasn't an area where you could comfortably climb off the bike and grab a snack. One mile. Give it one more mile. I watched ahead, counting off the blocks, 800 yards then that's it. It was becoming increasingly difficult to breathe, as with each breath came another sharp pain attack. Still sixty-fives miles to go today. Don't think about it, Jane.

Ryan and Martyn were talking to me but it seemed like a dream. I knew the ride was over, my body was broken and waves of pain rampaged through my stomach.

We'd been travelling about an hour.

'There's a McDonald's there,' Ryan said. 'Pull over, Jane, we'll stop here.'

We were just in Wilmington. It felt that this was the point where I had to make a decision on whether to keep going before we reached the suburbs of Philadelphia. It was clear even from Wilmington what today was going to bring. It was a rundown area which you'd see in old films about the Bronx. The broad streets were grimy, the buildings intimidating, the stares even more so. This was compounded by the stop-start nature of travelling on main roads through a town.

We ordered coffees and muffins and took them outside the restaurant. 'You don't have to continue for us,' Martyn said. 'We've crossed America.'

'Martyn's right, we've done what we set out to do.'

'We can see how much you're suffering, Jane. I've seen you lots of times on the bike in severe discomfort but nothing like this.' Martyn looked at Ryan.

'You know just the three of us getting to Baltimore was as good as it gets, Jane. You've ridden across the continent.' Another glance from Ryan to Martyn this time, who were they trying to convince? Martyn's camera was conspicuous by its absence.

'We've done the coast to coast, achieved the goal we set out to do. No one's going to be bothered, Jane. Everyone here can see how poorly you are. You don't have to put yourself through this,' Martyn said.

The food and coffee were welcome. McDonald's would normally be the last place I'd choose to eat but this was hitting the spot. I was just relieved not to be in as much pain. My mind worked furiously, trying to break down the remaining journey; fifty-five miles left today, probably the same tomorrow, then ten on Saturday. If I could summon up the strength to get through today then I knew tomorrow would be better.

We sat in silence for ten minutes. 'I know we've finished the coast to coast but that's not the ride we set out to do,' I said finally. 'We set out to cycle from Golden Gate to Brooklyn and if we don't do that we'll have failed even though we've travelled nearly four thousand miles. I can't give up now whatever it takes. Steven will be heartbroken. It's enough that I'm dying. He doesn't need to live with his mum failing as well. I promised him we'd get to New York.'

Martyn and Ryan didn't say a word.

'The fundraising's been abysmal,' I continued. 'We set out to raise a small fortune and we've achieved eighteen thousand pounds. We could have raised more doing jumble sales. The only way this ride's going to be a success is if I finish in New York. We all know it's the end when the funds will role in.

'I did this ride in the hope that we'd be able to put on the 10k in Leeds so that we can continue to raise money after I'm dead. I don't want others to have to live this life. To give up now so close to the finish would be too disappointing for everyone. But whatever happens to me, hospital or having to go home, I want you guys to finish.'

Both Martyn and Ryan were silent, there was nothing they could say to help. They knew the only way I wouldn't finish this ride would be if I collapsed.

'Come on,' I said.

The route took us into Chester, past the airport, where conveniently I got a flat which Ryan changed as if he was practising for a Formula One team. We travelled over Platt Bridge and the area became more industrial.

'Have you seen that salubrious joint, Jane?' said Martyn.

A seedy back street strip joint set back from the road advertised that it was a perfect location for 'Stag, stagette and divorce parties'.

'I wouldn't let Mike go to a divorce party anyway,' I said.

'He doesn't get away from you that easy then, Jane,' Martyn said.

'Not us, he can get out any time,' I said. 'I mean if one of his mates gets divorced he could forget going to one of those.'

The Oramorph had kicked in and was easing the liver pain, which in turn helped the breathlessness. As we moved into south Philadelphia so the suburbs became more intimidating. We were down deep in the ghettos, areas where three Lycra-clad Brits could not have been more out of place.

People gawped as we passed them. We were out of their faces before they realised who we were or what we were doing. Martyn was carrying a lot of camera equipment but I didn't feel comfortable for either of the guys. We were a comedy freak show but it was our eccentricity value that was our greatest protector. We just prayed that we wouldn't get a puncture.

Concentrating on the risk of being attacked diverted attention from the pain. As we cycled each block, I scanned the vicinity, sizing up the gangs standing on the corners looking threatening. Traffic lights and road junctions were worst, my heart pounded as we came to them and we tried to ensure that the timing of each approach was right. Only once did we feel that the perceived threat was so immediate that we had to turn back up a street and choose a different route. These were rough streets where the threats and menace clung to the atmosphere like a thick fog.

As we went down one particularly intimidating street, we attracted some comments about the Tour de France.

'I'm expecting some self-sacrifice from you two if needed,' I said. 'Some nice fresh meat for the boys in the hood.'

'You must be feeling a little better,' Ryan said.

'Yes, but you're sitting a little uncomfortably, I notice.'

We passed by the docks then underneath the Benjamin Franklin Bridge which at one point had been the world's longest suspension bridge. The roads were busy and wet from the rain.

Philadelphia was a hard industrial town, the airport, refineries and docks gave it a rough feel. There was so little pleasure, the only goal was to finish.

Progress north of the centre was slow and we were pleased to see another McDonald's, another safe haven. The area declined further, the streets looked like they'd just had a gangland feud, remnants of disorder scattered the pavements. My heart raced. I could see Martyn and Ryan's heads weave around 360 degrees as if they were child's toys. All of us were anticipating being attacked when I saw a tiny sign saying cycle path.

'Look, can we go down there?' At that moment an elderly guy on a bike came cycling down an opening in the opposite direction.

'Is that a bike route?' I called.

'Sure is,' he said.

Taking the detour was a godsend, our speed picked up as there were no more traffic lights. It was a major pickup. We eventually rejoined the highway in a leafier suburb before crossing the Calhoun Street Bridge over the Delaware River to Trenton.

Trenton was an old town and I was surprised to find that it was the state capital of New Jersey. In fact, we'd been through a lot of state capitals and I'd been surprised every time. Trenton was just as busy and as difficult to pick a route through. As we rode into town we spotted a cycle shop and decided to ask about the route ahead.

'I wouldn't cycle through the centre of town,' the young man said. 'I'll show you where's a good route.'

He pulled down a map from a stand and opened it out over the counter. 'You're here,' he pointed with his thumb; he edged his way out and around the outskirts of town.

'How much longer than if we went straight through?' I said.

'Oh, I'm guessing about fifteen miles.' I pulled a resigned look. 'I wouldn't recommend going the direct way, it's quite dangerous, the traffic's heavy and it really wouldn't be too much fun.'

'Thank you,' we said and exited the shop. 'I'm not up to a fifteen-mile detour,' I said. It was a physically demanding last fifteen miles, the shop assistant was right, it wasn't any fun.

'How are you?' Mike said as I pulled up. We'd phoned on several occasions so he knew how bad things had been.

'Weary, very weary.'

He grabbed the bike, swapping it for a recovery drink.

'Sorry, it's the only flavour left,' he said, handing me a strawberry-flavoured can. 'There's a few places to eat nearby, the room's average but if you get a shower and changed, Steven and I will sort everything else out.'

'I don't feel like eating, Mike.'

'Come on, Jane, you need something, even if it's soup and a roll. You're way too thin.'

'I feel thin, see-through thin.' I'd not been this light since my early twenties. 'I'll put this weight back on when I get home.'

My appetite had not been right since being at altitude and American cuisine didn't help. 'I'm shattered, Mike. I think I'll have to have tea lying down.'

Day 64 – Thursday, 31 August
Trenton, NJ to Staten Island, New York

MIKE

The sign for the motel at Trenton was six feet high and about as wide. It could not have been more blindingly obvious had it been flashing in pink neon. The entrance, however, was not. It took Steven and me thirty minutes and several attempts to finally find the junction which led us off the interstate and into the car park.

Still it could have been worse, I could have been with the Radio 5 Live crew who took seven hours to complete the same manoeuvre. At 9 p.m., while I was in the hotel lobby, the only spot in the vicinity where there was a wireless connection, with the laptop on my knees, two women from Radio 5 Live walked in. We sized each other up before one of them said, 'Is it Mike?'

'Yes,' I said. 'Please don't tell me you're just checking in.'

'I'm afraid so.'

'But you were just down the road.'

'I know.'

'Well, I'm glad I wasn't with you two. Was there much falling out over the directions?'

'A little,' said one.

I was surprised to see them both bright eyed and chirpy the next morning. They'd decided that rather than risk getting lost again they'd follow us. Within minutes we'd left the main road and were heading towards the university town of Princeton. The grey stone architecture was English in feel and the town could easily have slipped into the Cotswolds unnoticed. A small wisp of mist hung over the lake as two rowing crews glided through the water without rippling its surface. The water was still, the trees heavy with foliage. I was surprised by how tranquil it was compared to the urban conurbations a few miles down the road.

We caught up with Jane, Martyn and Ryan at New Brunswick, well into New Jersey. By now there were five TV crews and two radio crews with them on the road and there was an air of a travelling circus.

'Can I cycle along with you?' one of the reporters said to Jane. 'We'll find an old bike, it's just for a few yards.'

'Have you got a helmet?' Jane asked.

'No, but it's just a staged shot, it'll just be a bit of a laugh for the news.'

'That's what I thought,' Jane said. 'I've just cycled four thousand miles in nine weeks and you just want to make it some kind of cheap entertainment. It's been a real test of endurance for all three of us and you want us to cycle a hundred yards up the road and you haven't even got a helmet. You've got to be joking.' Jane turned away from the reporter and walked up to me. 'Did you hear that?'

'Yes, you're dead right. I'd already told them not to ask you.'

'She'd never get her fat arse over the crossbars anyway,' Jane said. 'Some media people are unreal.'

'Don't worry, there's no pampering to the media. I've already turned down two requests from other stations to go across Brooklyn Bridge with you tomorrow.'

'Yes, but I know what you're like,' she said, her eyes narrowing.

Unfortunately, we hadn't found a road on to Staten Island on which the cyclists could safely travel. So we agreed to meet everyone at East St Georges Avenue at Linden which was close to Goethals Bridge where the cyclists were loaded onto vehicles to cross it.

Michael, Steven and I didn't hang around after the cyclists had set off again at the other end as it was quite conceivable that if the traffic was busy, the cyclists could steal a march on us.

It surprised me how close we'd come to New York without feeling we were approaching one of the world's biggest cities. As we moved up New Jersey, so the areas became more built up.

We pulled up by a park opposite the Coliseum Diner, which looked more than suitable for some lunch. The first of the autumn leaves had begun to fall leaving a patchy brown carpet over the grassland. The skies were overcast but it certainly wasn't cold. Steven strolled along in T-shirt and shorts but his cowboy hat had been banished.

Jane was soon upon us. After a quick lunch we grouped outside. A chequered flag and a Stars and Stripes fluttered in the breeze.

'Can I have a photo with us and the flags, Jane?' I asked.

'Please, Mum,' Steven said.

The three of us went quietly across to the flags knowing that if any of the crews had spotted this perfect picture moment they would have descended upon us. Jane knelt down clutching the map holder, her fingerless gloves showing a glimpse of the eternity ring I'd given her five years ago when we renewed our marriage vows.

My mind sprung back to our wedding day, two decades earlier.

'You can't get out of this now,' said my best man Mick as I'd turned round to see Jane walking down the aisle, her arm linked with her dad's, who was in a neck brace, a physical reminder of his poor health. Jane looked fragile even then, her slender figure hugged in an ivory dress and a veil covering her long permed hair.

Temporarily dumbstruck I couldn't respond but merely watched transfixed as she walked slowly towards me as the Cat Stevens song 'How Can I Tell You?' played from a mobile tape player. For both of us, the vows we made that day were sacred, the commitment, total.

A year after Jane was told she would die, we had renewed our vows again, the words 'till death do us part' taking on a much greater significance.

Through the lens of the camera, the chequered flag fluttered behind Jane. Without saying it, we both knew that her life was moving towards the finish, a journey we were no longer steering.

After I'd taken the shot, we went back to the others.

'I'll see you at the start of the marathon,' she said, referring to Fort Wadsworth, the holding area for the New York marathon where ten months earlier we'd stood together.

'Take care,' I said.

An hour later, we were standing by the huge Verrazano Narrows Suspension Bridge waiting for Jane on the final full day of cycling. In front of us was a tranquil park, lush green surrounding a baseball pitch.

'Have you enjoyed America, Steven?' I asked.

'Not the RV or the poverty,' he said.

'What about the scenery?'

'It's okay.'

'Are you looking forward to going to school next week?'

'I want to see my friends . . . and my sisters.'

We grabbed a coffee and by the time we'd returned, the cyclists had arrived, having taken a detour to look across Upper New York Bay towards Manhattan. We quickly departed to our hotel before heading off into Brooklyn with Dave Harrison, Phil Iveson, Ryan and Jane.

All the cyclists had kept one new cycling top for the final day, so Ryan and Jane broke their packets open for an interview with Dave Harrison, looking across the East River under the shadows of Brooklyn Bridge towards Manhattan.

Jane was adamant that she didn't want to cross the bridge tonight, there was only one way she would be crossing that bridge – and that was using her own pedal power.

Day 65 – Friday, 1 September
Staten Island, New York – Battery Park, New York

JANE

I moved across the lobby, dragging my aching body through the doors and out on to the forecourt. The day was overcast though there seemed little chance of rain. I walked round the back of the hotel where the RV was parked. It was a hive of activity, suitcases piled outside, bikes propped against the framework. John Shanley from Sparks who'd flown out yesterday was talking to Cindy.

'Can I help you with your bags, Jane?' Michael asked, as helpful as ever.

'I think Mike could do with some help,' I said.

'No problem, what was your room number?'

'Three hundred and four. Thanks, Michael.' Michael moved off.

'Hi, Jane,' Ryan said. 'I can't believe this is it.' He was standing wiping down my bike ensuring the paintwork was spotless for the finish.

'Is everything ready, Ryan?' I said, attaching the Garmin GPS navigating unit to the handlebars.

'Yep, I've filled the bottles up, the brakes and tyre pressures are okay. Are you okay, Jane?'

'Hi, Jane,' John and Cindy said before I could respond.

'Good morning,' I said, and checked my watch. It was seven forty-five. 'We need to be off at eight at the latest. Are we ready?' We were due to finish at just after 10 a.m. New York time, 3 p.m. British time which would allow the TV crews to get footage organised for the evening news. It was the last day but we all had jobs to do and no one wanted to get caught in the morning rush hour into Manhattan. Unfortunately, we weren't going to be able to cycle over the Verrazano Narrows Bridge as it couldn't be crossed by cycles so Cindy would drive us across to Brooklyn then head off to return the RV before getting to the finishing point at Battery Park. The two Michaels would drive with Steven on to Manhattan and park somewhere near Battery Park.

'Morning, Jane,' Rob shouted across. Martyn followed him freewheeling on his bike.

'Come on, guys, let's get focused,' Mike began chivvying people along. 'Cindy, are we ready to go? Michael is everything loaded? Steven get in the car, come on.' He came across to me, 'Jane, we should be going, have you got everything?'

I nodded. 'Yes. Have you got all the travel documents, passports?'

'Yes, they're in with the laptop, where they've been all trip.'

'My medicines and the documentation?'

'What documentation?' His face looked puzzled.

'Mike! The documentation from Doctor Perrin explaining the medicines and my condition.' He smiled. 'Bastard.'

'Don't worry, everything is under control,' he said. 'But we need to get organised. Come on,' he bellowed to no one and everyone. 'Did you practise the route into Brooklyn last night, Cindy?'

'I'll be okay,' she responded.

Mike walked up to us. 'Have a good cycle. Enjoy Brooklyn Bridge and most of all enjoy the moment.'

He shook Ryan and Martyn's hands then gave me a big hug. We climbed in the RV, Cindy started the engine and immediately we took a wrong turn upon leaving the hotel car park and lost Michael's car.

Eventually, we got to Brooklyn and it was a relief to climb out of the RV and touch the pavement. Conscious that we needed to ensure that we hit the times we didn't hang around, but the pressure was off and we could tootle along enjoying a relaxed chat. Time permitted us to stop at a pavement café and enjoy a last coffee. Brooklyn is a beautiful spot to cycle through, the atmosphere colourful and friendly.

I recalled the moment I'd sat staring out of the plane window as we travelled from New York to San Francisco, the vast lands and the tears of fear I'd shed. If I'd known then what I knew now, I'd have been hysterical: Carson Pass, the crickets, the heat of the Colorado River, Monarch Pass, the winds of Kansas, Missouri, the dogs, my failing health. What had we done?

'Jane, Jane.' I heard a voice.

'What?'

'You were miles away,' Ryan said. 'Martyn was asking what was your highlight of the ride.'

'The ride down from Escalante to Escalante River without a doubt. Beautiful, peaceful and downhill. The low point was Chillicothe.'

'Are you glad you came?' Ryan said.

'No. I knew when Mike mentioned it, just how difficult it would be. It has been without doubt the worst nine weeks of my life, although a lot of that is down to my health. But . . .' I allowed a pause. 'I am looking forward to crossing Brooklyn Bridge.'

We set off at a slow pace, soaking in the moment, our senses heightened. As we approached the bridge a BBC reporter on a bike asked to join us, which I flatly refused. He looked a little crestfallen but this was an experience which should be enjoyed by the three of us without the media.

'Well done, Jane,' Martyn said, cycling alongside me, holding out his hand to shake mine as we reached the middle of the bridge. For us, this was the journey's end in every sense.

MIKE

'Mike, can we grab you for two minutes?' I jolted my head back as a microphone was thrust under my chin.

'Yes,' I said, just as my phone started to bleep in my pocket. 'But give me a minute . . .'

Turning my back on the group of journalists and cameras which had assembled at the finishing line, I answered the phone to Jane.

'Where are you?' I asked.

'Brooklyn Bridge, just on the Brooklyn side. Are you at the finish?'

'Yes, how long will you be?'

'We'll finish bang on time,' she said. I smiled. She knew the importance of timing when it came to British journalists needing to file copy or feeding their broadcasts.

'Enjoy the moment,' I said.

'We will,' she said. 'See you.'

I snapped the phone shut.

'Mike, are you ready?' The microphone reappeared.

'Just give me five minutes,' I said. 'Steven!' I shouted across to him. He was wearing his green fleece which he'd barely worn throughout our journey.

'What, Dad?' he said, bounding over.

'Come here, let's have five minutes alone,' I said. We wandered away from the media crews who were congregating by the promenade looking out to the Statue of Liberty. The sky was overcast, the weather damp and miserable. We walked across the grassland till there was just the two of us.

'Are you okay?' I asked.

'I'm good,' Steven said. 'How long will Mum be?'

'Twenty minutes,' I said and leant down towards him. He threw his arms around me.

'I love you, Dad,' he said. 'I'm glad Mum's finishing.'

'Me too.'

'Are we definitely going home today, Dad?'

'Yes, we'll be home by breakfast tomorrow.'

'What are we doing this weekend?'

'Resting. Then Monday we're back at work.'

'Okay. When am I at school?'

'Wednesday. Come on, little fella, let's get you back and see your mum.'

By the time we returned, the throng had grown. Representatives of the British Consulate had joined us as well as journalists who'd been out across on the other side of Brooklyn Bridge.

Within minutes the three cyclists arrived amid a cacophony of cheers and claps from the assembled crowd. Behind them a river cruise ship obscured the view of Jersey City. Within seconds Jane had freewheeled in, stopping right in front of the Sky News crew. In no time her head disappeared and her small frame was swamped by the crowd of journalists. I moved away and saw Ryan standing alone.

'Well done, Ryan,' I said.

'Thank you, sir, it's been an awesome trip. It's been a real privilege to be with such a good crew.'

'Thanks for everything, Ryan. I never thought we'd get here. The laughs, rows, emotion and everyone still smiling.'

'Awesome, just awesome.'

We shook hands and I went to search for Martyn. He was standing on the grass, observing the media scrum from a distance. 'Mike,' he shouted. 'Thank you so much for inviting me on this trip, it's been amazing.'

'We wouldn't have come without you.'

'What a journey!' His smile was contagious. There was nothing else to do but wear the most enormous of grins.

'Mike! Mike!' I turned. Dave Harrison was shouting, a gap had opened up in the crowd and there was Jane. I walked over and leant forward and put my arms around her neck. She reached up to hug me and moved her lips to my ears, but there was nothing to say.

Called away for another interview, Jane beamed. She looked tanned, happy and alive. Dried sweat cracked her cheeks and her hair was straggly. But she looked like she'd given every ounce of energy to this trip. As she stood, microphone in hand, recording another live interview to the UK, her toned legs, muscled arms, slender physique hid a body that for the last six weeks had been killing her from within. Martyn was grinning like a Cheshire cat, but Ryan's face portrayed little emotion. I knew that she'd never get on the bike again.

'What's the plan, Mike?' she asked, taking a seat next to me on a wooden bench. Around us, various members of the wider team were recording interviews.

'Here's some food,' I said, passing her a brown bag. 'Fruit and drink, from the nice deli you remember from when we stayed here.'

'Jane! Mike!' Ryan shouted. 'A group photo!' The others were gathering with their backs to the Statue of Liberty, the bikes were racked against the seafront railings, empty drink bottles littered the streets. Apart from me, everyone looked a stone lighter but the image was little different to that taken three and a half years earlier at Land's End when Jane had completed her John o'Groat's to Land's End journey.

'We need to be off, Mike,' Dave Harrison said, approaching us. 'The car's waiting.'

And so, with little formality, we shouted goodbye to Martyn, Rob, Ryan, Michael and Cindy. Ten weeks of companionship gone in a second and a wave.

Within minutes, Dave had taken us to the terraced rooftop garden of the Associated Press building overlooking Madison Square Garden. It was neither square nor a garden. To the left end of the terrace was a shed-like building set up as a TV studio, though instead of a photographic backdrop there was a stunning open vista of New York. As she gave another interview, Jane stood on a foot high wooden box while bright white arc lights accentuated her white cycling top.

'Are you sure you don't fancy staying in New York, Mike?' Dave said.

'No, I can't wait to leave. Suzanne's due soon, Jane is desperately ill and we need to get to see Doctor Perrin as soon as possible.'

I looked up at Dave. After calling Suzanne, Becca and our parents I had switched the phones off. It was clear that the news coverage in the UK was extensive as messages of congratulations were flooding in. We were also being inundated with calls from the American media, all now anxious to cover Jane's story.

'The phones have gone mad,' I said to Dave. 'All the networks want interviews. We'd have had loads of coverage doing the rounds if we'd stayed a week but they've had ten weeks to contact us.'

'They love a success story over here though.'

'It's too late.'

'How much have you raised so far?'

'About £18,000, it's shockingly bad.'

Dave's face fell, impossible to hide the disappointment for all the effort everyone had given over a year in the planning.

'We'll see what today brings,' he said. 'You'll have a great show. It's all over the media in the UK.'

Within twelve hours we were pulling in at home, the adventure over.

Thursday, 27 September
Leeds

MIKE

'Mike, there's Jane on the phone,' David, my boss, said.

'Hello, Grandad.'

'Fucking hell, when?'

'Fifteen minutes ago. She's called Emily. Congratulations, Mike. Suzanne's well.'

My eyes watered. I bowed my head but most of my colleagues were now looking on.

'Congratulations, Jane,' I said. 'I'm so pleased. I'll get off straight away. I'll pick up some flowers on the way.'

'Mike,' Jane said.

'What?'

'I love you.'

'Me too, although I can't say I'm chuffed at being married to a grandma.'

'You should just be lucky to be married to anyone.'

Within the hour we were sitting in the maternity ward at St James's Hospital with Suzanne and Tom. Jane sat in the corner, cuddling Emily. I'd not seen her so happy in years. It had been just over three weeks since we'd stood in Battery Park but it seemed a lifetime ago.

Twenty-four hours later we were at St James's again seated in front of Dr Perrin, about to hear the scan results that had been conducted immediately upon our return from the USA.

'How have you been, Jane?' he said.

'I'm getting quite a lot more pain in my liver,' she said. 'But generally the bony pain is much better controlled with the Fentanyl patches. It feels as though I'm getting a little of my life back.' Jane had always been reluctant to increase the amount of pain control medication until she found it impossible to function on a daily basis.

'Well, I'm pleased that we're getting you a little bit more comfortable,' he said. 'You did look in great discomfort before your scans. You won't be surprised to know though that the scan results are pretty dreadful.'

Jane dabbed her eye. But it was not enough to stop other tears rolling. Dr Perrin moved across and grabbed some tissues, holding them out to her.

I sat about a yard away. Experience told me to do and say nothing.

'Would you like to read the report?' said Dr Perrin. He passed across the sheet of paper to Jane who read it intensely.

'Do you want to see it, Mike?'

I shook my head. Seeing Jane's and Dr Perrin's reaction was sufficient.

'If I had seen this for a patient I'd think, "You poor cow",' said Jane.

Dr Perrin looked grave. 'Your disease has advanced quite a lot,' he said. 'All the markers are poor.'

For the next half hour we discussed treatment options. When Jane had first been diagnosed, the experts had likened it to having a medicine cabinet from which we could pick treatment. Once a drug had been removed and used, it could never be replaced. Now it felt that the shelves were empty and we were scraping our hands on them to find any scrap that had been overlooked.

As we left the consultation room Jane was inconsolable. Thanks to the media coverage of the trip, every pair of eyes in the large waiting room was upon her. She scuttled off to the ladies' while Sue Hector, a sister who'd worked in the Oncology Department when Jane's dad had been poorly twenty years ago, came up to me.

'Is everything all right?' she asked softly. I screwed up my face and shook my head. She was too experienced to try any platitudes. She just squeezed my forearms.

'Bastard disease,' Jane said as she came out and we walked across the road after leaving St James's. 'Bastard fucking disease.'

EPILOGUE

MIKE

Although the sun wasn't shining it was warm, especially in the south-facing living room. The patio doors were slightly ajar, not enough to let the cats in, but sufficiently to admit some air. Steven ran into the room.

'Is it okay if I go on the computer, Dad?'

'Don't you want to come and help in the kitchen?' He put on a forced sad face.

'Let him,' said Jane. She rose slowly to her feet, leaving the crutches redundant at her side. 'Do you want a drink, Mike?'

I jumped up. 'I'll do it.' I moved quickly past her and entered the kitchen, moving the dining chair out of the way so she could manoeuvre unencumbered.

'I'm not a child, Mike, I can manage.'

She moved slowly into the kitchen. Her liver had swollen considerably, making her look several months' pregnant, a trap into which a young shop assistant at Marks & Spencer had fallen into a few days before. Apart from that and a slight loss of colour in her face, Jane looked well and you wouldn't have guessed that she'd arrived home on a weekend visit from the hospice a few hours earlier.

'Save your energy for when everyone comes,' I said. 'Is it strange to be home?'

'A little. You need to keep on top of the watering, it'll be better when Luke puts in the irrigation system to the pots at the front. I think he's going to do it this afternoon.' She moved to the back door. 'I'm just popping out for a minute.'

She stumbled over the lip of the back door but soon steadied herself. It had been a whirlwind two weeks; we'd arrived home from a holiday from hell in Ireland with Jane in desperate pain. For once, we didn't need the scans to tell us the prognosis. Since her first diagnosis, Jane had always pondered whether to continue treatment. It was never an easy decision to make, knowing as we did that treatment might extend the quantity – but not the quality – of her life. It's a situation that all terminal cancer patients find themselves in, one where there's no right or wrong answer, just an individual choice.

The choice ten days ago, however, was as stark as it was clear – the treatment had as much chance of killing Jane as the disease. For the first time in six years, we'd left the consulting room with no treatment options available. We simply had to await a call from a hospice in the hope that a bed could be found.

I watched Jane as she carefully picked a path to the bottom of the garden and to her favourite bench under an arbour, upon which a clematis and hop were battling for space. She sat leaning forward as she had done almost daily for the last seven years but she couldn't keep still for long. She was soon up and dead-heading a rose.

The front door opened. Suzanne walked into the kitchen. Behind her, Tom was holding Emily in his arms.

'Hi, Dad.' She walked over and gave me a hug. 'The joint smells nice. I've brought the veg.'

'Good, because your mum's beginning to wear me out. She won't keep still. Hi, Tom.'

'All right, Mike,' said Tom.

Suzanne walked out of the back door and I watched as she went over to Jane and gave her a long hug. Despite being similar heights, Suzanne seemed to tower over her mum. They held each other for a long time before drawing back slightly and sizing one another up.

Jane had entered the hospice ten days earlier to control the acute pain and nausea. The experts' view was that once they were under control, Jane would be able to return home for a couple of months before end care was required.

But while her symptoms were eased, the disease had taken control more rapidly. I'm not sure why this had surprised me as for years I'd lived with the knowledge that Jane was much more poorly than she'd ever alluded to.

Within half an hour, Jane's brother Luke and his family arrived. Despite everyone's protestations, Jane wouldn't release control over the cooking, but still took time out to watch over Luke as he tended to the irrigation system.

'Becca, will you set out the plates?' Suzanne asked. Becca scowled at her sister, biting her tongue, finding it difficult to accept her sister's bossiness without response. There were shouts from Steven and his two cousins Pete and Tom from the computer. Prudence the cat lazily walked across the kitchen and jumped on a chair.

'Becca! Get Prudence away from the table,' said Suzanne. Becca scrunched up her face.

I went outside where Karen, Luke's wife, was sitting at the table reading the morning's *Guardian*.

'Where's Jane?' I asked.

'I'm here.' Jane walked around from the side of the house, holding some secateurs in one hand while leaning on her crutch with the other. 'Stop fussing, Mike.'

Carefully, she moved forward on to the garden, which was a raised brick bed, tricky at times for even the nimble footed. Within a second, in slow motion, she was going down, the crutch dropping as she clumsily hit the ground.

'See, you could tell that was going to happen,' I said, moving closer to help her up.

Jane looked up and gave the same face that Becca had chucked at Suzanne moments earlier.

'Is the syringe driver okay?' she asked. The syringe driver was a device that ensured that the supply of Jane's drugs was evenly spread over time so avoiding the peaks and troughs she got with tablets. It was held in a little cotton bag hanging by

Jane's side but was hooked over her shoulder. We'd affixed a similar, but smaller one to Lamby, a toy who was Jane's hospice bedtime companion.

'Mike, you're not helping,' Jane said. 'I'm fine, I'm not a child and don't look like that.'

She rose slowly, checked the driver, gave me a quizzical look and smiled and sat down next to me.

Luke came over.

'It's working, Jane,' he said, referring to the newly installed irrigation system. 'Do you want to have a look?'

'Two ticks,' she said, heading back towards the shed. She turned to look at me and made a funny face, then went inside the shed and appeared a minute later.

'I bought these,' she held out a set of topiary shears. 'Expensive but why not?'

The two of them disappeared around the path to the front garden while I went back inside to check on tea. Jane was soon back, mixing the Yorkshires. After tea, we all decamped to the garden, where unusually for an August Bank Holiday the late afternoon was warm and pleasant. Jane had lit the stove she'd bought for my birthday. Luke stoked it with logs. Two wine bottles adorned the patio table, one finished, the second just opened.

'All right, love?' Terry from next door arrived clutching some cans of bitter, followed by his wife Cynthia, wine glass in hand. 'You've got the garden looking right.'

'Thanks for keeping on top of the watering.' Jane stood up. 'I think the baskets are about finished.'

Cynthia came forward, her emotions taking over, she started to sniffle. 'Have you seen the pears?' Jane said, diverting the attention.

It had been seven years to the weekend since Jane had been told her cancer was incurable, just before the Sydney Olympics which she'd watched throughout the night as she'd come to terms with her illness. Back then, who would have thought she would have been an ambassador for the London 2012 bid?

Over the last few years, Jane's life had taken her in a direction that the greatest of fantasists couldn't have imagined. As for those of us close to her, we couldn't have begun to dream.

Jane, though, hadn't been affected one bit by the time. She remained essentially the same person, her sense of joy in life and family untainted.

We sat enjoying a beer and chat as the night drew in. 'Jane's been a while,' Karen said. 'Is she all right?' Jane had gone inside twenty minutes earlier, heading off to see Steven and put some hand cream on.

'I'll go and check,' I said. I got up and a blast of warm air felt good on my skin as I walked past the stove. I bent down to pull a little piece of camomile from Jane's herb garden and smelt the fragrance. The opening bars of 'Hotel California' came wafting over from a neighbour's garden.

My mind switched back to last summer to California, Missouri, and a warm feeling of nostalgia made me smile as I remembered the ride. It's funny how, with the passage of time, the whole journey is one long vivid and beautiful memory. I'd spoken to Martyn only a couple of times since we returned, but on each occasion, it had been hard not to burst out into laughter, giggling like schoolboys as we recalled some of the more 'interesting' moments.

Ryan had been a more constant fixture in our lives. He'd helped us put on the first Leeds 10k run in June. Striding out immediately prior to the race, he'd started from the VIP area, leading out the celebrity runners. I remember him looking up to the starters' podium where Jane was standing and he waved. To see 8,000 runners lined down the Headrow took my breath away, a sea of humanity.

Strangely, it was only after the run had taken place that each of us experienced the post-ride euphoria that had been lacking at the actual finish.

'We did it, sir.' Ryan came up to me after the race and shook my hand. He walked up to Jane and gave her a huge hug. 'This has been the most incredibly awesome run.'

Jane, despite being desperately ill, had stood and watched everyone return, her mum, sisters, brothers, friends and colleagues all crying, cheering and clapping. The American ride had raised only £150,000 but it had provided the launch pad to set up the run which had raised £500,000 in year one. Jane looked at Ryan, tears streaming down her face.

'I told you finishing would make all the difference,' she said. 'Never give up in life. You give up one day, you give up for ever.'

I opened the kitchen door and Jane was sitting at the table, the 'Review' section of the *Guardian* laid out as a double page in front of her, the coffee espresso machine on it and a spanner in her right hand. She'd half disassembled the machine: screws, pieces of metal and assorted bits were laid out in neat rows.

'What are you doing?' I asked.

'I fancied a coffee and the machine hadn't been cleaned for a while, the gunge has made the nozzle stiff.' She looked up at me. 'You'll need to get Becca to do this.'

'It doesn't matter, love, I don't use it.'

'You don't, but you might have visitors who'd like a coffee.'

'Whatever.'

'Oh, you know how much I hate that word. Listen, I've written out instructions for the washing machine, they are on the top of it.'

'Thanks, love,' I said. 'Why don't you come out and say goodbye to people, they'll be leaving soon.'

I made to go back outside.

'Mike,' Jane said and I turned. 'I love you.'

'I love you too.'

Jane had one more night at home and died in St Gemma's Hospice, Leeds, eight days later.